MAGNETO-ENCEPHALOGRAPHY

Edited by **Elizabeth W. Pang**

Magnetoencephalography
Edited by Elizabeth W. Pang

Published by InTech
Janeza Trdine 9, 51000 Rijeka, Croatia

Technical Editor Sonja Mujacic

Cover Designer InTech Design Team

Additional hard copies can be obtained from orders@intechopen.com

Magnetoencephalography,
Edited by Elizabeth W. Pang
p. cm.
ISBN 978-953-307-255-5

Meet the editor

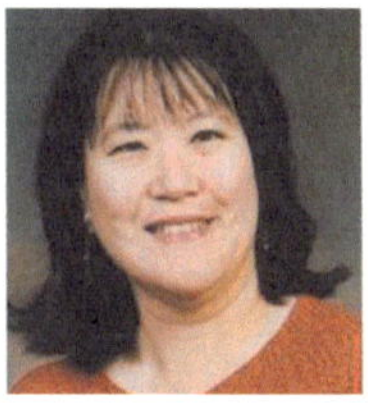

Dr. Elizabeth W. Pang, Ph.D. is the Director of the MEG Functional Mapping Lab and a Neurophysiologist in the Division of Neurology at the Hospital for Sick Children, Toronto, Canada. She is also an Associate Scientist in the SickKids Research Institute. She holds appointments at the University of Toronto in the Department of Paediatrics, Faculty of Medicine and the Institute of Medical Science, School of Graduate Studies. The Hospital for Sick Children was the first institution in the world to install an MEG dedicated to the study of children. As Director of the lab, Dr. Pang established the protocols used for their paediatric functional mapping studies. Dr. Pang also maintains an active research lab where she uses MEG to examine the neural underpinnings of language development.

Contents

Preface

Since the first single sensor magnetoencephalographic (MEG) recording in the 1960s, MEG has experienced a steady expansion in a number of directions. The most obvious is the increase in numbers of sensors available in whole-head MEG systems; currently, 300+ channels are the norm allowing high density, high spatial resolution recordings. With less expensive and more powerful computer processors, MEG computational methods for source analysis, signal processing, and data reduction have also been increasing. This is allowing for more accurate source localization and improved methods for data visualization and comparison. As well, more computing power has allowed exploration into new facets of brain activity; for example, studies of neural oscillations, brain synchrony, and neural networks. Finally, the numbers of applications for MEG use have also been increasing steadily. MEG is being used, increasingly, to examine different clinical cohorts or different population demographics; as well, MEG is being applied to diverse research questions ranging from basic neural function to the cognitive neurosciences. With its excellent temporal and spatial resolution, MEG is an excellent complement to the other non-invasive neuroimaging modalities, such as event-related potentials (ERP) or function magnetic resonance imaging (fMRI).

In this book we bring together MEG scientists and clinicians. Some chapters look back to review the MEG research literature. Some chapters look at the present to portray the current state of the art with regards to MEG. And some chapters look ahead to describe innovative new methods for MEG systems and data.

The first section contains a trio of reviews. Chapter One by Prendergast and Hymers is an eloquent and thorough discussion of clinical approaches to the study of epilepsy, Parkinson's Disease, and Alzheimer's Disease using MEG. These authors chart how the method and analyses have developed in the study of these populations, and they end the chapter with some thoughts on the utility of MEG as a biomarker in other diseases. Chapter Two by Silva Nunes and colleagues continues to describe studies in clinical populations, but shifts focus to examine changes in cognitive function as a function of disease. Specifically, they look into two important cognitive functions, memory and language. They describe memory and language studies that have included patients with Alzheimer's Disease, depression, mild cognitive impairment, reading disabilities and dyslexia. Having reviewed the literature, they end by setting the stage for the future by stating that clearly the next step is to move beyond studying neural activations and to move towards studying the neural connectivity of cognitive functions. The third Chapter by Moses, Hanlon and Ryan builds on the previous two by focusing specifically on MEG applications to the study of human memory. This readable chapter describes the technical challenge of using MEG to image the hippocampal activity associated with memory, then proceeds to highlight the plethora of innovative MEG studies that have studied memory, and in particular, its relation to the hippocampus. This comprehensive chapter includes work on both clinical and healthy populations, and across the life span from children to older adults.

The second section contains a trio of chapters all of which attempt to address one of the most important current issues in MEG studies: how to deal with the inverse problem. Chapter Four by Quraan assesses the advantages and limitations of a newer technique, the use of beamforming for source localization. The chapter provides the theory behind scalar and vector beamformers and compares their performance using both simulated and experimental datasets. The chapter ends with some caveats which is a must-read for all researchers using, or contemplating using, beamforming methods. The next two chapters describe two types of parametric models for solving the inverse problem. Chapter Five by Pascarella and Sorrentino presents a concise description of statistical approaches to the inverse problem, detailing both imaging and parametric methods. Specifically, there is a focus on parametric methods and a thorough account of the use of one particular dynamic parametric method, multi-dipole particle filtering that allows automated dipole estimation. Details for implementing this method are given in this chapter also. Chapter Six by Nara describes a novel solution that incorporates the advantages of both parametric and imaging approaches to inverse problem. By modelling the source as an equivalent current dipole plus quadrupole, this accounts for the spatial extent of the current source. This chapter introduces the rationale for the dipole plus quadrupole model and then demonstrates its accuracy and utility with a series of simulations.

The third section contains two papers that describe the analysis of MEG phase information. Chapter Seven by Dammers and Schiek reports a potentially promising method for extracting brain signal from artefact by examining phase in the independent components. This chapter presents examples of successful extractions of brain data despite cardiac and ocular artifacts. Chapter Eight by Matani and colleagues introduce the concept of epoch filtering, as an addition to the traditional temporal and spatial filters. They present simulation data and experimental data from a semantic priming experiment to demonstrate the applicability of epoch filters for the analysis of phase information, and the use of this in understanding long-distance brain synchrony.

Chapter Nine by Ochi, Go and Otsubo stands on its own. This is a practical, step-by-step account of how to use and interpret dipole source results in pediatric patients with intractable epilepsy. With concise instructions and many diagrams, the reader will be led in the process of detecting and selecting appropriate epileptic spikes, applying a single moving dipole analysis, selecting and rejecting appropriate dipoles to interpret whether there is an epileptic cluster that predicts an epileptogenic zone. Case studies are included to illustrate the process.

The last section again contains a trio of papers, all of which look toward future advances. Chapter Ten by Takeda and colleagues addresses an issue facing all MEG users, that of helium consumption. Maintaining the MEG system at appropriate temperatures requires large amounts of helium. This is costly in terms of operating expenses, and it has an immediate environmental impact and a broader environmental impact, that is with regards to transportation and containment. Takeda presents a fascinating and innovative plan for building a system that re- uses and re-cools the helium so that re-fills are no longer necessary on a weekly basis. This chapter contains practical instructions with diagrams. If this idea is implemented on a wide basis, this will have a tremendous impact. Institutions that were reluctant to purchase MEG systems because of the high operating costs would no longer face this obstacle. MEG use would increase even further and this technology would continue to expand and grow. Chapter Eleven by Foldes and colleagues presents the innovative concept of online MEG. Traditional MEG data are processed off-line with the interpretation of MEG results occurring after the subject has left the lab, or the patient has left the hospital. These authors introduce the idea that, with current computing capabilities, MEG data can be processed on-line and even in real time; however, there are a multiplicity of challenges and concerns. The authors describe and address these challenges, leaving the reader optimistic that this can become a reality and speculating as to new possibilities for future research and clinical applications. The last chapter in this book by Walla is a provocative chapter that urges the reader to think "outside the box". This chapter presents the possibility and evidence that MEG can be used to examine non- conscious brain processes. The author asserts that 80% of one's daily activities are performed outside one's awareness, thus, these studies would contribute insightful information on an infrequently studied, difficult to access, but ubiquitous and powerful domain.

Clearly, we are at an exciting time for MEG research and clinical applications. The MEG community has made huge strides to advance from systems with one single channel to systems with hundreds of channels. Currently, new advances continue to be made with regards to source localization, signal processing and data visualization and reduction. The future is bright with innovations that will broaden the scope of research and make MEG use more widely available and accessible. This book covers the breadth of these developments and I hope the reader finds these chapters thought-provoking and informative.

Elizabeth W. Pang
The Hospital for Sick Children
Toronto, Ontario,
Canada

Part 1

Looking Back: Review of the Literature

1

Past, Current and Future Clinical Applications of MEG

Garreth Prendergast and Mark Hymers
York Neuroimaging Centre, University of York
United Kingdom

1. Introduction

Magnetoencephalography (MEG) is a technique which detects weak magnetic fields from above the surface of the head produced by electrical activity within the brain (Hämäläinen et al., 1993). It is non-invasive, acoustically silent and able to measure a direct correlate of neuronal activity with sub-millisecond resolution. The technique is therefore well suited to clinical applications as it can readily be used in children and other populations who may not tolerate more demanding procedures such as fMRI or PET. Clinical applications of MEG, although currently limited, have developed in parallel with advances in hardware, software, analysis tools and general understanding of the technique as a non-invasive measure of biomagnetic neuronal activity. The goal of this review is to describe the advances made to date regarding the clinical applications of the technique and the potential areas for expansion and application in the future.

Although much MEG research has been conducted in clinical populations, helping to provide an understanding of the pathology and manifestation of various categories of illness, it generally remains a technique used in the research laboratory rather than as a routine part of clinical evaluations. MEG is routinely used in research to investigate the dynamic neuronal processes involved in the representation of sensory systems such as vision, audition, somatosensation and movement. The technique is also readily applied to experiments studying more cognitive processes such as language perception, memory encoding and retrieval and higher level tasks. Non-invasive imaging of the human brain is potentially a very useful diagnostic tool in the identification, prevention and treatment of numerous disease and illnesses as it is able to study a range of cerebral functions.

The main clinical application of MEG remains in the pre-surgical evaluation of patients suffering from epilepsy. In recent years, the technique has been applied to the study of a much broader range of symptoms and pathologies, however this is almost exclusively in the context of research on clinical populations rather than being a routinely used diagnostic procedure. The aim of this chapter is not to provide an exhaustive review of all studies which report the use of MEG scanning techniques on individuals from a clinical population. The aim is to give an overview of how the clinical applications of the technique have developed in parallel with purely methodological and empirical research applications and to highlight steps which are necessary for the technique to be more readily applied to a wider range of clinically relevant problems. The first part of this chapter gives on overview of the early uses of MEG in the patient care and treatment plan of individuals suffering from epilepsy. Again, rather than focusing on the many studies published in this area which provide evidence for the usefulness of MEG as a diagnostic tool, the chapter will focus on describing how the use of MEG in the epilepsy field has continued to evolve and develop in conjunction with the methodological and cognitive applications of the technique. In many ways, the use of MEG in the epilepsy population represents a bench-mark for what may be possible in other clinical populations. The chapter will then describe preliminary results from patient groups suffering from a range of diseases including Parkinsonism, Alzheimer's disease, cortical lesions, and Autism. The main theme of the chapter will be that it is essential that high-quality, robust and rigorous research studies precede any advances towards using MEG as a clinically useful tool and that these studies must be performed by multi-disciplinary research teams combining methodological and technical expertise with clinicians willing to strive towards faster, more objective and robust diagnostic methods. The chapter concludes that, although currently the application of MEG as a diagnostic tool to many types of illness is premature, the potential uses of MEG as a clinically accessible technique are vast. Due to large steps forward in the understanding of MEG signals and the proliferation of specific and flexible analysis techniques, the effectiveness of MEG now extends far beyond that of epilepsy and the next 5-10 years could see MEG become a diagnostic tool for a great many conditions.

2. Epilepsy research

Epileptic seizures are caused by spontaneous and uncontrolled electrical activity within the brain. Although there are many different sub-types of epilepsy, many of these manifest themselves as spontaneous, high-amplitude electrical activity and therefore are particularly well suited to detection via MEG. There are a number of excellent reviews of the role of MEG in the diagnosis and pre-surgical evaluation of epilepsy patients (for example da Silva, 2005; Knowlton, 2003; Tovar-Spinoza et al., 2008). As outlined in the introduction, the aim of this chapter is not to exhaustively describe the evidence for the effectiveness of MEG in the diagnosis of epilepsy, but to outline the progression of the analyses and methods used in the study of epilepsy and to highlight where this has been successful.

2.1 Early epilepsy research

Initial studies utilising MEG to measure magnetic field distributions from epilepsy patients treated the technique as a subtle variation on electroencepahlography (EEG). EEG has been a widely used technique with which to categorise various types of epilepsy and to determine the best course of treatment for a given pathology for many decades (Abbott & Schwab, 1948; Parker, 1947). EEG is still the most commonly used tool in hospitals to determine the focus of an individuals epilepsy. Initially MEG was used in a similar way, with the magnetic fields being analysed in much the same way as the EEG waveforms. The standard method was to visualise the waveforms on the electrodes or sensors and describe the scalp locations which showed slow, or spike-wave activity. Rose et al. (1987) used MEG, EEG and electrocorticography to measure inter-ictal spikes from three young adults suffering from epilepsy. It was found that MEG dipoles could be calculated from the scalp topography and a simple dipole fitting algorithm localised these to the anterior-temporal lobe. This localisation showed good concordance with the intra-operative electrode recordings from various surfaces of the temporal lobe, whereas the mapping of EEG spikes showed a localisation either anterior or posterior to the location identified by MEG. This was one of the first examples of a case where the localisation of high-amplitude inter-ictal activity in MEG not only appeared possible, but was also more closely related to the data collected by electrodes placed on the cortical surface during neurosurgery than the localisation achieved via EEG.

Following these early studies there were a number of validatory experiments which compared the localisation capabilities of MEG to those of EEG and intra-operative recordings (for example Knake et al., 2006; Rose et al., 1991). The consensus was that MEG provided a viable alternative to the invasive procedure of electrocorticography for pre-surgical localisation of epileptogenic zones and, due to the spatial smearing of electrical signals caused by the conductivity of the dura and skull, MEG provided a potentially more reliable and accurate signal than EEG on which to base the localisation of epileptiform activity (Nakasato et al., 1994). The primary analysis tool for analysing these high-amplitude, transient bursts of energy was the equivalent current dipole (ECD). Ebersole (1997) provides an introduction to the concept and implementation of dipole models to epilepsy data, but the technique is simply a fitting procedure in which an algorithm determines the location, orientation and strength of a dipole which minimises the error between the observed field and the field topography produced by the model. The head is assumed to be a sphere and the ECDs calculated are typically considered valid if the correlation between the modelled and observed field patterns is greater than 98% and have a physiologically realistic magnitude (Otsubo & Snead, 2001).

The field of epilepsy research using MEG then moved from simply identifying the irritative zone (region of the brain which generates interictal epileptogenic discharges), to delineating regions of eloquent cortex. The term eloquent cortex is used to define cortical locations that if removed or damaged would result in a loss of sensory processing, linguistic ability or the ability to make controlled movements. Many cases of epilepsy are concurrent with some form of structural deficit, such as a tumour, an infarction or focal cortical dysplasia. It is these types of cases that are particularly suitable for surgical re-section if the structural deficit is shown by some other technique (typically EEG) to also form the epileptogenic zone. These regions are often in or very close to language areas and the sensorimotor cortex. MEG thus became a tool for not only lateralising and localising epileptogenic cortex by measuring spontaneous magnetic fields when the patient was at rest, but also for measuring fields generated during a task in order to allow the localisation of specific perceptual functions.

Primary sensory regions (for example, motor, somatosensory, auditory, visual) can be localised in MEG with relative ease. The tasks are typically simple, the protocols are short and the analyses often a straight-forward extension of the dipolar techniques used to localise spontaneous spike activity. Hund et al. (1997) introduced a measure of surgical risk for cortical lesions located adjacent to the motor cortex. They use the minimal distance between the lesion and sensory and motor cortex as defined by MEG to calculate a functional risk profile. Of the forty patients in the study, 11 patients with gliomas showed a high risk profile and 6 of these individuals underwent non-operative treatment. Of the 28 patients with a low functional risk profile, none showed any neurological deficit postoperatively. Ganslandt et al. (1999) investigated 50 patients who had a tumour resected from around the motor cortex. The sensorimotor cortex was defined in all patients using MEG in conjunction with dipolar modelling techniques. The central sulcus was identified intra-operatively and this localisation was compared with the MEG results with the two showing excellent concordance. The efficacy of localising sensorimotor cortex via MEG has also been compared to electrocorticography recordings. Roberts et al. (2000) compared the mapping of somatosensory motor cortex with intra-operative cortical stimulation and found that the results were concordant in 90% of cases, with a high level of concordance in 77% of cases. One of the reasons for the success of MEG in being able to accurately identify the location of primary sensory areas such as primary auditory, somatosensory, motor and visual cortex is the fact that these are well defined cortical regions. From electrophysiological studies, the cytoarchitecture of these areas in the normal population is known. Not only is the location of these primary cortices well established, but they represent relatively discrete processing modules. The other function most commonly localised pre-surgically to reduce the risk of removing eloquent cortex is language processing. However, the language network does not have a primary cortex of representation and is more accurately described as a distributed neuronal network.

Simos et al. (1998) introduced a method via which language laterality could be determined in MEG. Individuals were placed in the scanner and the tasks used were a word-matching and a tone matching task. In each task, the portion of the response that was analysed was after the onset evoked from primary sensory cortices which typically occurs between 80 and 150 ms. The latter portion of the response was analysed and ECDs were used to compute an interhemispheric laterality index. A greater number of dipole solutions were found in the left hemisphere in 87% of subjects in response to the word-matching task. This study demonstrated that it was feasible to place an individual in the MEG scanner whilst performing a language task and the event-related fields produced during this task could be modelled using the now well established dipole techniques, and that the results could reveal information regarding the underlying hemispheric dominance. This protocol was then developed and optimised and the next step was to compare the ability of MEG to determine language function with an independent, established technique.

The Intra-carotid Amobarbital Procedure (IAP) (Wada & Rasmussen, 2007) has been a standard pre-operative diagnostic tool in epilepsy patients since its inception in the 1960's. The test involves injection of a barbiturate into one cerebral hemisphere in order to anesthetise it. A language and memory task is then conducted in order to determine the language capabilities of the non-injected hemisphere. The process is then repeated with the other hemisphere injected. The scores from each of the two tests are then used to determine if either cerebral hemisphere shows dominance for language or memory or if the result is a bilateral representation of function. The results of the test are often used to confirm whether or not a patient is suitable for surgical re-section. The procedure is sensitive to differences in vasculature, has strict time constraints which limit the amount of testing possible and is also associated with risk of morbidity. It is therefore desirable to replace this procedure with a non-invasive alternative which is able to provide the same information regarding hemispheric dominance for language function.

Breier et al. (1999) extended the initial implementation of the language lateralisation paradigm in MEG described by Simos et al. (1998) and investigated concordance levels between the IAP and MEG lateralisation metrics in 26 patients suffering from intractable epilepsy. The results confirmed that there were high levels of agreement between the two metrics. This template of performing non-invasive MEG tests of language dominance in parallel with IAP tests (which patients were having regardless) in order to reach a conclusion regarding their suitability for surgical re-section became widely used in order to provide mounting evidence for the ability of MEG to be used as a pre-operative diagnostic tool. Papanicolaou et al. (2004) measured signals in MEG from 100 epilepsy surgery candidates ranging from 8-56 years of age in response to a word recognition task. Single ECDs were used to model the activity and compute a laterality index. The MEG and IAP lateralisations were concordant to a level of 87%. This study was replicated by Doss et al. (2009) using a cohort of 35 surgery candidates. The MEG and IAP laterality results were concordant in 86% of cases, with high levels of sensitivity (80%) and specificity (100%). Breier et al. (2001) performed a similar comparison of MEG and IAP measures of language laterality in children, demonstrating excellent levels of concordance in 17 out of 19 patients. Studies such as these were essential in determining objective criteria with which to improve data quality and the robustness of analysis techniques in order to allow MEG to be used for mapping language functions in a clinically relevant manner.

2.2 Summary

Since its inception, Magnetoencephalography has been used to investigate the underlying cortical activity related to epilepsy. This began by using MEG as a basic extension of EEG and simply identifying atypical, epileptiform traces of activity. However, with the introduction of the equivalent current dipole, the field rapidly moved to performing source modelling in order to localise the irritative zone. Before MEG was able to be used clinically it required validation by comparing the results to standard, existing methods. The MEG results were rigorously compared to those from EEG and intra-operative recordings. As the field of MEG as a whole began to use the technique to look at the response of specific perceptual and cognitive systems, the field of epilepsy research continued to develop. Pre-surgical mapping was performed on primary sensory areas and to derive estimates of language laterality. Again, at each stage the results from MEG were compared with established techniques such as electrocorticography recordings and the intra-carotid Amobarbital procedure.
As stated previously, there have been many excellent reviews on the role of MEG in the localisation of both irritative zones and regions of eloquent cortex (Frye et al., 2009; Simos et al., 2000). The purpose of the the brief review presented in this chapter is to use the application of MEG to the diagnosis and treatment of epilepsy as a template with which to evaluate progress in other clinically relevant areas. The clinical needs prior to surgical re-section are clearly defined in epilepsy; it is necessary to define the irritative onset zone and if a cerebral lesion is associated with the seizures, to what extent does this area interact with regions of eloquent cortex. MEG measurements combined with dipole modelling are sufficient to be able to provide an answer to these questions in order to allow progression toward rendering a patient seizure free. However, despite the tools existing to allow MEG to be used in the pre-surgical evaluation of these patients, the development of new methods and techniques did not cease. The next section considers more recent advances in signal processing techniques that have been used to further enhance the ability of MEG to non-invasively inform the treatment and management of epilepsy. What becomes clear is that the study of epilepsy via MEG has continued to grow and develop at a similar pace to the development of new technologies and methods within the broader field. Due to this fact, the speed at which the scans can be performed has increased as knowledge about the most effective protocols grows. As confidence in the diagnostic abilities of the technique grows, more and more clinicians become aware of its utility, resulting in MEG being performed routinely at various epilepsy centres around the world, not as an an innovative and exploratory technique but as a valued and essential step in determining the most appropriate intervention (Ray & Bowyer, 2010; Schwartz et al., 2008). If other conditions are to use MEG as part of a routine diagnostic procedure, then it is necessary not only to apply standard analysis techniques, but to use studies of these conditions to drive forward novel and innovative statistical and modelling techniques.

2.3 Recent epilepsy research

The field of MEG research has continued to grow over the past decade, with new methods, analyses and statistical approaches being developed and rapidly applied to the investigation of a vast array of sensory and cognitive systems. The clinically relevant applications of MEG in epilepsy research were initially developed using the ECD, and this analysis method for the localisation of the irritative zone and of eloquent cortex has been shown to be effective. However, when new techniques were developed, rather than the epilepsy research persisting with what was already shown to work, researchers embraced these new approaches and worked to obtain more robust, more accurate localisations of function and a better understanding of the underlying pathology associated with the illness.

The ECD approach has a number of weaknesses in that it assumes the activity being modelled is a point-like source of activity. It is also a full inverse solution in that each sensor contributes equally to the fit. For example, a current source emanating from the frontal lobe will be best represented on the sensors in the anterior portion of the sensor array. However, the fields measured on the posterior sensors still contribute to the final fit, and it is possible that excluding this information from the model would result in a more accurate inverse estimate. As the activity is treated as a point-like source, there is no estimate of the extent of activation, or in the case of epilepsy data, the extent of the irritative zone or of eloquent cortex. The two other commonly used inverse methods are Minimum Norm Estimation (MNE) (Hämäläinen et al., 1993) and Beamforming (Van Veen et al., 1997). MNE is a distributed source model which estimates the current density at many thousand locations. The locations are fixed to the cortical surface and the orientation of the signals are fixed to be tangential to this surface. The amplitude of these thousands of sources are then estimated from the data. However, MNE can only be applied in a stable manner to averaged data and, as stated, is restricted to the cortical surface. Beamforming is an adaptive spatial filtering technique which assesses the contribution of each voxel within the brain volume to the measured field. Spatial filtering approaches are now common in research that measures signals via MEG and it is a process which can be highly flexible. Beamformer solutions are able to perform whole-head analyses and can also be used to reconstruct the estimated neural time course at any point within the head. These so-called Virtual Electrodes (VE) have the potential to estimate the electrical activity of a source at a specific location with the temporal resolution of the original signal.

These more advanced modelling techniques have been used on data from epilepsy patients and they are potentially able to provide a more satisfactory description of the underlying pathology than ECD techniques alone. Bowyer et al. (2005) used a current density modelling approach termed MR-FOCUSS (Bowyer et al., 2005) to estimate cortical regions of language activation in 27 patients with localised intractable epilepsy. Verb generation and picture naming tasks were used and a laterality index was calculated for each task and three different latencies. One latency captured all language processing (150-550 ms) while the other two focused on activation of Wernicke's area (230-290 ms) and Broca's area (396-460). In 23 of the 24 patients in which a successful IAP measurement was obtained, the laterality of the activity in the 396-460 ms window was in agreement with the IAP result. Three patients showed either a bilateral or undetermined language representation on the IAP, and in one of these patients the lateralisation obtained by the current density estimate was in agreement with intra-cranial measurements. The results of this study suggest that MNE is able to provide information regarding the lateralisation of function in a cohort of patients. Give that the technique estimates neuronal activity at many thousands of cortical locations, and that laterality is calculated over a number of these estimates, it perhaps allows a more stable estimate of laterality than using the number of single location, point-like sources from dipolar models.

Spatial filtering approaches have also been shown to be effective in the localisation of eloquent cortical function. Beamformers typically focus on the total power of a response (Hymers et al., 2010), however in recent years there has been an increase in the number of variations of specific filter implementations. Cheyne et al. (2006) introduced a novel, event-related beamformer (ERB) based on an implementation initially described by Robinson

(2004). Cheyne et al. (2007) investigated the ability of an event-related beamformer to localise somatosensory and auditory cortices in participants with metallic dental implants and controls. The ECD model and ERB technique produced comparable localisations in control participants, but in patients with metallic implants the ECD method was unable to localise the activity whereas the ERB produced results consistent with expected anatomical regions of activation. The event-related beamformer has been shown to reliably localise the motor cortex in paediatric epilepsy patients (Gaetz et al., 2009) and has also been validated against direct cortical stimulations and the results confirm that it is a viable and robust framework with which to perform non-invasive preoperatve investigations (Pang et al., 2008). Robinson et al. (2004) further refined the spatial filtering approach to bias it toward scanning the head for detection of epileptogenic activity. The electrical time series of activation is estimated at many thousands of points within the volume and at each location the excess kurtosis is calculated to give a metric of the "spikiness" of the data. The advantage of these higher level analyses is that they are more robust to low signal-to-noise ratios and provide a better estimate of the spatial extent of these regions. The ECD models the activity as a single point-like source, whereas MNE and beamformer estimates give a greater indication of the extent of activation. These techniques are also more suited to inferential statistical thresholding than the ECD. The MNE and, in particular, beamformer analyses are tools which can be implemented in a number of different ways in order to optimise the analysis to focus on the specific response of interest. When investigating complex and dynamic processes such as language processing and higher cognitive mechanisms, these are highly desirable facets of an analysis. It is likely that the application of MEG to clinical populations other than epileptics will be dependent on the power and flexibility of these techniques being fully exploited.

The MEG community now also benefits from time and the fact that it is no longer a new technique with a relatively small amount of expertise and knowledge within the field. In recent years there has been a rapid increase in the amount of theoretical and methodological work in order to really push the boundaries of what types of analyses are possible with MEG data. The purpose of this section is to outline how these recent advances have already been applied to the study of epilepsy and how the proliferation of novel and specific analysis techniques means the potential of MEG to be used in a wide range of clinical setting becomes very real.

Previously, one logistical downside of MEG was the amount of data acquired, with modern scanners having in excess of 200 sensors and a default sampling frequency of around 600 Hz, the amount of data collected in a single study can be vast. However, with modern computing power now more affordable and more efficient, there are many fewer constraints on the type of analyses it is possible to perform. The fact that data storage and transfer is now much easier to implement and manage allows even more data to be collected. It is therefore now possible to collect data at much higher sampling frequencies and these large datasets can still be manipulated with ease. One area in which there is unexplored potential is in the acquisition of MEG signals in the upper parts of the frequency spectrum. Typically MEG signals are acquired at 300-600 Hz, and for many studies which investigate human neural processes the analyses focus on biological signals below 100 Hz. Recent work however has shown that there may be reliable diagnostic information represented in high frequency oscillations produced by epileptogenic cortex. The presence of fast oscillations, or ripples, at 100-250 Hz and also fast ripples between 250-500 Hz has been demonstrated in depth electrode recordings made from patients suffering from epilepsy (Bragin et al., 1999; 2002). Urrestarazu et al. (2006) investigated high-frequency activity that occurred during the slow wave immediately after an inter-ictal event and found that in patients suffering from epilepsy there was a decrease in the energy content at frequencies above 100 Hz. Further work demonstrated that ripples were seen in all epilepsy patients in a group of seven and fast ripples were found in five of these patients (Urrestarazu et al., 2007). Furthermore, there was a higher incidence of ripples measured from inside the irritative zone compared to outside it and this effect was even stronger for the incidence of fast ripples. Therefore the existence of high-frequency oscillations could be used to delineate the irritative zone and epileptogenic zone from other regions of cortex.

High frequency oscillations have been detected in MEG and these signals are potentially a more accurate and robust indication of the extent of the epileptogenic zone. Xiang et al. (2009) collected MEG signals at a sampling frequency of 4 kHz from 30 paediatric epilepsy patients. 86% of patients showed high frequency oscillations and 63% showed more than one high frequency component. The range of frequencies varied across patients with a peak of 910 Hz. Localisation of this high-frequency activity was performed with a beamformer and the sites of activation identified were concordant with cerebral lesions in 70% of cases. Eleven of these patients went on to have surgery and the MEG localisations were concordant with intra-operative recordings in 82% of patients. The combination of high frequency data with a spatial filtering approach is therefore potentially more reliable than standard dipolar techniques in the pre-surgical evaluation of epilepsy patients (Xiang et al., 2010). Although there is still much validation work to be done, for example it may be desirable to combine high frequency data with the excess kurtosis beamformer, it is clear that the clinical efficacy of MEG regarding the treatment of epilepsy continues to develop and evolve.

3. Parkinsonism research

Parkinson's disease is a degenerative disorder of the central nervous system with symptoms typically including tremor, rigidity, slowness of movement and postural instability. The current pathophysiological concept of Parkinsonism is that due to a loss of dopaminergic connections from the substantia nigra to the striatum there is abnormal functionality in the basal ganglia (Obeso et al., 2000). This hyperactivity in the subthalamic nucleus leads to inhibition of the thalamus and subsequently the sensorimotor cortex which leads to a loss of bodily movement, known clinically as hypokinesia. This altered connectivity affects the entire motor network, and evidence for the concept was found when high frequency stimulation of the subthalamic nucleus caused a reduction in Parkinsonian symptoms (Krack et al., 1998). As Parkinson's disease is the manifestation of altered connectivity, which causes a change in oscillatory dynamics in cortical areas, it is potentially well-suited to study and detection via MEG. This section aims to outline the advances made, and analyses used in the application of MEG to the identification of this disease. Specific studies are highlighted to show the progression and development within the field (see for example Berendse & Stam, 2007; Stam, 2010; Timmermann et al., 2007, for a more exhaustive review of the literature).

Volkmann et al. (1996) provide one of the earliest studies using MEG to investigate Parkinsonian tremor. As with much of the early epilepsy research, a single ECD model was used to localise activity. The data analysis was biased to focus on oscillatory activations that were concurrent with the observed Parkinsonian tremor. The dipole models showed activity at the diencephalic level and in pre-motor and sensorimotor cortices accompanied the resting tremor. Since it became clear the MEG could be used to investigate the underlying pathology associated with Parkinson's disease there have been a number of follow-up studies. Although the volume of studies is far fewer for Parkinson's disease than for epilepsy, a similar pattern can be seen in the types of studies performed and the progression in complexity of analysis approaches. As was described earlier in the context of epilepsy diagnosis, more recent investigations of Parkinson's disease using MEG have utilised more specific analysis techniques which are more suitable to studying the disease than the simple ECD.

Many of the analysis methods used focus on characterising the oscillatory dynamics associated with Parkinson's disease at the level of the sensors rather than performing source modelling. Kotini et al. (2005) measured spontaneous MEG signals from 9 Parkinsonian patients with minimal tremor. Each recording was 2 minutes in duration and the eyes remained closed in order to reduce artefacts and increase the alpha rhythm. The power spectrum for each each sensor was calculated by means of a Fast Fourier Transform (FFT) and the first dominant frequency was extracted. In a comparison of controls versus patients, the patients showed a prominent frequency which was lower than the 6 Hz typically observed in the healthy controls. The spatial distribution of power in these patients tended to be over a wide region in the low-frequencies whilst healthy controls showed a more focal topography for their higher frequency predominant activity. Bosboom et al. (2006) used similar techniques to investigate oscillatory differences between demented and non-demented Parkinsonian patients. Spontaneous neuronal signals were measured via MEG from 13 demented and 13 non-demented patients whilst off medication. Two 13-second epochs were used for data analysis and the data filtered in to delta, theta, alpha, beta and gamma bands of activity. The MEG sensors were also grouped into regions of interest i.e. frontal, central, parietal and occipital on both side of the sensor array. Non-demented patients showed a diffuse increase in theta power and a decrease in beta power relative to controls in central and parietal channels. Demented Parkinson's disease sufferers showed a diffuse increase in delta and theta power and a simultaneous decrease in relative alpha and beta bands when compared to the non-demented controls. Stoffers et al. (2007) used the same technique to show that the slowing of oscillatory dynamics is a feature of non-demented Parkinson's patients from a very early stage in the disease and this is independent of disease duration, severity and dopaminergic treatment. Stoffers et al. (2008) also investigated differences between patients in the early and later stages of the disease. In this study, the same frequency bands and sensor topography was used but instead of calculating changes in total power, or changes in relative power between two populations of patients, synchronisation likelihood (SL) was calculated. SL is used to to estimate both linear and non-linear correlations between time-series. SL was calculated both within and between specific topographic regions within the sensor array. The results showed that early-onset, drug naive patients showed an increase in SL in the 8-10 Hz band relative to controls whilst disease duration was positively related to 10-13 and 13-30 Hz. The 8-10 Hz was therefore thought to represent increased resting-state cortico-cortical connectivity from the onset of the disease and this altered connectivity extends to neighbouring frequency regions as the disease progresses.

It is highly encouraging that differences between patients suffering from Parkinson's disease and healthy controls can be observed at the level of the sensors. Furthermore, differences between demented and non-demented, early and late onset sufferers can also be detected. These studies suggest that the underlying pathology of the disease may have specific representations in certain frequency bands and in specific parts of the sensor array. The clinical utility of these observations is that MEG could be used to obtain an objective measure of the specific nature of Parkinson's disease and also when diagnosed, the technique may be used to provide an estimate as to the duration of the disease and to provide a measure of the rate of decline. Although it is encouraging that differences can be seen at the sensor level in a population of Parkinsonian patients, the analyses in some cases are highly rudimentary. It may be that specific types of Parkinson's disease can be identified via the oscillatory activity measured at the MEG sensors without any inverse modelling, and that this framework can be extended to other neurodegenerative disease. It is not the case that the more complex and mathematically intricate an analysis is the more accurate or robust it becomes, and therefore constraining analyses to the sensor domain may be entirely appropriate in some cases and extremely effective. However the method of peak-picking in the spectral domain is highly simplistic as well as being statistically weak. For example it is unclear if this type of activity is associated with other illnesses, or how prevalent such activity is the normal population. The use of synchronisation likelihood is a more powerful technique, but it is still limited to the analysis of data on the sensors. Parkinson's disease is thought to manifest as the altered connectivity between cortico-cortical connections and thus what the MEG is able to measure is how these changes in connectivity affect the global brain dynamics. There are a number of problems associated with performing connectivity analyses at the level of the sensors, and these issues all essentially stem from the issue of field spread. Due to the fact that a neuronal source is measured by a number of sensors it is possible to observe long-range interdependencies between MEG sensors and any change seen in the specific connectivity measure chosen could be due to a number of reasons (Schoffelen & Gross, 2009). Therefore, although the initial results are promising in that differences between clinical populations can be observed, the techniques and analyses require more robust validation. One method for mitigating the effect of field spread to some degree is to perform the analyses in source space rather than sensor space. As discussed earlier, the spatial filtering framework is a flexible approach which can be tailored to focus on specific responses, and even with the relatively small number of studies on Parkinson's disease patients, at least compared to epilepsy studies, already the field has start driving forward innovative and specific analysis approaches.

Gross et al. (2001) introduced a specific beamformer implementation to focus on cortico-cortical connectivity. The Dynamic Imaging of Coherent Sources (DICS) approach is a frequency-domain spatial filter implementation that allows coherence to be estimated throughout the brain volume. Each location within the brain is compared to a reference measure of coherence, which can be taken from an external source such as an electromyogram (EMG) or from a specific region of interest within the brain volume. In a single patient suffering from idiopathic Parkinson's disease, spontaneous activity was recorded for 5 minutes in conjunction with an EMG. Cortico-muscular coherence was estimated in the 9-12 Hz frequency band as this range contained the largest component in the power spectrum of the EMG. The resultant volumetric image showed peak levels of coherence in the contralateral primary motor cortex. This approach was shown to be more robust than using signals recorded on the sensors. Timmermann et al. (2003) extended this case study example to a cohort of 6 individuals suffering from tremor-dominant Parkinson's disease in order to better characterise the oscillatory network involved in Parkinson's disease. When off medication patients showed a dominant 4-6 Hz tremor which cohered strongly with the EMG. The main frequency of cerebro-cerebral coherence was at double this tremor frequency. Thalamic and cerebellum activity showed a broad peak of coherence around 20 Hz. They reported a bi-directional coupling between the EMG and cortical areas such as the posterior parietal cortex and secondary somatosensory cortex.

Litvak et al. (2010) used a spatial filter analysis to analyse MEG recordings from patients with electrodes inserted into the subthalamic nucleus to allow deep brain stimulation of the structure. Such a procedure can be used to treat Parkinson's disease by electrically stimulating the subcortical structure in an attempt to realign the oscillatory dynamics of the cortico-cortical loop. In many ways this is analogous to the comparison of electrocorticography recordings in epilepsy patients and ascertaining to what extent the MEG can be an accurate and reliable measure of the underlying neuronal activity. The inserted electrode not only has the ability to deliver a current to the area, but to also record signals. MEG data were acquired from a single Parkinsonian patient and a healthy control whilst at rest and also whilst performing a simple, and then a more complex motor task. An electro-oculargram and EMG were acquired simultaneously. The inherent noise-cancelling effect of a beamformer was used to localise source activity despite the large signals produced by the implanted electrodes and associated hardware. The DICS beamformer was used to localise cortical sources that were coherent with signals in the subthalamic nucleus detected by the inserted electrode, to estimate the time course of cortical activity using a virtual electrode and to uncover volumetric regions associated with movement-related power changes. Litvak et al. (2011) extended this use of the DICS beamformer into a larger cohort of 13 Parkinson's disease patients with a view to describing the dynamics of the cortico-subthalamic loop rather than focusing on methodology. Two different networks were identified which were distinct both in spectral power and spatial location. A temporoparietal-brainstem network was coherent with recordings from the subthalamic nucleus in the 7-13 Hz frequency range, whilst a frontal network was coherent with subthalamic recordings in the 15-35 Hz range. It was also noted that dopamine levels increased the coherence of this frontal network. It is possible that these networks represent distinct manifestations of the disease and if they can be better characterised may lead to a more successful diagnosis of the different Parkinsonian subtypes to ensure that patients receive the correct treatment at the earliest possible stage in the disease onset.

The other potential clinical utility of MEG in the diagnosis and treatment of Parkinson's disease is to quantify the affects that external cortical stimulation has on a patients symptoms. Mally & Stone (1999) describe a study in which the application of transcranial magnetic stimulation (TMS) was shown to alleviate Parkinsonian symptoms in a group of 10 patients. TMS is a technique whereby a focused, high-amplitude magnetic field is produced by a coil positioned outside the head which induces electrical activity within the brain. The therapeutic effects of TMS and direct current stimulation (a technique which also induces electrical activity within the brain) have been demonstrated to be long-lasting (Lefaucheur et al., 2004; Wu et al., 2008). However, it can clearly be seen in a systematic review of the literature by Fregni et al. (2005) that the mechanisms by which symptoms are alleviated as well as the optimal parameters of stimulation duration, frequency etc are unknown. MEG has been used to try and uncover the reasons why techniques such as TMS are able to alleviate symptoms. If this can be uncovered then it would greatly enhance the efficacy of this intervention and also allow it to become more commonly used. Anninos et al. (2007) recorded one minute of MEG data from 30 patients diagnosed with idiopathic Parkinson's disease both before and after the application of TMS. Patients were divided into two group of partial responders and favourable responders. Partial responders were patients whose tremor or dyskinesia returned within 12 months and showed a low-amplitude alpha rhythm in their subsequent EEG. Favourable responders showed no Parkinsonian symptoms for a year and showed a high-amplitude alpha rhythm. The only MEG analysis performed in this study was to label the pre and post stimulation recording as one of normal, abnormal or partially normal. Therefore the analysis allows no insight into how the intervention alters the cortico-cortical network in order to alleviate symptoms. A more systematic study could use MEG to quantify the oscillatory dynamics of the network before and after TMS is applied with a number of different sub-groups, each one receiving a different set of parameters. In such a study MEG may be able to provide a clear insight as to why the TMS has such a profound benefit, and then efforts can be focused on optimising the magnitude and duration of any alleviation from symptoms.

3.1 Summary

Numerous studies have provided evidence for the fact that MEG is able to measure oscillatory dynamics related to Parkinson's disease at the levels of the sensors. Differences have been seen not only between recordings from patients and healthy controls but also between different phenotypes of the disease. Further validatory studies are needed to build on the evidence for the ability of MEG to to accurately observe the effects of altered connectivity between subcortical and cortical structures. However, the initial work is promising and suggests that the technique may well have a role to play in improving diagnosis of the disease, monitoring specific interventions and evaluation of the effect of specific pharmacological treatments. MEG can potentially provide an objective means by which to determine the specific type of Parkinson's disease, which may lead to the most effective treatment being administered quickly. The technique may also be able to be of predictive value in determining the likelihood of severe and rapid dementia being co-morbid with the disease. The progression of analysis techniques in many ways matches that of epilepsy research, with initial studies using the ECD before more specific analysis tools were adopted that are more appropriate to the response of interest, such as a spatial filter that is sensitive to coherence. Spontaneous recordings are often made, but movement tasks are also used as it is known that the motor network is involved in the disease. As the range of statistical analyses grow and are developed with the specific goal of characterising cortico-cortical loops, the clinical application of MEG to populations of Parkinsonian patients in a routine and systematic way is likely to move from possessing great potential to a real possibility.

4. Alzheimer's disease

Alzheimer's disease is the most common neurodegenerative disease and detecting individuals who are susceptible to the condition and achieving an accurate and early diagnosis is an essential step in developing and quantifying effective therapies. As with previous sections, the aim is to not to provide an exhaustive review of the literature to date (for such a review see Criado et al., 2006), but to give an overview of the progress made in the uses of MEG to investigate Alzheimer's disease. Berendse et al. (2000) provided an initial description of the oscillatory changes involved in Alzheimer's disease by measuring the resting-state MEG from a group of 5 patients and 5 age-matched controls. Power and coherence were calculated in a number of frequency bands and the patients showed a greater magnitude and diffusion of low-frequency signals, predominantly in the frontal regions. Higher frequency power was decreased in patients over temporal and occipital regions. In patients, the coherence values at all frequencies were found to be lower than in controls. which suggests that there may be readily available metrics with which to quantify the extent of the condition. Fernández et al. (2006) extended this into a more thorough analysis of the spectral content of MEG data acquired from Alzheimer's patients and reported that oscillatory activity in the 2-4 Hz and 16-28 Hz ranges showed high degrees of sensitivity and specificity when classifying data as from a patient or a control. When measuring signals from patients suffering from Alzheimer's disease, it is common to not only acquire resting-state oscillatory changes, but also those involved in a task. For example Pekkonen et al. (1996) noted that in patients, the auditory response to simple tones was delayed when compared to age-matched controls. The P50 and N100 are standard responses that occur originate from primary auditory cortices in response to tones with simple pitch and amplitude characteristics. The study demonstrated that if the sound was played to a single ear, these early sensory responses were delayed in the ipsilateral but not contralateral hemisphere of patients. Pekkonen et al. (2001) extend this finding to look at the process of performing auditory discriminations, i.e. a task with some decision process and active listening rather than looking at passive, automated responses. The results confirmed that ipsilateral auditory areas showed a delayed response, although this did not affect the patients' ability to perform the auditory discrimination task. These findings suggest that it may be possible to use abnormal processing in sensory systems to perform an objective assessment of Alzheimer's disease and that these changes need not necessarily be associated with impaired cognitive or sensory percepts. Of course the difficulty is then to determine whether delayed auditory processing points to the onset of Alzheimer's disease or the onset of some other condition.

Another task which is used to investigate cortical dynamics in Alzheimer's disease is a memory task, which is concordant with one of the prominent features of the disease being impaired memory. Maestú et al. (2001) used a high load probe task in which targets needed to be remembered and distinguished from distractors. Control subjects were reported to show an increased number of sources over temporal and parietal regions 400-700 ms after the stimulus onset, whereas Alzheimer's patients showed a greater number of sources over frontal motor areas. The number of sources in patients' left parietal regions was also predictive of their performance on clinical scales of cognitive functioning. In a second study, these left parietal sources were also found to be correlated with the level of hippocampal atrophy (Maestú et al., 2003). One of the potential clinical applications of MEG in the diagnosis and treatment of Alzheimer's disease is to be able to predict which individuals are susceptible to the disease and how rapid their decline may be. Alzheimer's disease has a long pre-clinical stage and Mild Cognitive Impairment (MCI) is often used to describe individuals who are declining from normal cognitive function to dementia. There is a conversion rate of MCI to Alzheimer's disease of around 10-15% per year (see Shah et al., 2000, for a review). Fernández et al. (2006) assessed the ability of MEG to determine the risk factor associated with individuals with MCI developing Alzheimer's disease. Dipoles were fitted to the low-frequency regions of the spectrum of resting-state recordings. Dipole density in the left parietal regions fitted over the delta frequency band were found to provide a reliable classification of Alzheimer's and MCI patients. MCI patients were also categorised as being at either low or high risk based on the observed magnetic fields. A follow-up clinical examination occurred 2 years later and the fact that more patients in the high MCI group had developed Alzheimer's disease than the low MCI group suggests that MEG can be a useful clinical utility for identifying risk factors for individuals. Osipova et al. (2006) conducted a study with a similar goal of predicting transition from MCI to Alzheimer's disease, and reported that the source distribution of the alpha rhythm was abnormal in Alzheimer's patients but not MCI patients when compared to controls, and so the changes in neuronal processes associated with MCI may be more subtle and more complex than those associated with other neurodegenerative diseases. Of course more longitudinal studies are required and, like other techniques discussed in this chapter, it may be desirable to move away from a simple dipolar technique and investigate the dynamics using other methods, but the initial results are promising.

Spatial filtering approaches have also been applied to Alzheimer's disease data which, as previously discussed, offers a more complete description of the data as it treats the activity as a distributed network rather than point-like bursts of activity. Alzheimer's, MCI and control patients were scanned and the two patient groups were noted not to show any slow-wave MEG activity in conjunction with the task, which was simply closing the eyes and opening them at 10 second intervals. The beamformer analyses revealed all three groups had increased activity in posterior regions when the eyes were closed in the 8-15 Hz band. Patients suffering from Alzheimer's disease showed greater activity in frontal regions in this frequency band when the eyes were closed compared to controls, whereas MCI patients showed no such difference. This finding was taken to show that alpha activity is found in frontal regions for Alzheimer's patients across a cohort, whereas the same is not true for MCI patients or controls. These findings, both in the spectral frequencies involved and the volumetric locations are consistent with previous results. Further analyses also confirmed that these changes in activity were correlated with clinical examinations of the mental state of the Alzheimer's disease patients (Ishii et al., 2010).

Dipolar and beamformer approaches have been shown to provide an objective measure which can categorise an individual as suffering from Alzheimer's disease. Such a technique could be valuable in the treatment of a disease that is difficult to diagnose and categorise. However, as the disease affects cognitive function in a general way, and in a manner that is only broadly consistent across individuals, applying these analyses to resting-state data may not be the best use of the technique. A number of higher-level techniques have been applied to MEG data acquired from Alzheimer's disease patients. Poza et al. (2008) used techniques from information theory to discriminate the resting-state data from a group of individuals and age-matched controls. Power spectral densities were calculated from the data and three different methods were used to compute the spectral entropy of the signals. Entropy can be thought of as a measure of uncertainty and it was demonstrated that Alzheimer's patients showed significantly lower levels of entropy than control participants. On the basis of these entropy measures, data from individuals were accurately identified as from patient or controls to a level of 87% and suggest a loss of irregularity in the dynamics of Alzheimer's patients. A similar finding, that data from Alzheimer's patients is more regular than that from controls, was reported using approximate entropy (Gomez et al., 2010). It is therefore possible that higher level statistical analyses may be more robust to detecting the signature oscillatory characteristics of Alzheimer's disease. It is these types of innovative, robust approaches that, when developed with specific clinically relevant questions in mind can allow MEG to be applied reliably to groups of patients suffering from illness and disease. Although much more is needed, both in terms of basic research and clinical trials in the efficacy of MEG in the identification and monitoring of neurodegenerative disease, the clinical applications are clear and the benefits are potentially vast.

5. Future applications

Specific diseases have a well defined biomagnetic representation. For example epileptogenic activity is typically high amplitude and can be characterised as slow wave activity or "spike-and-wave" activity. It has a strong dipolar representation on the sensors and is therefore readily identified both visually and statistically. Other types of illness such as Parkinson's disease show more complex temporal dynamics in the measured MEG, however there are still typical spectral shapes which can be used to identify the illness, for example diffuse and exaggerated low-frequency information. Parkinson's disease is also known to affect connectivity related to motor cortices and so there is a priori information regarding sensors and cortical regions of interest. There are however, numerous diseases which do not have such clearly defined neuromagnetic representations. However, some of these illnesses are still suitable to diagnosis and detection via MEG. Detection of certain illnesses is possible via a neural system largely unrelated to the symptomatic manifestation of the disease. "Biomarker" is a term often used to describe the observation of altered or atypical processing in one domain which provides an independent measure of another function, in this case an objective measure related to an illness or disease. Such a measure may allow early and effective diagnosis, to evaluate different interventions or to predict an individuals responsiveness to a drug or their rate of decline. This final section gives a brief overview of some of the recent applications of MEG in the identification of biomkarkers for specific conditions.

The application of MEG measurements to patient populations is clearly still developing and evolving. One of the biggest risk factors in developing neurodegenerative disorders is age and although, as previously discussed, MEG is able to provide a measure of the underlying neuronal activity associated with these diseases, the changes in oscillatory dynamics in the normal aging population are still poorly understood. Rossini et al. (2007) note that MEG can be used in conjunction with other imaging modalities in order to distinguish between physiological and pathological aging. In order to more robustly identify neurodegenerative disease it is essential that the aging brain is more fully characterised. This needs to be done not purely in terms of the dominant spectral frequencies of the data, but also using higher-level metrics such as coherence, entropy etc. The statistical robustness of diagnosing diseases such as Parkinson's and Alzheimer's will then increase as the distribution of the normal population can be characterised and these conditions may be more clearly identified.

MEG has been used to investigate responses associated with schizophrenia and schizoaffective disorder. Uhlhaas et al. (2008) provide a review of the role of oscillatory rhythms in cortical networks in relation to the illness. The role of delta, theta, alpha, beta and gamma rhythms are often discussed in relation to a range of neural processes such as memory, language, auditory and visual processing. The synchrony and amplitude of these rhythms during a range of behavioural tests are seen to be altered in patients suffering from Schizophrenia, and so investigation of these processes via MEG may provide an insight into the development and manifestation of the disease. More specific examples include altered auditory processing in response to deviant sounds. The Mismatch Negativity (MMN) paradigm is often used to investigate automatic auditory processing. A sequence of identical stimuli are played and a deviant stimulus is inserted at random. For example, in the middle of a train of 500 Hz tones, a 550 Hz tone is heard. The response to this deviant is amplified and an insight into the auditory system can be obtained. Näätänen & Kähkönen (2009) describe data which demonstrates that in schizophrenic individuals the MMN is attenuated. The MMN in response to frequency deviation is also found to be attenuated in a manner that reflects the progress of the disease as measured by disease duration. There is also evidence that specific characteristics of the MEG measured in response to auditory stimulation may implicate the patients possessing positive or negative symptoms. Reite et al. (2010) retrospectively investigated differences between the auditory steady-state response of patients with schizoaffective disorder and schizophrenia and suggest that whereas the amplitude and phase of the response is atypical in schizophrenia sufferers, the schizoaffective disorder patients are more similar to controls. Differentiating between schizophrenia and schizoaffective disorder is a difficult and unclear process, however differential diagnoses lead to different interventions and different paths of pharmacological treatment. Therefore the potential ability of MEG to differentiate between the two could have great clinical utility. Ince et al. (2008) used a working memory task and demonstrated differences between schizophrenic patients and controls in specific parts of the sensor array and in specific frequency bands.

Autism spectrum disorder (ASD) is another condition that has received interest from researchers who use MEG as a measure of neuronal functioning. ASD encompasses a number of illnesses including Autism disorder and Asperger's syndrome. The conditions are most commonly diagnosed in childhood and therefore early detection may be able to limit the impact they have on development into adulthood. Again, the auditory system appears to be reliably associated with the underlying nature of the conditions, with ASD patients showing both delayed and attenuated responses to simple sounds when compared to age-matched controls. Roberts et al. (2010) presented tones of different frequencies to a group of ASD and healthy controls and analysed the M50 and M100 response from both left and right superior temporal gyri. No differences were seen between groups for the amplitude or latency of the M50 but the M100 response was delayed in ASD patients by an average of 11 ms across the entire group. One clear difference between ASD and the other conditions discussed in this chapter is that ASD is a neurodevelopmental disorder, and therefore by its very definition affects the paediatric population. This therefore amplfies some of the inherent challenges of scanning patients in MEG, such as movement of the head and trunk and also stresses the need to design protocols that can be easily understood and tolerated by young individuals. Scanning children in MEG is a time consuming and difficult process, and the data are more susceptible to artefacts. However, given the prevalence of ASD, the potential benefits of using MEG as a screening tool to allow early identification of the illness make the technique a valuable one.

Georgopoulos et al. (2007) made MEG recordings from 142 individuals whilst they fixated on a spot of light for 45-60 seconds. The analysis stream utilised the sensor information and assessed zero-lag cross-correlations in order to provide an estimate of synchronous coupling. The analyses appear to provide some insight regarding which subset of clinical conditions each participant could be categorised as matching. Patients with multiple sclerosis, Alzheimer's disease, schizophrenia, Sjogren's syndrome, alcoholism, and facial pain as well as a group of control participants were reliably identified. A second study by the same group applied similar techniques to a group of patients suffering from post-traumatic stress disorder (Georgopoulos et al., 2010). Although a study which attempts to differentiate so many different conditions is susceptible to limitations in the analysis and a lack of statistical robustness, the results are extremely promising and highlight the powerful nature of MEG as a non-invasive tool with which to objectively evaluate clinical populations.

MEG has also been found to have a clinical utility unrelated to measures of functional mechanisms. Martino et al. (2011) used MEG to look at the functional connectivity of the so called "resting-state network". The resting-state network is used to describe the cortical dynamics that can be observed in the absence of any task. Functionally connected regions still communicate with each other and decreased levels of connectivity in this network are expected in many types of illness and disease. Functional connectivity is an umbrella term used to describe a series of analysis methods which focus on measures of coherence, correlation and synchronisation. A brief overview of some of these metrics has been given in previous sections of this chapter, however it is worth noting that measures of connectivity are becoming more and more sought after by researchers of human brain function. The advantage of studying the resting-state connectivity of areas is that no task is required, which means the recodring can be short and can be carried out in patients who may struggle to perform a language, memory, or movement task. Martino et al. (2011) created functional connectivity maps using imaginary coherence and the aim was to determine if this information could predict the results of intra-operative electrical stimulation (IES) carried out to identify eloquent regions of cortex. 57 patients with tumours in or near motor, sesnory or language areas were studied. A lesion-related area of cortex was identified and compared to a representative number of points taken from the whole of the brain, as a control the lesion-related area was compared to the same area in the contralateral hemisphere. The results revealed MEG functional connectivity maps to have a 100% negative predictive value, which means that when the connectivity in the lesion-related area was lower than the contralateral volume in each of these patients (a total of 7), no functional areas were idenitied

in the lesion via IES. In 42 subjects, at least some voxels in the lesion-related area showed increased connectivity and in 64% of these patients, IES revealed a functionally active area. The authors stress that the study must be repeated on a larger sample of patients but, as they also note, the potential clinical utility of such information has a potentially huge impact upon pre-surgical planning and investigation. These recordings are very short and require no active participation in a task, or any attentional processes. The study presented attempts to use robust statisatical analyses to evaluate the responses, a facet which is missing from MEG studies in a number of areas. The resting-state network, also known as the default-mode network, has become a hot topic in both fMRI and MEG in recent years.
Currently, a large number of metrics are used to obtain an estimate of so-called functional connectivity. Methods such as coherence, imaginary coherence, phase lag index and synchronisation likelihood are currently being applied to MEG recordings from both patients populations and healthy controls. Although they differ in their underlying mathematics, their specific assumptions are the same, that distant brain regions that are communicating with each other will have an observable MEG signal which is very similar. The main problem for all the methods is also the same, that of field spread. This results from the fact that any inverse estimate is calculated using only the sensor data, and this information is the same when estimating activity coming from region *A* and region *B*. Therefore spurious connectivity becomes highly likely given that the same sensor data is used to obtain both inverse estimates. It is likely that in the coming years a number of these methods will emerge as being favoured. This must be because they are 1) the most robust to spurious connectivity and 2) they are suitable for statistical interrogation. If the application and devlopement of these connectivity measures can be done in clinical populations in parallel with healthy controls then the resting-state network, and estimates of the connectivity present within the network, has the potential to be a clinically relevant tool which is not limited to a specific sub-type of illness. Such a measure could be used a a preliminary screening tool for a range of conditions, however if the clinical utility of such an approach is to be maximised, it is essential to fully characterise the network in the normal population and then develop statistically viable ways of identifying how different diseases affect the network.

6. General summary

This chapter has outlined the current clinical utility of MEG by charting the progression of analyses and methodologies in a range of different clinical populations. What is striking is the similarity which exists in the progression of the technique across different sub-types of illness and disease, despite the fact that these advances were made at very different moments in time. Epilepsy is by far still the area which is able to obtain the most clinically relevant information from MEG scans. The initial role of MEG in epilepsy diagnosis and management was to identify atypical waveforms, much in the same way as EEG was used. This was then followed by the use of dipole fitting techniques to estimate the brain location responsible for the epileptogenic activity. Dipolar techniques were then applied to various perceptual and cognitive functions in the epileptic population to delineate eloquent cortex before more advanced modelling techniqes such as minimum-norm estimation and spatial filters were used to better characterise the dynamic changes in neuronal activity. These advances took somewhere in the region of two decades, as the field of epilepsy research via MEG managed to maintain pace with the general field of MEG research. Subsequently, MEG has been used to investigate the underlying dynamics of a range of illness and disease, and although the developments have occurred at a greater pace, the general pattern persists; dipole fits are first applied to passive resting data, they are then applied to more complex perceptual and cognitive tasks before more complex modelling criteria are used altogether. MEG has been shown to be able to reliably distinguish the length of onset of a disease, to accurately identify an individual as being a patient or a healthy control, and to predict the probability of a patient suffering further decline. The type of illness and disease that these effects have been shown for are typically difficult to detect clinically until relatively late in the progression of the disease. Therefore the early, accurate and reliable diagnosis of these conditions can allow patients to receive the appropriate intervention as soon as possible.

The methodological advances in MEG now occur at a rapid pace, with ever more eloquent and complex measures of coherence and correlation applied to investigate mechanisms of functional connectivity. Many of these measures have been shown, in small samples, to have a potential clinical utility. Due to MEG now being more widely used and better understood than in the early days of epilepsy research the field is in an extremely promising position. Much work is needed over the coming years to validate these initial clinical findings. Independent clinical tests are needed to support the information obtained via non-invasive biomagnetic measurements. Longitudinal studies are required to determine the accuracy and sensitivity with which MEG is able to predict the onset and development of certain conditions. Comprehensive and thorough research studies are needed to determine the most robust algorithms with which to measure coherence between different brain regions, and there needs to be clear bi-directional communication between scientists and clinicians to establish what the clinically relevant questions are and if MEG is technique which is able to add extra information to the diagnosis of a range of conditions. There is no doubt that the evidence for the clinical utility of MEG is compelling, It is no longer a technique reserved for identifying epileptiform activity, it is now a technique with the potential to provide an insight into the underlying neuronal activity of pathologies which currently no other invasive or non-invasive method can. There is much confirmatory work to be done but, MEG clearly does have the potential to become a routinely used method to aid in the diagnosis and treatment plan of a range of diseases which manifest themselves as cerebral deficits.

7. References

Abbott, J. A. & Schwab, R. S. (1948). Some clinical aspects of the normal electroencephalogram in epilepsy., *N Engl J Med* 238(14): 457–461.
URL: *http://dx.doi.org/10.1056/NEJM194804012381401*

Anninos, P., Adamopoulos, A., Kotini, A., Tsagas, N., Tamiolakis, D. & Prassopoulos, P. (2007). Meg evaluation of parkinson's diseased patients after external magnetic stimulation., *Acta Neurol Belg* 107(1): 5–10.

Berendse, H. W. & Stam, C. J. (2007). Stage-dependent patterns of disturbed neural synchrony in parkinson's disease., *Parkinsonism Relat Disord* 13 Suppl 3: S440–S445.
URL: *http://dx.doi.org/10.1016/S1353-8020(08)70046-4*

Berendse, H. W., Verbunt, J. P., Scheltens, P., van Dijk, B. W. & Jonkman, E. J. (2000). Magnetoencephalographic analysis of cortical activity in alzheimer's disease: a pilot study., *Clin Neurophysiol* 111(4): 604–612.

Bosboom, J. L. W., Stoffers, D., Stam, C. J., van Dijk, B. W., Verbunt, J., Berendse, H. W. & Wolters, E. C. (2006). Resting state oscillatory brain dynamics in parkinson's disease: an meg study., *Clin Neurophysiol* 117(11): 2521–2531.
URL: *http://dx.doi.org/10.1016/j.clinph.2006.06.720*

Bowyer, S. M., Fleming, T., Greenwald, M. L., Moran, J. E., Mason, K. M., Weiland, B. J., Smith, B. J., Barkley, G. L. & Tepley, N. (2005). Magnetoencephalographic localization of the

basal temporal language area., *Epilepsy Behav* 6(2): 229–234.
URL: *http://dx.doi.org/10.1016/j.yebeh.2004.12.003*
Bowyer, S. M., Moran, J. E., Weiland, B. J., Mason, K. M., Greenwald, M. L., Smith, B. J., Barkley, G. L. & Tepley, N. (2005). Language laterality determined by meg mapping with mr-focuss., *Epilepsy Behav* 6(2): 235–241.
URL: *http://dx.doi.org/10.1016/j.yebeh.2004.12.002*
Bragin, A., Engel, J., Wilson, C. L., Fried, I. & BuzsÃąki, G. (1999). High-frequency oscillations in human brain., *Hippocampus* 9(2): 137–142.
URL: *http://dx.doi.org/3.0.CO;2-0*
Bragin, A., Mody, I., Wilson, C. L. & Engel, J. (2002). Local generation of fast ripples in epileptic brain., *J Neurosci* 22(5): 2012–2021.
Breier, J. I., Simos, P. G., Wheless, J. W., Constantinou, J. E., Baumgartner, J. E., Venkataraman, V. & Papanicolaou, A. C. (2001). Language dominance in children as determined by magnetic source imaging and the intracarotid amobarbital procedure: a comparison., *J Child Neurol* 16(2): 124–130.
Breier, J. I., Simos, P. G., Zouridakis, G., Wheless, J. W., Willmore, L. J., Constantinou, J. E., Maggio, W. W. & Papanicolaou, A. C. (1999). Language dominance determined by magnetic source imaging: a comparison with the wada procedure., *Neurology* 53(5): 938–945.
Cheyne, D., Bakhtazad, L. & Gaetz, W. (2006). Spatiotemporal mapping of cortical activity accompanying voluntary movements using an event-related beamforming approach, *Hum Brain Mapp* 27(3): 213–229.
Cheyne, D., Bostan, A. C., Gaetz, W. & Pang, E. W. (2007). Event-related beamforming: a robust method for presurgical functional mapping using meg., *Clin Neurophysiol* 118(8): 1691–1704.
URL: *http://dx.doi.org/10.1016/j.clinph.2007.05.064*
Criado, J. R., Amo, C., Quint, P., Kurelowech, L. & Otis, S. M. (2006). Using magnetoencephalography to study patterns of brain magnetic activity in alzheimer's disease., *Am J Alzheimers Dis Other Demen* 21(6): 416–423.
URL: *http://dx.doi.org/10.1177/1533317506293502*
da Silva, F. H. L. (2005). What is magnetoencephalography and why it is relevant to neurosurgery?, *Adv Tech Stand Neurosurg* 30: 51–67.
Doss, R. C., Zhang, W., Risse, G. L. & Dickens, D. L. (2009). Lateralizing language with magnetic source imaging: validation based on the wada test., *Epilepsia* 50(10): 2242–2248.
URL: *http://dx.doi.org/10.1111/j.1528-1167.2009.02242.x*
Ebersole, J. S. (1997). Magnetoencephalography/magnetic source imaging in the assessment of patients with epilepsy., *Epilepsia* 38 Suppl 4: S1–S5.
Fernändez, A., Hornero, R., Mayo, A., Poza, J., Maestü, F. & Ortiz, T. (2006). Quantitative magnetoencephalography of spontaneous brain activity in alzheimer disease: an exhaustive frequency analysis., *Alzheimer Dis Assoc Disord* 20(3): 153–159.
Fernändez, A., Turrero, A., Zuluaga, P., Gil, P., Maestü, F., Campo, P. & Ortiz, T. (2006). Magnetoencephalographic parietal delta dipole density in mild cognitive impairment: preliminary results of a method to estimate the risk of developing alzheimer disease., *Arch Neurol* 63(3): 427–430.
URL: *http://dx.doi.org/10.1001/archneur.63.3.427*
Fregni, F., Simon, D. K., Wu, A. & Pascual-Leone, A. (2005). Non-invasive brain stimulation for parkinson's disease: a systematic review and meta-analysis of the literature., *J*

Neurol Neurosurg Psychiatry 76(12): 1614–1623.
URL: *http://dx.doi.org/10.1136/jnnp.2005.069849*

Frye, R. E., Rezaie, R. & Papanicolaou, A. C. (2009). Functional neuroimaging of language using magnetoencephalography., *Phys Life Rev* 6(1): 1–10.
URL: *http://dx.doi.org/10.1016/j.plrev.2008.08.001*

Gaetz, W., Cheyne, D., Rutka, J. T., Drake, J., Benifla, M., Strantzas, S., Widjaja, E., Holowka, S., Tovar-Spinoza, Z., Otsubo, H. & Pang, E. W. (2009). Presurgical localization of primary motor cortex in pediatric patients with brain lesions by the use of spatially filtered magnetoencephalography., *Neurosurgery* 64(3 Suppl): 177–85; discussion 186.
URL: *http://dx.doi.org/10.1227/01.NEU.0000316433.10913.32*

Ganslandt, O., Fahlbusch, R., Nimsky, C., Kober, H., Mller, M., Steinmeier, R., Romstck, J. & Vieth, J. (1999). Functional neuronavigation with magnetoencephalography: outcome in 50 patients with lesions around the motor cortex., *J Neurosurg* 91(1): 73–79.
URL: *http://dx.doi.org/10.3171/jns.1999.91.1.0073*

Georgopoulos, A. P., Karageorgiou, E., Leuthold, A. C., Lewis, S. M., Lynch, J. K., Alonso, A. A., Aslam, Z., Carpenter, A. F., Georgopoulos, A., Hemmy, L. S., Koutlas, I. G., Langheim, F. J. P., McCarten, J. R., McPherson, S. E., Pardo, J. V., Pardo, P. J., Parry, G. J., Rottunda, S. J., Segal, B. M., Sponheim, S. R., Stanwyck, J. J., Stephane, M. & Westermeyer, J. J. (2007). Synchronous neural interactions assessed by magnetoencephalography: a functional biomarker for brain disorders., *J Neural Eng* 4(4): 349–355.
URL: *http://dx.doi.org/10.1088/1741-2560/4/4/001*

Georgopoulos, A. P., Tan, H.-R. M., Lewis, S. M., Leuthold, A. C., Winskowski, A. M., Lynch, J. K. & Engdahl, B. (2010). The synchronous neural interactions test as a functional neuromarker for post-traumatic stress disorder (ptsd): a robust classification method based on the bootstrap., *J Neural Eng* 7(1): 16011.
URL: *http://dx.doi.org/10.1088/1741-2560/7/1/016011*

Gomez, C., Abasolo, D., Poza, J., Fernandez, A. & Hornero, R. (2010). Meg analysis in alzheimer's disease computing approximate entropy for different frequency bands., *Conf Proc IEEE Eng Med Biol Soc* 2010: 2379–2382.
URL: *http://dx.doi.org/10.1109/IEMBS.2010.5627236*

Gross, J., Kujala, J., Hamalainen, M., Timmermann, L., Schnitzler, A. & Salmelin, R. (2001). Dynamic imaging of coherent sources: Studying neural interactions in the human brain., *P Natl Acad Sci USA* 98(2): 694–699.

Hämäläinen, M., Hari, R., Ilmoniemi, R. J., Knuutila, J. & Lounasmaa, O. V. (1993). Magnetoencephalography—theory, instrumentation, and applications to noninvasive studies of the working human brain, *Rev. Mod. Phys.* 65(2): 413–497.

Hund, M., Rezai, A. R., Kronberg, E., Cappell, J., Zonenshayn, M., Ribary, U., Kelly, P. J. & LlinÃąs, R. (1997). Magnetoencephalographic mapping: basic of a new functional risk profile in the selection of patients with cortical brain lesions., *Neurosurgery* 40(5): 936–42; discussion 942–3.

Hymers, M., Prendergast, G., Johnson, S. R. & Green, G. G. R. (2010). Source Stability Index: a novel beamforming based localisation metric., *Neuroimage* 49(2): 1385–1397.

Ince, N. F., Goksu, F., Pellizzer, G., Tewfik, A. & Stephane, M. (2008). Selection of spectro-temporal patterns in multichannel meg with support vector machines for schizophrenia classification., *Conf Proc IEEE Eng Med Biol Soc* 2008: 3554–3557.
URL: *http://dx.doi.org/10.1109/IEMBS.2008.4649973*

Ishii, R., Canuet, L., Kurimoto, R., Ikezawa, K., Aoki, Y., Azechi, M., Takahashi, H., Nakahachi, T., Iwase, M., Kazui, H. & Takeda, M. (2010). Frontal shift of posterior alpha activity is correlated with cognitive impairment in early alzheimer's disease: a magnetoencephalography-beamformer study., *Psychogeriatrics* 10(3): 138–143.
URL: *http://dx.doi.org/10.1111/j.1479-8301.2010.00326.x*

Knake, S., Halgren, E., Shiraishi, H., Hara, K., Hamer, H. M., Grant, P. E., Carr, V. A., Foxe, D., Camposano, S., Busa, E., Witzel, T., HÃd'mÃd'lÃd'inen, M. S., Ahlfors, S. P., Bromfield, E. B., Black, P. M., Bourgeois, B. F., Cole, A. J., Cosgrove, G. R., Dworetzky, B. A., Madsen, J. R., Larsson, P. G., Schomer, D. L., Thiele, E. A., Dale, A. M., Rosen, B. R. & Stufflebeam, S. M. (2006). The value of multichannel meg and eeg in the presurgical evaluation of 70 epilepsy patients., *Epilepsy Res* 69(1): 80–86.
URL: *http://dx.doi.org/10.1016/j.eplepsyres.2006.01.001*

Knowlton, R. C. (2003). Magnetoencephalography: clinical application in epilepsy., *Curr Neurol Neurosci Rep* 3(4): 341–348.

Kotini, A., Anninos, P., Adamopoulos, A. & Prassopoulos, P. (2005). Low-frequency meg activity and mri evaluation in parkinson's disease., *Brain Topogr* 18(1): 59–63.
URL: *http://dx.doi.org/10.1007/s10548-005-7901-4*

Krack, P., Benazzouz, A., Pollak, P., Limousin, P., Piallat, B., Hoffmann, D., Xie, J. & Benabid, A. L. (1998). Treatment of tremor in parkinson's disease by subthalamic nucleus stimulation., *Mov Disord* 13(6): 907–914.
URL: *http://dx.doi.org/10.1002/mds.870130608*

Lefaucheur, J.-P., Drouot, X., Raison, F. V., MÃl'nard-Lefaucheur, I., Cesaro, P. & Nguyen, J.-P. (2004). Improvement of motor performance and modulation of cortical excitability by repetitive transcranial magnetic stimulation of the motor cortex in parkinson's disease., *Clin Neurophysiol* 115(11): 2530–2541.
URL: *http://dx.doi.org/10.1016/j.clinph.2004.05.025*

Litvak, V., Eusebio, A., Jha, A., Oostenveld, R., Barnes, G. R., Penny, W. D., Zrinzo, L., Hariz, M. I., Limousin, P., Friston, K. J. & Brown, P. (2010). Optimized beamforming for simultaneous meg and intracranial local field potential recordings in deep brain stimulation patients., *Neuroimage* 50(4): 1578–1588.
URL: *http://dx.doi.org/10.1016/j.neuroimage.2009.12.115*

Litvak, V., Jha, A., Eusebio, A., Oostenveld, R., Foltynie, T., Limousin, P., Zrinzo, L., Hariz, M. I., Friston, K. & Brown, P. (2011). Resting oscillatory cortico-subthalamic connectivity in patients with parkinson's disease., *Brain* 134(Pt 2): 359–374.
URL: *http://dx.doi.org/10.1093/brain/awq332*

Maestü, F., Arrazola, J., Fernändez, A., Simos, P. G., Amo, C., Gil-Gregorio, P., Fernández, S., Papanicolaou, A. & Ortiz, T. (2003). Do cognitive patterns of brain magnetic activity correlate with hippocampal atrophy in alzheimer's disease?, *J Neurol Neurosurg Psychiatry* 74(2): 208–212.

Maestú, F., Fernández, A., Simos, G, P., Gil-Gregorio, P., Amo, C., Rodriguez, R., Arrazola, J. & Ortiz, T. (2001). Spatio-temporal patterns of brain magnetic activity during a memory task in alzheimer's disease., *Neuroreport* 12(18): 3917–3922.

Mally, J. & Stone, T. W. (1999). Improvement in parkinsonian symptoms after repetitive transcranial magnetic stimulation., *J Neurol Sci* 162(2): 179–184.

Martino, J., Honma, S. M., Findlay, A. M., Guggisberg, A. G., Owen, J. P., Kirsch, H. E., Berger, M. S. & Nagarajan, S. S. (2011). Resting functional connectivity in patients with brain tumors in eloquent areas., *Ann Neurol* 69(3): 521–532.
URL: *http://dx.doi.org/10.1002/ana.22167*

Näätänen, R. & Kähkönen, S. (2009). Central auditory dysfunction in schizophrenia as revealed by the mismatch negativity (mmn) and its magnetic equivalent mmnm: a review., *Int J Neuropsychopharmacol* 12(1): 125–135.
URL: *http://dx.doi.org/10.1017/S1461145708009322*

Nakasato, N., Levesque, M. F., Barth, D. S., Baumgartner, C., Rogers, R. L. & Sutherling, W. W. (1994). Comparisons of meg, eeg, and ecog source localization in neocortical partial epilepsy in humans., *Electroencephalogr Clin Neurophysiol* 91(3): 171–178.

Obeso, J. A., Rodriguez-Oroz, M. C., Rodriguez, M., Macias, R., Alvarez, L., Guridi, J., Vitek, J. & DeLong, M. R. (2000). Pathophysiologic basis of surgery for parkinson's disease., *Neurology* 55(12 Suppl 6): S7–12.

Osipova, D., Rantanen, K., Ahveninen, J., Ylikoski, R., HÃd'pplÃd', O., Strandberg, T. & Pekkonen, E. (2006). Source estimation of spontaneous meg oscillations in mild cognitive impairment., *Neurosci Lett* 405(1-2): 57–61.
URL: *http://dx.doi.org/10.1016/j.neulet.2006.06.045*

Otsubo, H. & Snead, O. C. (2001). Magnetoencephalography and magnetic source imaging in children., *J Child Neurol* 16(4): 227–235.

Pang, E. W., Drake, J. M., Otsubo, H., Martineau, A., Strantzas, S., Cheyne, D. & Gaetz, W. (2008). Intraoperative confirmation of hand motor area identified preoperatively by magnetoencephalography., *Pediatr Neurosurg* 44(4): 313–317.
URL: *http://dx.doi.org/10.1159/000134923*

Papanicolaou, A. C., Simos, P. G., Castillo, E. M., Breier, J. I., Sarkari, S., Pataraia, E., Billingsley, R. L., Buchanan, S., Wheless, J., Maggio, V. & Maggio, W. W. (2004). Magnetocephalography: a noninvasive alternative to the wada procedure., *J Neurosurg* 100(5): 867–876.
URL: *http://dx.doi.org/10.3171/jns.2004.100.5.0867*

Parker, M. M. (1947). The clinical utility of electroencephalography in idiopathic epilepsy., *Health Cent J* 1(1): 13–17.

Pekkonen, E., Huotilainen, M., Virtanen, J., NÃd'Ãd'tÃd'nen, R., Ilmoniemi, R. J. & Erkinjuntti, T. (1996). Alzheimer's disease affects parallel processing between the auditory cortices., *Neuroreport* 7(8): 1365–1368.

Pekkonen, E., JÃd'Ãd'skelÃd'inen, L. P., Erkinjuntti, T., Hietanen, M., Huotilainen, M., Ilmoniemi, R. J. & NÃd'Ãd'tÃd'nen, R. (2001). Preserved stimulus deviance detection in alzheimer's disease., *Neuroreport* 12(8): 1649–1652.

Poza, J., Hornero, R., Escudero, J., FernÃąndez, A. & SÃąnchez, C. I. (2008). Regional analysis of spontaneous meg rhythms in patients with alzheimer's disease using spectral entropies., *Ann Biomed Eng* 36(1): 141–152.
URL: *http://dx.doi.org/10.1007/s10439-007-9402-y*

Ray, A. & Bowyer, S. M. (2010). Clinical applications of magnetoencephalography in epilepsy., *Ann Indian Acad Neurol* 13(1): 14–22.
URL: *http://dx.doi.org/10.4103/0972-2327.61271*

Reite, M., Teale, P., Collins, D. & Rojas, D. C. (2010). Schizoaffective disorder - a possible meg auditory evoked field biomarker., *Psychiatry Res* 182(3): 284–286.
URL: *http://dx.doi.org/10.1016/j.pscychresns.2010.02.007*

Roberts, T. P., Ferrari, P., Perry, D., Rowley, H. A. & Berger, M. S. (2000). Presurgical mapping with magnetic source imaging: comparisons with intraoperative findings., *Brain Tumor Pathol* 17(2): 57–64.

Roberts, T. P. L., Khan, S. Y., Rey, M., Monroe, J. F., Cannon, K., Blaskey, L., Woldoff, S., Qasmieh, S., Gandal, M., Schmidt, G. L., Zarnow, D. M., Levy, S. E. & Edgar, J. C.

(2010). Meg detection of delayed auditory evoked responses in autism spectrum disorders: towards an imaging biomarker for autism., *Autism Res* 3(1): 8–18.
URL: *http://dx.doi.org/10.1002/aur.111*

Robinson, S. E. (2004). Localization of event-related activity by SAM(erf)., *Neurol Clin Neurophysiol* p. 109.

Robinson, S. E., Nagarajan, S. S., Mantle, M., Gibbons, V. & Kirsch, H. (2004). Localization of interictal spikes using sam(g2) and dipole fit., *Neurol Clin Neurophysiol* 2004: 74.

Rose, D. F., Sato, S., Ducla-Soares, E. & Kufta, C. V. (1991). Magnetoencephalographic localization of subdural dipoles in a patient with temporal lobe epilepsy., *Epilepsia* 32(5): 635–641.

Rose, D. F., Sato, S., Smith, P. D., Porter, R. J., Theodore, W. H., Friauf, W., Bonner, R. & Jabbari, B. (1987). Localization of magnetic interictal discharges in temporal lobe epilepsy., *Ann Neurol* 22(3): 348–354.
URL: *http://dx.doi.org/10.1002/ana.410220311*

Rossini, P. M., Rossi, S., Babiloni, C. & Polich, J. (2007). Clinical neurophysiology of aging brain: from normal aging to neurodegeneration., *Prog Neurobiol* 83(6): 375–400.
URL: *http://dx.doi.org/10.1016/j.pneurobio.2007.07.010*

Schoffelen, J.-M. & Gross, J. (2009). Source connectivity analysis with meg and eeg., *Hum Brain Mapp* 30(6): 1857–1865.
URL: *http://dx.doi.org/10.1002/hbm.20745*

Schwartz, E. S., Dlugos, D. J., Storm, P. B., Dell, J., Magee, R., Flynn, T. P., Zarnow, D. M., Zimmerman, R. A. & Roberts, T. P. L. (2008). Magnetoencephalography for pediatric epilepsy: how we do it., *AJNR Am J Neuroradiol* 29(5): 832–837.
URL: *http://dx.doi.org/10.3174/ajnr.A1029*

Shah, Y., Tangalos, E. G. & Petersen, R. C. (2000). Mild cognitive impairment. when is it a precursor to alzheimer's disease?, *Geriatrics* 55(9): 62, 65–62, 68.

Simos, P. G., Breier, J. I., Zouridakis, G. & Papanicolaou, A. C. (1998). Assessment of functional cerebral laterality for language using magnetoencephalography., *J Clin Neurophysiol* 15(4): 364–372.

Simos, P. G., Papanicolaou, A. C., Breier, J. I., Fletcher, J. M., Wheless, J. W., Maggio, W. W., Gormley, W., Constantinou, J. E. & Kramer, L. (2000). Insights into brain function and neural plasticity using magnetic source imaging., *J Clin Neurophysiol* 17(2): 143–162.

Stam, C. J. (2010). Use of magnetoencephalography (meg) to study functional brain networks in neurodegenerative disorders., *J Neurol Sci* 289(1-2): 128–134.
URL: *http://dx.doi.org/10.1016/j.jns.2009.08.028*

Stoffers, D., Bosboom, J. L. W., Deijen, J. B., Wolters, E. C., Berendse, H. W. & Stam, C. J. (2007). Slowing of oscillatory brain activity is a stable characteristic of parkinson's disease without dementia., *Brain* 130(Pt 7): 1847–1860.
URL: *http://dx.doi.org/10.1093/brain/awm034*

Stoffers, D., Bosboom, J. L. W., Deijen, J. B., Wolters, E. C., Stam, C. J. & Berendse, H. W. (2008). Increased cortico-cortical functional connectivity in early-stage parkinson's disease: an meg study., *Neuroimage* 41(2): 212–222.
URL: *http://dx.doi.org/10.1016/j.neuroimage.2008.02.027*

Timmermann, L., Florin, E. & Reck, C. (2007). Pathological cerebral oscillatory activity in parkinson's disease: a critical review on methods, data and hypotheses., *Expert Rev Med Devices* 4(5): 651–661.
URL: *http://dx.doi.org/10.1586/17434440.4.5.651*

Timmermann, L., Gross, J., Dirks, M., Volkmann, J., Freund, H.-J. & Schnitzler, A. (2003). The cerebral oscillatory network of parkinsonian resting tremor., *Brain* 126(Pt 1): 199–212.

Tovar-Spinoza, Z. S., Ochi, A., Rutka, J. T., Go, C. & Otsubo, H. (2008). The role of magnetoencephalography in epilepsy surgery., *Neurosurg Focus* 25(3): E16.
URL: *http://dx.doi.org/10.3171/FOC/2008/25/9/E16*

Uhlhaas, P. J., Haenschel, C., NikoliÄĞ, D. & Singer, W. (2008). The role of oscillations and synchrony in cortical networks and their putative relevance for the pathophysiology of schizophrenia., *Schizophr Bull* 34(5): 927–943.
URL: *http://dx.doi.org/10.1093/schbul/sbn062*

Urrestarazu, E., Chander, R., Dubeau, F. & Gotman, J. (2007). Interictal high-frequency oscillations (100-500 hz) in the intracerebral eeg of epileptic patients., *Brain* 130(Pt 9): 2354–2366.
URL: *http://dx.doi.org/10.1093/brain/awm149*

Urrestarazu, E., Jirsch, J. D., LeVan, P., Hall, J., Avoli, M., Dubeau, F. & Gotman, J. (2006). High-frequency intracerebral eeg activity (100-500 hz) following interictal spikes., *Epilepsia* 47(9): 1465–1476.
URL: *http://dx.doi.org/10.1111/j.1528-1167.2006.00618.x*

Van Veen, B. D., van Drongelen, W., Yuchtman, M. & Suzuki, A. (1997). Localization of brain electrical activity via linearly constrained minimum variance spatial filtering, *IEEE T Bio-med Eng* 44(9): 867–880.

Volkmann, J., Joliot, M., Mogilner, A., Ioannides, A. A., Lado, F., Fazzini, E., Ribary, U. & LlinÃąs, R. (1996). Central motor loop oscillations in parkinsonian resting tremor revealed by magnetoencephalography., *Neurology* 46(5): 1359–1370.

Wada, J. & Rasmussen, T. (2007). Intracarotid injection of sodium amytal for the lateralization of cerebral speech dominance. 1960., *J Neurosurg* 106(6): 1117–1133.
URL: *http://dx.doi.org/10.3171/jns.2007.106.6.1117*

Wu, A. D., Fregni, F., Simon, D. K., Deblieck, C. & Pascual-Leone, A. (2008). Noninvasive brain stimulation for parkinson's disease and dystonia., *Neurotherapeutics* 5(2): 345–361.
URL: *http://dx.doi.org/10.1016/j.nurt.2008.02.002*

Xiang, J., Liu, Y., Wang, Y., Kirtman, E. G., Kotecha, R., Chen, Y., Huo, X., Fujiwara, H., Hemasilpin, N., Lee, K., Mangano, F. T., Leach, J., Jones, B., DeGrauw, T. & Rose, D. (2009). Frequency and spatial characteristics of high-frequency neuromagnetic signals in childhood epilepsy., *Epileptic Disord* 11(2): 113–125.
URL: *http://dx.doi.org/10.1684/epd.2009.0253*

Xiang, J., Wang, Y., Chen, Y., Liu, Y., Kotecha, R., Huo, X., Rose, D. F., Fujiwara, H., Hemasilpin, N., Lee, K., Mangano, F. T., Jones, B. & DeGrauw, T. (2010). Noninvasive localization of epileptogenic zones with ictal high-frequency neuromagnetic signals., *J Neurosurg Pediatr* 5(1): 113–122.
URL: *http://dx.doi.org/10.3171/2009.8.PEDS09345*

2

The Role of MEG in Unveiling Cognition

M.V. Silva Nunes[1], F. Maestú[2] and A. Castro Caldas[1]
[1]*Institute of Health Sciences of The Catholic University of Portugal,*
[2]*Laboratory of Cognitive and Computational Neuroscience, Centre for Biomedical Technology, Complutense University of Madrid*
[1]*Portugal*
[2]*Spain*

1. Introduction

As Dolan (2008) has suggested, to measure brain activity associated with discrete states of mind is the Holy Grail of cognitive neuroscience. Fortunately, and as pointed by several authors, the techniques and analitic tools to study the living brain have greatly evolved. In fact, since 1970 there have been remarkable advances in the way we study human brain thought imaging and, as Raichle (2001) has pointed out, the results of this work constitute a strong argument for the development of new imaging methods to try to overcome the weakness of data gathering or data analysis. In conjunction, new hardware and signal processing methods, are also addressing the weaknesses of data gathering and data analyses.

In his 1998 book, Papanicolau compares imaging with the process of taking photographs and makes the argument that all imaging is mediated rather than direct. Whether one is talking about photography or brain imaging, all images are partial, not complete models of the reality imaged, and the accuracy with which they represent reality varies. Though it might seem obvious, it is important to reinforce that all imaging is mediated rather than direct, in order to emphasize that although one of MEG's advantages is that it "measures directly" brain activity, as with every other technique, the obtained imaging is mediated by processes of recording and registration of a form of energy and processes of development or construction of a representation or a model of the object. Because virtually an infinity of different models can be constructed based on the same reality, functional brain imaging is a "mixed blessing: it renders functional imaging valuable and promises tools for new discoveries, while it entails the perils of deception, error and disappointment" (Papanicolau, 1998).

Regarding the importance that imaging now has in the study of cognition, it is also worthwhile to note that sometimes the advances were not only methodological. For instance, *f*MRI, in comparison with PET: "democratized access to a powerful technology for investigating the living human brain, allowing a broad cross-section of academic disciplines to pursue new agendas" (Dolan, 2008). These disciplines, like cognitive psychology or neuropsychology, with their specific contributions, brought to the fore questions related to human cognition in the development of the field of neuroimaging. The same is happening with MEG.

2. Studying cognition

Cognition can be understood not as a single process, but as several performances and behaviors in a well designed task or in daily living activities that always come from the activity of the brain (Dixon & Nilsson, 2004). Therefore, it seems possible to clearly state the task of functional brain imaging as: identifying regions and their temporal relationships associated with the performance of a well designed task (Raichle, 2001).

However, there are several caveats in this approach. Brain activation patterns captured by functional brain imaging are assumed to reflect aspects of neuropshysiological mechanisms necessary to a function. If we understand a function as a process of production of a set of similar phenomena that serve a common purpose or accomplish a common goal, and consider each phenomenon in the set as a token or an instance of the function, then when we are studying cognition we must provide a way to trigger the phenomena tokens of the function, the stimulus and instructions that constitute the experimental task (Papanicolau, 1998). However, tasks are never pure and always involve a complex blend of different cognitive operations. In functional neuroimaging studies this implies that the set of brain regions associated with a particular task may reflect not only the cognitive operation that we are interested in studying but any of the cognitive operations engaged by the task.

Several approaches have been used to tackle this difficulty. First with PET, neuroimaging was based in subtraction techniques derived from a concept from Donders (see Raichle, 2001, for a more detailed description). Here different blocks of stimuli were presented to subjects, one block representing the condition of interest (task state) and another block associated with a control condition (control state). In the beginning of *f*MRI these block designs were also common. (Aguirre & D'Esposito, 2000; Donaldson & Buckner, 2001). However, as suggested by Stufflebeam and Rosen, with the implementation of event-related fMRI, a procedure similar to the measuring of evoked responses in electrophysiology (Aguirre & D'Esposito, 2000; Donaldson & Buckner, 2001), it was possible to overcome the limitations of a more rigid block design and, at same time, use the knowledge of the properties of neurons to enhance both spatial and functional sensitivity (Stufflebeam and Rosen, 2007).

In the modern imaging methods currently available, functional magnetic resonance imaging (fMRI) is still one of the most frequently used techniques. Many investigators have aimed at localizing function, identifying the brain areas that are responsible for cognitive tasks. However, these techniques have not clearly identified which properties of the brain are responsible for cognition (Douw et al., 2011).

As Dolan (2008) points out, although many of the findings resulting from the extensive study of cognition by means of neuroimaging reproduced what was discovered using lesion-based models, there were also unexpected results. According to Dolan, these findings have to do with the fact that sophisticated perspectives on the impact of a lesion suggest that cognition arises not just out of functional differentiation, but also from functional integration. This implies that the impact of a localized lesion is likely to reflect both local and distributed effects, evidenced by more widespread activations seen with neuroimaging than was predicted by a lesion-deficit model. Besides that, cognitive functions require precise coordination of neural activity across long distances in the brain (Stufflebeam & Rosen, 2007).

3. Why use MEG to study cognition?

Each of the several available imaging techniques has its own individual strengths and weaknesses. Some are particularly useful in temporal resolution (generally understood as the smallest time period of brain activation that can be distinguished), others in spatial resolution (generally understood as the smallest area of brain activation that can be distinguished). The electromagnetic imaging techniques include MEG and EEG, and they might not be thought of as imaging at all (Stufflebeam & Rosen, 2007). However, they possess excellent temporal resolution since they measure the underlying neural currents directly (although requiring the processes of acquisition and development) on the order of milliseconds, albeit with limited spatial resolution.

Hari et al. (2000) suggest that this is a major advantage since the brain is a real-time processor, which implies that its functions can best be studied with tools that allow tracking of neural activation within the millisecond time scale. Only EEG and MEG are capable of providing information at such a high temporal resolution, and in a non-invasive manner, necessary for the study of brain dynamics. According to Stam (2005), two major sources for a renewed interest in MEG and EEG can be identified as "1) the realization that a full understanding of the neuropshysiological mechanisms underlying normal and disturbed higher brain functions cannot be derived from a purely reductionist approach and requires the study of emergent phenomena such as large scale synchronization of neuronal networks in the brain 2) the introduction of new techniques, concepts and analytical tools which make it possible to extract more and more meaningful information from recordings of brain activity." A cited example of these analytical tools is the application of time series analysis techniques derived from nonlinear dynamics to the study of MEG and EEG. Although it lies outside the scope of this chapter, it is nevertheless important to understand that nonlinear time series analyses, when applied to time series of brain activity, allow us to better understand the dynamics of the underlying system. This is particularly true at the level of functional connectivity, a concept referring to any type of correlation between time series of brain activity. The underlying assumption is that functional connectivity reflects, at least to some extent, functional interactions between different brain regions (see Stam, 2005 for a detailed description), and this represents a major step forward, passing from localization to connectivity.

There are several detailed descriptions of the underlying phenomena measured by MEG. It is usually said that MEG measurements are sensitive to postsynaptic currents in the dendrites of cortical pyramidal neurons (Hämäläinen et al., 1993). These changing synaptic currents of cortical pyramidal neurons give rise not only to an electric field but also to a magnetic field, since changes in an electric field induce a magnetic field. When a large set of cells that are typically not synchronized begin to signal in unison, their combined electric currents will create a large deviation. With MEG we record the surface distribution, that is the magnetic flux or the magnetic fields, that arises from the primary or source currents overcoming the EEG limitations since, unlike with electrical signals, tissues do not distort magnetic signals. MEG can be used to detect spontaneous as well as evoked brain activity (see Hari, 1998; Hämäläinen and Hari, 2002; & Papanicolau, 1998 for detailed descriptions).

In a review article Zamrini et al. (2011) identify other advantages of MEG, specifically over other measures of electrical activity of the brain, including its freedom from the requirement for a reference electrode which has the potential to improve calculations of the electrical power and source localization of the signal. Also, because MEG normally uses many more detectors than traditional EEG, it allows for better spatial resolution. Because there is no need for a reference point in MEG studies, this facilitates synchronization and coherence analyses, which is increasingly important in order to understand the relations between brain and cognition. Another important factor in the study of cognition is that MEG is more sensitive to the gamma band and, as pointed out by Zamrini (2011), there is increasing evidence of the relations between gamma band and cognition. Hari et al. (2000) identify other specific advantages of MEG in the study of human brain functions, reinforcing that it is noninvasive, with excellent temporal resolution, reflecting neural activation directly (mainly postsynaptic currents), and it is selective to activation of fissural cortex which is difficult to access with other techniques. Another important claim is that MEG allows the study of individual processing strategies because conclusions can be made on the basis of a single subject. This is particularly important because each brain is unique, and the active areas can differ between individuals in similar tasks, with the expectation that these differences can become clearer in the timing than in the sites of cortical activation (He & Liu, 2008). This further reinforces the unique contribution made by MEG to the understanding of cognitive strategies, in normal as well as in clinical populations. Hari et al. (2000) also mention that MEG does not require subtraction between conditions, which makes cognitive experiments more flexible.

Synthesizing MEG is appropriate for studies of fast activation sequences of human cortical activation. It also allows comparisons of timing between distinct brain regions, being capable of capturing small time differences. In fact, as pointed out by several authors in several studies, MEG can detect fast switching on the different brain regions as they become active with a time resolution in the order of ms.

However, as with all the other techniques MEG has some disadvantages. The recorded magnetic field is much more difficult to measure than the electric currents recorded by EEG, particularly because they are of very low field strength when compared to the surrounding magnetic fields, namely the magnetic field of the earth. This implies that in order to be able to capture these magnetic distributions several technological advances were needed and a very expensive apparatus is required. In Stam's description the requirement is for "Cooled conductive coils in order to make them superconductive which allows the current to flow without resistance. Magnetic fields can induce currents in theses coils, and thanks to superconductivity very weak magnetic fields can be measured. Converting the currents in the coils to a signal that can be measured requires the SQUID (superconducting quantum interference device): very small rings with a very small interruption which can be crossed by electrons thanks to the quantum effects. SQUIDS are the key elements in the MEG system. Further improvement of signal-to-noise ratio is achieved by measuring only local gradients (gradiometers) instead of the absolute field. Finally the whole MEG recording system is shielded from the magnetic fields of the surroundings by placing it in a magnetically shielded room (MSR) …. The stimulation apparatus that gives rise to electromagnetic fields has to be placed outside the room and has to be transferred to the subject inside the MSR in an appropriate way" (see Stam, 2010). All of this apparatus is responsible for one of its major drawbacks, the price. It also requires the subject to cooperate and to keep the head immobile during the recording, which makes it difficult to use this technique with all populations, as it will be important for a range of cognitive studies. Another often pointed disadvantage is that deep and radial sources are largely neglected since magnetic flux deriving from deep sources will reach the head surface with difficulty and those derived from the radial source will not be captured.

Besides that, the data interpretation on MEG is hampered by the non-uniqueness of the inverse problem. As stated previously, MEG field patterns recorded outside the head are interpreted in terms of current distribution in the brain. The characteristics of the source inside are estimated on the basis of the regular features of the recorded distribution. This solution results in a hypothetical distribution. From perfectly known phenomena are derived the imperfectly known causes of the phenomena (the five parameters of the source, strength, orientation and location, X, Y, Z) (see Papanicolau, 1998). As suggested by Hauk (2004), several efforts have been made to tackle this problem, but explicitly or implicitly it is recognized that according to the Helmholtz principle the bioelectric inverse problem has no unique solution. In fact, whatever result is obtained with one method there are still infinitely other possible solutions equally compatible with the recorded signal, which implies the question: Which method yields the correct answer for the bioelectromagnetic inverse problem? In Hauk's opinion this is a futile question: "it's like reconstructing a three-dimensional object from its shadow because those data simply don't exist."

Aside from these difficulties, and in general, MEG, with its ability to follow the course time of brain activation, has been proven increasingly useful in the study of cognition. Several advances are being made in the understanding of oscillatory and synchronized brain activity and it is now assumed that synchronization of neural activity between different brain regions may reflect functional interactions between these regions, which will reinforce the ability of MEG to respond to the new focus on functional neuroimaging - no longer where but how.

4. Memory and MEG

Because of its role in cognitive functioning, and by the salience of its change across a lifetime with normal as well with pathological aging, memory has been a field of interest for neuroimaging, and MEG is no exception. As we shall see, because it is of extreme importance to implement techniques that are able to distinguish normal brain aging from abnormal and degenerative processes as early as possible, there is a great amount of work being done that addresses memory networks in pathological groups. However, there are also several projects trying to apply MEG techniques to a better understanding of the organization of memory networks. For example, MEG has been used to better understand the relative contributions and relations among different memory systems. Standing beyond the scope of this brief review concerning memory, since the seminal work of Scoville and Milner (1957) two areas have been consistently associated with memory processing, namely the medial temporal lobe (MTL) and the prefrontal cortex (PFC), with the medial temporal lobe being consistently associated with long-term memory, and the prefrontal being associated with working memory. However, with the advancement of imaging techniques there is growing support for the hypothesis that both structures are part of a unified memory network, challenging a more localizationist and segregated approach. As pointed out by Anderson et al. (2010), although functional connectivity analysis of *f*MRI data has revealed correlations between the lateral PFC and MTL in several types of memory, hemodynamic data does not provide an insight into the underlying neuronal processes. Using implanted electrode grids, these authors showed that the values of theta coherence between these two brain areas are task modulated, which in their opinion constitutes evidence of MTL-PFC interaction during memory tasks and points to the relevance of the role of theta activity in mediating this interaction. The point here is that previous results, specifically with MEG, found support for the idea that the increase of working memory load can lead to the increase of functional connection of extended regions (Tanaka et al., 2003). Results with MEG seem to reinforce the concept of a neural network shared by both types of memory (Campo et al., 2005). In a recent study of working memory, where MEG signals were recorded while subjects were performing a verbal working memory task with parametric load manipulation, results led the authors to propose an alternative principle of theta functionality, showing that the oscillatory mechanisms of verbal working memory comprise interacting processes across a distributed network and, more importantly for the present point, that capacity limitations are associated with both increased and decreased frequencies in the 4-12 hertz range (Moran et al., 2010).

In terms of the role of MEG in studying pathological memory networks, the great bulk of the research has been on Alzheimer's disease (AD). Alzheimer's disease (AD) is one of the major concerns of developed nations, being frequently cited as the main drawback of the advance in life expectancy. In fact, the incidence and prevalence of AD rises as individual's age. On the other hand, because of the nature of the signal measured by MEG the neurons affected by the pathological processes underlying AD can be measured directly. In concordance with this, and as summarized by Rossini et al. (2007), different types of neuropshysiological techniques have demonstrated abnormalities in AD during memory tasks, namely hyperactivation of prefrontal and midline activity, functional disconnection between prefrontal cortex and hippocampus, and stronger activation of the left temporal cortex, concluding that there is evidence for the importance of neuroelectric measurements in AD. In a MEG study examining focal slow wave generators they were found to be abnormally frequent in the cortical structures, particularly in the parietal and temporal lobes of patients with an AD diagnosis. The authors interpreted such an enhanced density of focal slow wave generators as the functional counterpart of the neurodegenerative process associated with the disease. The AD patients exhibited more MEG delta and theta activity than healthy aged control subjects because the focal slow waves would be focused on temporal and parietal structures, which is in accordance with previous results using EEG analyses. They also found that temporoparietal dysfunction can predict the cognitive and functional status of patients with AD (Fernandez et al., 2002).

It is known that physiological aging affects resting, but also event-related alpha rhythms. In a MEG study specifically addressing event-related desyncronization (ERD) in demented patients (compared with a group of normal young people and a group of normal elderly) in a two-task paradigm with different loads, it was shown that during the delay period of both tasks, the alpha ERD was stronger in demented patients than in the other groups (Babiloni et al., 2005). This suggests an abnormal increase of cortical excitation or disinhibition in dementia, generally compatible with differences in neurotransmission systems, namely at the cholinergic level. It is interesting to note that MEG in AD seems to be sensitive to changes in early cortical processing. For instance, in a study aimed at investigating the auditory-steady state response (SSR) in mild to moderate non-medicated AD patients as recorded by MEG it was found that the amplitude of auditory SSR is significantly increased in AD as compared to normal controls. This is interpreted by the authors as an impaired adaptation of auditory neurons to repetitive stimuli and decreased inhibition, probably due to changes in the acetylcholine system. These results seem then to reflect changes in the

primary cortex, showing that stimuli deficit processing can be present at an early cortical stage (Osipova, 2006).
Although the majority of the conditions, and Alzheimer's disease in particular, are determined by several interrelated factors, it is also true, and a result of several constraints, that the majority of the studies rely on a single technique. As pointed out by Fernandez at al. (2003) in a brief review, each technique has been able to identify features of AD. For instance, several studies using metabolic methods, namely PET and SPECT, evidenced features of AD, particularly hipometabolism-hipoperfursion in the temporoparietal and hipocampal. Similarly, with EEG an increase in slow activity, usually focused in the temporoparietal regions, together with decreased activity in the alpha band are considered the prototypical features of AD. Structural volumetric measurements obtained a reduced volume of temporaparietal and hipocampal formation volume, etc. The point the authors make is that magnetic source imaging can overcome some difficulties of previous approaches combining high temporal and high spatial resolution in detecting focal neural activity. One important aspect when using any imaging method is the coherence with the findings obtained by other methods. So, correlating volumetric MR data and MEG data of probable AD patients and a control group, they report that the higher the number of low frequency activity sources in left temporal and parietal areas, the higher the atrophy in the mesial aspects of the left temporal lobe. They conclude by proposing that "MTL atrophy and temporoparietal hypofunctioning may be considered complementary pictures of the same involutive process," but more than that, they reinforce the role of MEG as an important tool for a complementary techniques approach, overcoming in particular several EEG limitations concerning its precision. Several others works have directly addressed the importance of the concurrent validity of the various measurements. For instance, one of the first works to our knowledge specifically addressing the spatio-temporal patterns of brain magnetic activity in AD, in a memory task, not only showed that this pattern was different among AD and elderly controls, with AD patients displaying reduced activation in temporal and parietal areas between 400 and 700 ms in late phases of stimuli processing, but, more importantly, the number of activity sources in the left parietal areas was a predictor of the scores on the cognitive and functional measurements that were used (Maestú, 2001). Subsequent work with the same subjects specifically examined the complementarily between functional measurements obtained with MEG and MRI volumetric measurements and neuropsychological data (Maestú, 2003). They found, among other results, that the degree of left hippocampal atrophy strongly correlates with the activation of left temporal areas, corroborating the existence of a relation between the structural integrity of the mesial temporal cortices, i.e. degree of atrophy, and the functional status of temporal and parietal regions i.e. lack of late brain magnetic activity. In a later study a specific pattern of changes was shown in resting state functional connectivity in AD patients. Synchronization likelihood (SL) was increased in the theta band over the central and parietal areas and in the beta band over the parietal and occipital areas. Coherence showed a similar pattern of parieto-occipital increase in AD in alpha 2, beta, and gamma bands. SL decreased in the alpha 1 band for long distance intrahemispheric sensor pairs, and both SL and coherence were decreased in the beta band for long distance frontal temporal parietal and short distance left temporal sensor pairs (Stam, 2006).
MEG seems also to be able to distinguish between AD and major depression in old people, with no differences being found between normal control subjects and elderly depressed

patients in a working memory task. This reinforces the claim that memory deficits in depressed patients are more closely linked to emotional factors than substantial differences in neuronal activation. The fact that the AD group in this study displayed the expected pattern with a small number of activity sources in the left temporal region when compared with the other participants (with or without depression) reinforces this interpretation, as well as the claim that MEG has the potential to be useful in diagnosing AD (Maestú et al., 2004). Generally speaking, although it is not a very old technique, when MEG started to be used with AD patients it soon showed a promising potential to identify these patients and characterize their brain dynamics. In a recent review, Stam identifies the different contributions of spectral analysis, source analysis, task data, nonlinear analysis, and functional connectivity, concluding that since the first studies in 2000 MEG studies in AD have increased rapidly. The author suggests that there is now strong evidence that AD is characterized by a general slowing of background activity, reflected by increased power in delta and theta bands as well as a decreased power of alpha and beta bands, among other differences (Stam, 2010). The same author emphasizes that, despite improvements in the understanding of oscillatory and synchronized brain activity that can help to study disturbances such as AD, as a large-scale network it is still lacking a proper theoretical framework to deal with the data obtained using these advanced techniques, proposing that focus should be placed instead on the small-world network, a combination of high clustering and short communication pathways, as one possible framework for the advancement of the study of AD.

However, MEG may have an important role not only in characterizing AD, but also in detecting the neuropathological process prior to its clinical manifestations. This necessity is acutely felt, since, as stated by several authors, there is a general agreement that the treatment strategies and interventions, ranging from cognitive stimulation to daily life changes as well as pharmacological approaches, should be as precocious as possible in order to maximize the impact of several groups of strategies in the delay of the symptoms and progression. However, that not only requires methodological and technical advancements but also conceptual ones. In fact, although it is also well known that pathological processes underlying Alzheimer's clinical onset start several years before, there are several difficulties in identifying subclinical Alzheimer's patients.

One of the most successful approaches in identifying these subjects, and one that is used in several clinical, behavioral, and neuroimaging studies, is the concept of Mild Cognitive Impairment (MCI). MCI patients are subjects who present memory impairment beyond that expected for age and education, yet are not demented, and who are at increased risk of progressing to AD (Petersen et al., 1999). In subsequent work it was pointed out that the construct of MCI, with its subtypes, namely the amnestic subtype, has evolved to capture what can be seen as a pre-dementia phase of cognitive dysfunction (Gauthier et al., 2006). However, because many of them will not advance to AD, it may not be accurate to label participants at the aMCI stage as having AD or even prodromal AD (Petersen et al., 2009). There are still important sources of variability in MCI studies, such as source of the participants, clinical heterogeneity, neuropsychological normative data, etc.; however, the concept has been important because among other reasons it provides a framework for imaging and biomarkers, better characterizes those who will progress to AD, helps to identify risk factors, and increases predictability (Petersen et al., 2009). However, although there is great interest in adding biomarkers to the confirmation of an AD diagnosis, the final diagnosis of definite AD is still reliant on neuropathological examination (Mirra, 1991).

Nevertheless, despite the aforementioned sources of variability in MCI patients, the sensitivity of MEG in detecting features related to preclinical changes has been assessed in several previous studies. In a study comparing MCI patients and 10 normal controls assessed by means of MEG, the time course and the *loci* of brain activity in a deep encoding (semantic) and shallow encoding (nonsemantic) condition followed by a recognition task of previously presented words (Puregger et al., 2003), the mean recognition performances of MCI and controls were similar. Normal controls displayed no differences in the magnetic field distribution related to both encoding conditions. However, in the MCI the shallow encoding was associated with higher brain activity, mainly over left temporal and left frontal sensors rather than in the deep encoding condition. According to the authors, the results demonstrate that MCI patients showed significantly higher brain activity during shallow word encoding than deep word encoding between 250-450 ms after stimuli onset in the left medial temporal brain area. For the authors, this means that shallow encoding condition distinguishes neuropshysiological aspects of the groups, suggesting that nonsemantic new information may have this increased activation in MCI as a result of a compensatory process. It is worthwhile to note that all subjects displayed better performance after deep encoding (semantic), as predicted by the depth of processing background. Specifically investigating the power profiles and distribution of oscillatory sources of spontaneous MEG activity in MCI, and trying to gain advantage from the fact that it is a technique that has a better spatial resolution both at the sensor and source level compared to EEG, another study showed that the cerebral source of alpha activity is not changed in MCI when compared to normal controls (Osipova et al., 2006b). Subsequent work, clearly assuming that MCI patients represent an intermediate state between normal aging and dementia, tried to capitalize on MEG advantage for the acquisition of temporal courses of activation over high spatial resolution techniques, and tried to investigate the existence of a spatio-temporal memory profile that could discriminate between MCI and age-matched normal controls in a memory task. It was shown that the MCI subjects evidenced time-modulated increased activity in the ventral pathway during performance of a memory task, which was interpreted as a compensatory mechanism that allowed MCI patients to achieve behavioral results similar to the normal group (Maestú, 2008). Analysis of functional networks could also contribute to early detection of both MCI and AD. It seems that, in order to compensate for the loss of the segregation and integration balance, MCI subjects tend to increase their long-range synchronization, which could be underlying the increased blood flow showed in *f*MRI studies during memory tasks (Buldu et al., 2001). A network analysis, based on graph theory, revealed an important piece of information. Although MCI participants showed higher synchronization values than controls, they showed lower clustering values as well as higher values on the outreach parameters (physical distance between sensors), which in combination with other parameters is an indication of a loss of small-world architecture leading the MCIs to a more random structure. These findings argue against the compensatory hypothesis in the sense that the reorganized network does not lead to greater efficiency for information processing. In fact a more random network, compared to the controls, revealed a clear inefficiency in information processing even in the presence of higher synchronization, which can be recognized as spurious mechanisms (Bajo et al., JAD, 2010)

In another study, the MEG scans of an initially normal elderly group (according to a careful neuropsychological, psychological, and medical evaluation) were obtained for a memory task. In a two-year follow up, when all the evaluation protocols were repeated, it was possible to identify decliners and non-decliners. When analyzing whether there were differences among early brain magnetic profiles between those two groups it was shown that brain activity at late latencies increased in those MCI patients that developed AD in comparison to non-decliners (Maestú et al, 2011), reinforcing MEG potential for the early prediction of dementia before symptoms are so clear that a conventional prognosis can be made. The same use of MEG as a possible method to estimate the risk of developing AD was assessed with AD patients, MCI patients, and healthy elderly controls when MEG recordings were obtained during a 5-minute resting period. Their results showed that high left parietal α dipole density is a possible marker of the risk of converting from MCI to AD within two years and, according to the authors, corroborated the interpretation that there is not a clear transition between MCI and AD (Fernandez, 2006).

Another important scenario where MEG may be an important tool is helping to clarify the clinical significance of subjective memory complaints (SMC), which is still a subject of debate. In a recent study, Maestu et al. (2011) specifically addressed this issue by comparing brain magnetic activity in three groups of elderly subjects: volunteers with SMC (memory complaints with a normal score in objective memory tasks), MCI (objective and subjective memory impairments), and a third group of normal subjects (neither objective nor subjective memory impairments). MEG scans were obtained in the context of a letter recognition task. When comparing the SMC and the MCI group no significant differences in brain activity were found. This is attributed to one of two possible scenarios: assuming that that SMC and MCI arise from similar neurophysiologic changes, the results may reflect lack of sensitivity of cognitive tests to detect the memory impairment in SMC. Alternatively, assuming that SMC and MCI have different etiologies, MEG may not be sensitive enough. The comparison between the SMC and the control group showed higher activation for the SMC in ventral posterior regions bilaterally and the dorsal pathway bilaterally between 200 and 900 ms. When comparing MCI with the control group, they displayed greater activation, again between 200 and 900 ms, mainly in areas similar to those found in previous work (Maestu et al., 2008); particularly in the ventral pathway (inferior parietal lobe), temporal lobe, and ventral prefrontal region. For late latency windows a bilateral increase in activity was also found in the dorsolateral prefrontal cortex. In a broad interpretation the bilateral activation is attributed to a compensatory mechanism in SMC and MCI, similar to that proposed by the HAROLD (Hemispheric asymmetry in older adults) Model (Cabeza, 2002). Generally speaking, these results reinforce MEG ability to identify physiological differences between healthy elders and elders with complaints. Recognizing the necessity of further research, namely longitudinal research, for the authors the results suggest that SMC and MCI can be two stages in a cognitive *continuum*. In another study of SMC with MEG by the same research group, and with the same three groups of carefully selected subjects, i.e. SMC, MCI, and normals, and the same task, the functional connectivity (which, as stated previously, is regarded simply as a measure of the statistical interdependencies between two brain signals and seems to relate to the brain's ability to communicate information between brain regions) was specifically addressed, trying to determine if functional connectivity was, or was not, spared in the subjects with no objective memory deficit (Bajo et al., 2011). They found different profiles of functional connectivity, suggesting that the SMC profile, in comparison with the MCI subjects, was very similar to the one displayed when MCI and controls are compared. They point out that, taking as a standard the functional connectivity of normal elderly subjects, SMC subjects showed a hypo-synchronization of their memory-related networks, while MCI subjects showed an increased synchronization as a result of a compensatory process and as a means to increase communication; finally with AD this compensatory mechanism is no longer available. The point here is that the use of MEG can help us to describe profiles of prediction no longer only from MCI to AD, but also from SMC to MCI. Additionally, the number of activity sources on the left MTL at the late latency window differed between those control subjects that subsequently developed MCI and those that did not (Maestú, 2006).

In a recent review, Zamrini et al. (2011) state that "biomarkers measured at the time of AD are excellent in predicting the presence of pathology at the time of autopsy, 8-10 years later. However they are less efficient at detecting the presence of pathology prior to the onset of clinical symptoms .... It seems necessary to have a biomarker that (1) measures neuronal activity directly, (2) has good temporal and spatial resolution, and (3) is able to evaluate functional networks and the associated neuronal code (i.e. oscillatory activity)." The same authors point out that electrophysiological / biomagnetic changes in the brain were not sufficiently explored as biomarkers bearing the potential of being the best indicator of the earliest functional changes secondary to the neuropathological process but prior to the clinical onset, and specifically discuss the MEG advantages over other AD biomarkers, namely EEG and *f*MRI.

5. Language and MEG

Language is a distinctive function of human cognition, of extreme importance. Therefore, and trying to prevent the deleterious consequences of brain surgery, preoperative determination of language areas is a long recognized clinical application of neuroimaging of cognition and several and important MEG studies were done with this purpose. Since the first language MEG studies it was recognized that, since MEG information's can be used in surgical planning it is of extreme importance to establish its capacity to reveal the location of brain areas that show activity uniquely related to key language functions.

Language requires a distributed network, that was first addressed by lesions studies, wich comprises, among others, the classical language systems as well as other areas related to other involved cognitive functions. To use MEG to study language, as with other imaging techniques, we need well designed tasks in order to activate language areas. Besides specific language processes that include phonological, lexical, syntactic, and semantic processing, concurrent cognitive processes, for example concurrent memory processes, occur with any language paradigm. As previously stated, there are no pure tasks - and language paradigms are no exception.

MEG temporal resolution can also be used to better understand language. In an important MEG study where right-handed normal subjects where scanned during a memory recognition task for words in a visual and in an auditory task, the spatial outline of brain activation observed was in accord with previous findings using a variety of methodologies that suggest that temporoparietal and basal temporal areas, predominantly in the left hemisphere, are involved in reading. In addition they obtained evidence for activation in medial temporal areas consistent with previous findings implicating the hippocampus and the entorhinal cortex in memory function. They also took advantage of the unique spatio-temporal resolution of MEG to obtain information regarding the relative timing of association in these areas, showing that occipital lobe activity, generally associated with primary visual processing, was present in all the participants and was solved 100 ms after stimulus onset. As expected, the activity was bilateral – basal temporal areas next became active around 100 to 200 ms and were resolving by approximately 350 ms – and seemed to be specific to visually presented verbal stimuli. Temporoparietal areas of the dominant hemisphere are involved in a variety of language tasks, and activation of these areas was consistently observed after the activity in the basal temporal areas began to resolve. Activity in the medial temporal areas was concurrent with that in the temporoparietal areas. These results indicate a consistent temporal relationship between activity in the ventral pathway and temporoparietal cortex that supports a hypothesis regarding the functional specialization of these areas for different aspects of reading. To the authors these data suggested that MEG, by capturing the temporal as well as the spatial aspects of task-specific brain activity, had a promising role as an adjunct to other functional imaging modalities, serving to complement and extend their findings, particularly in language mapping (Breier et al., 1998). Other results reinforced the MEG role as a promising tool for identifying brain regions involved in the analysis of linguistic stimuli, in addition to the visual encoding of stimulus features (Simos et al., 1998).The number of left sources was greater than the number of right hemisphere sources in both tasks. In the word tasks the vast majority of sources were localized in temporal and temporo-parietal areas during latter portions of the waveform. In another study (Breier et. al, 1999) with epilepsy patients, an excellent agreement was found between the data obtained with magnetic source imaging and Wada indices.

A very important consideration is that MEG allows the component of sensory input to be excluded from the process. The temporal discrimination of MEG also allows us to study early components. Walla et al. (1999) confirmed that cognitive processes within word recognition tasks can be associated with different brain activities as early as under 200 ms after the stimulus onset, providing a distinction between the processes of encoding and the processes of retrieval attempts of verbal information. Because of its temporal resolution it can be used in studies specifically comparing early and late theories. For instance, to shed light on the time course of processing in visual word recognition, visual recognition of heteronymous- phonological and semantically distinct words that share a common orthography, providing a unique opportunity to distinguish between lexical and word form properties, were examined with MEG, finding results that suggest that true lexical access does not occur prior to 200 ms, but rather at a latter stage of processing (Solomyak & Marantz, 2009). A covert name and covert reading task concluded that MEG is a valuable tool to investigate both the time course of speech-evoked cortex activation as well as the localization of the main speech areas (Kober et al., 2001). The N400 component has also been addressed with MEG. This is an EEG-evoked response to the presentation of words and other meaningful stimuli that appear as a negative deflection in the ERP waveform, finding results that support a view in which the N400 effect observed in ERP reflects facilitated access of stored information rather than relative difficulty of semantic integration, "renewing the hope of a true top down effect on access" (Lau et al., 2009).

Several other works specifically addressed the determination of the language dominant hemisphere, which is critical for many clinical applications. But it is not an easy task to find a comprehensive protocol. In 2001, Breier et al. evaluated the validity of data derived from magnetic source imaging regarding hemispheric dominance for language in children and adolescents with intractable seizure disorders by a comparison with results of the intracarotid amobarbital procedure (IAP) showing that the laterality indices obtained by both procedures were highly correlated. They also found that independent clinical judgments based on both procedures to identify the lateralization of language function in individual patients were highly correlated. A 2002 study (Maestu et al., 2002) of Spanish-speaking patients with intractable epilepsy compared MEG data with IAP (intracarotid amytal procedure; see Maestu et al., Brain and Language, 2004 for a comparison with electrocortical stimulation). The results obtained closely parallel the original findings with English speakers and seem to support the cross-language generalization of the protocol used. This receives further support by the anatomical location of activity that shows the highest correlation with IAP data. To the authors these results confirmed the impression that these procedures are easy to implement, reliable, and valid, and may be used routinely to provide clinical information to increase the efficiency of pre-surgical evaluation. However, it is interesting to note that these patterns seem not to generalize for Chinese speakers (Valaki et al., 2004).

A 2009 paper by Frye et al. reviewed the functional neuroimaging of language using MEG and its importance as a functional neuroimaging technique for mapping the language-specific cortex. Referring to the assessment of cerebral dominance, they suggest that the WADA procedure, while it is the most commonly used method for assessing cerebral dominance for language during pre-surgical evaluation of patients, has several limitations, namely concerning the invasiveness of the technique, but also its lack of regional specificity needed to determine the precise location and extent of the language-specific cortex. As these authors point out, many of their own works over the past decade, some of which are cited in this chapter, have included considerable efforts to develop a reliable MEG language-mapping protocol that could be used instead of more invasive procedures with no health risks, adaptable to test-retest reliability studies and able to be used in different tasks of extended duration. They point out that mapping of the language-specific cortex has been achieved using a variant of the Sternberg task for short-term memory known as the continuous recognition memory paradigm (CRM). Synthesizing several studies, they indicate that a stable feature of MEG-derived cortical activation maps in the context of CRM is a greater degree of activity in the left perysilvian region, in accordance with the expected left hemisphere dominance for receptive language in the majority of neurologically intact individuals. In a normative study of language profiles with MEG (Papanicolau et al., 2006) it was shown that brain activation profiles featured two components, an early and a late, but more importantly those features remained constant across task parameters, stimulus modality age, and gender of the participants, indicating that they constitute the basic aspects of the language perception mechanisms.

However, the main problem of MEG protocols in determining hemispheric dominance, when compared with Wada procedures, is that MEG protocols usually only test receptive language (reading and listening to single words), and there is a need to develop more robust paradigms capable of recording and modeling brain activity in anterior speech regions. There are already some expressive paradigms. In a study with a verb generation task it was possible to identify language lateralization by analyzing frequency specific spectral power changes (Fisher et al., 2008). Another MEG expressive language task successfully identified neural regions involved in language production showing high concordance with *f*MRI verb generation to pictures and verb generation to words) but they all possess some caveats, namely, and according to the authors "the need for MEG users to be cognizant of the effects of task choice, threshold selection, MEG latency window and frequency band selections for data analyses" (Pang et al., 2011).

MEG has also proven its value with special populations. It was previously reported that several differences in brain functioning could be attributed to the absence of knowledge of orthography (Castro Caldas, 2004). Another study with MEG was done with subjects that learned to read and write during childhood (literates) and subjects who learned to read and write late in life (late literates). It was found that while subjects were visually recognizing previously presented words, late literates showed more late sources in right temporoparietal areas compared to controls, and controls showed more left inferior frontal sources. There is evidence that the right hemisphere plays a more important role in language processing in illiterate subjects. It is possible that the differences that arise after a 400 ms period can be attributed to a biased processing towards the right hemisphere. The interpretation proposed to explain the fact that late literate controls have fewer fonts in the left inferior frontal cortex is that control subjects have quicker access to the result of the visual decoding than late literates. Visual decoding gives access to the phonological form of the words, which is related to left IFG. Therefore this difference may reflect articulatory rehearsal. The general interpretation that we suggest for this group of results is that the process of learning to read and write during adulthood differs significantly from the process of learning to read and write in childhood (Castro Caldas et al., 2009). Ex-illiterate subjects also exhibited less brain functional asymmetry during an auditory recognition task with MEG (Silva Nunes et al., 2009) reinforcing the interpretation that education influences brain organization.

Other MEG studies involving children showed that compared to good readers, poor readers delayed and reduced left hemisphere activation to the most demanding phonological contrast and the overall sustained bilateral activation may reflect their greater difficulty with phonological processing (Wehner et al., 2007). As suggested by Frye et al. (2009), the bulk of MEG studies of children with dyslexia have shown that they exhibit a reduced ability to discriminate the phonological units of speech that contain fast auditory transients, such as syllables, displaying different spatio-temporal patterns of activation during the execution of reading tasks, and consistently exhibiting a reduced activation of the left posterior superiortemporal / supramarginal gyri, accompanied by hyper-activation of the right-homotopic regions and compensatory increases in pre-frontal activity. In a recent review of the contributions of MEG to reading it is pointed out that in order to read properly the brain is required to recruit distant cortical areas to function in highly complex and dynamic ways (Pammer, 2009), features that are well captured with EEG.

More recent work seems to be more theoretically driven and has isolated more specific aspects of language processing. For instance, Barca et al. (2011) studied Right Visual Field advantage in reading with MEG. RFV has been known about for more than 50 years, with the explanation that it has to do with language dominant hemisphere, which is for most right handers the left hemisphere. They found that activity in the speech motor area was lateralized to the left hemisphere and stronger for RVF than LVF words, which is interpreted as the proximal cause of the RFV advantage for the naming of written words. They also found that there were faster, stronger responses of the left midfusiform gyrus (Visual Word Form Area) to RVF than LVF words. Hirschfield et al. (2011) studied the effects of language comprehension on visual processing, taking advantage of MEG temporal resolution to conclude that while a perceptual match is detected a mere 120 ms after stimulus onset, overall semantic match between sentence content and pictures is indexed by a modulation of the N400. Another study looked at category-specific spatio-temporal representations, showing the importance of understanding not only the spatial but also the temporal representation of semantic categories using multivariate techniques (Chan et al., 2011).

Generally speaking, and despite the limitations raised; in terms of language study MEG is a valid tool for assessing cerebral dominance, elucidating temporal-spatial patterns of activation, and distinguishing between typical and atypical populations and between different components of language theories.

6. Conclusion

Because MEG is sensitive to the spatial and temporal properties of cortical signs, it can provide a valuable contribution to the study of cognition. As suggested by Rossini et al. (2007), "a major challenge of modern neuroscience is to identify patterns of neuronal activity underlying cognitive functions and to disentangle these actions from ongoing electromagnetic brain signals unrelated to task performance, background activity and function related activity," and there is now a growing awareness that a more complete understanding will only come through integration of different imaging technologies (Stufflebeam and Rosen, 2007). As an example, a recent study of visual short-term memory aimed to observe directly the relationship between the BOLD activation in intra-parietal and intra-occipital cortex and the electrophysiological component (Sustained Posterior Contralateral Negativity) and the Magnetoencephalographical marker (Sustained Posterior Contralateral Magnetic field) of the maintenance of information in visual short-term memory, specifically testing the hypothesis that both physiological markers (BOLD and SPCN/SPCM) reflect the same underlying neural processes. They tested the same subjects with fMRI, EGG, and MEG in very similar experiments of laterally-encoded stimuli in order to allow comparison between different techniques and with varying memory load (see Robitaille et al., 2010). However, contrary to what was expected the BOLD signal in IPS was the same in the left and right hemispheres regardless of the visual space where the stimuli was encoded; this is contrary to what happens with EEG and also, to a lesser extent, with MEG. The authors concluded that "despite the numerous advances in source localization of MEG signals, the use of multiple methods is still advised, along with careful interpretation of the results." Nevertheless, they point out that MEG was the only method capable of detecting cerebral activations bilaterally and contralaterally. Freeman et al. (2009) show that the brain as a thermodynamic system consumes energy at rates roughly tenfold greater than any other organ of comparable mass and that in the continuous interactions of excitatory and inhibitory currents in the same dendritic trees must at least partially cancel the extracellular electric and magnetic fields, but the metabolic needs must still be met for both forms of activation and for all frequency ranges. These authors point that, because inhibition is a process that requires expenditure of metabolic energy, activation and deactivation are radically different from excitation and inhibition. Multivariate approaches for characterizing and decoding local and distributed neuronal activity patterns in fMRi have been receiving increased attention in recent years. The integration of fMRI and EEG/MEG has received the most interest. MEG holds the promise of revealing dynamic connectivity since it is sensitive to transient neural activities occurring on the order of milliseconds. Cerebral functions are simultaneously localized and distributed (functional integration), which as pointed out above is important for the relevance of functional connectivity (Flecther et al., 1996). Also of importance is the investigation of the relationships between the functional connectivity as derived from fMRI data and from MEG/EEG data. Due to the different time scales and spatial resolutions of these two modalities there has not been a clearly established consistency between the results obtained with fMRI data and EEG/MEG alone.

As suggested by A. Ya. Kaplan et al. (2005), the search to understand how human beings create intentional behavior and how the mental world emerges within the human brain on the basis of neuronal activity inevitably leads researchers to study neuronal co-operation. Modern theoretical and experimental work suggests that the assemblies of couples and synchronously active neurons represent the most plausible candidates for the understanding of brain dynamics. Multimodal neuroimaging is becoming increasingly important (He and Liu, 2008).

As a final word, with all the recent and expected advances, there is no doubt that room for improvement still exists in functional neuroimaging. MEG can have an increased importance in the study of the functional connectivity, which is of pivotal importance in the study of cognition.

One of the aspects we consider to be of major importance is the study of individual activations. Although usually stated as a MEG advantage, individual differences are often "justified," perhaps because there is no integrated conceptual framework to accommodate the diversity. There is also, particularly for the study of cognition, room for improvement in the study of individual activations - once again, MEG can play an important role.

7. References

Aguirre, G. K. & D'Esposito, M. Experimental design for brain fMRI. In *Functional MRI* ((2000). C.Moonen & T. W. Bandettini (Eds.), Heidelberg: Springer-Verlag Berlin. pp. 369-380.

Anderson, K. L., Rajagovindan, R., Ghacibeh, G. A., Meador, K. J., & Ding, M. (2010). Theta oscillations mediate interaction between prefrontal cortex and medial temporal lobe in human memor. *Cerebral Cortex,* Vol. 20, No. 7 (2010): p. 1604.

Babiloni, C., Cassetta, E., Chiovenda, P., Percio, C., Ercolani, M., Moretti, D., Moffa, F., Pasqualetti, P., Pizzella, V., Romani, G. L., Tecchio, F., Zappasodi, F., & Rossini, P. M. (2005). Alpha rhythms in mild dements during visual delayed choice reaction time tasks: a MEG study. *Brain Research Bulletin,* Vol. 65, No. 6 (2005): pp. 457-470.

Bajo, R., Castellanos, N. P., López, M. E., Ruiz, J. M., Montejo, P., Montenegro, M., Llanero, M., Gil, P., Yubero, R., Baykova, E., Paul, N., Aurtenetxe, S., Del Pozo, F., & Maestu, F. (2011). Early dysfunction of functional connectivity in healthy elderly with subjective memory complaints. Age (Dordr), (6 April 2011) [Epub ahead of print].

Bajo, R., Maestú, F., Nevado, A., Sancho, M., Gutiérrez, R., Campo, P., Castellanos, N. P., Gil, P., Moratti, S., Pereda, E., & Del-Pozo, F. (2010). Functional connectivity in mild cognitive impairment during a memory task: Implications for the disconnection hypothesis. *J Alzheimers Dis.,* Vol. 22, No. 1 (2010): pp. 183-193.

Bandettini, P. A. (2009). What's new in neuroimaging methods? *Annals of the NY Academy of Sciences: The Year in Cognitive Neuroscience,* Vol. 1156, No. 1 (2009): pp. 260-293.

Barca, L., Cornelissen, P., Simpson, M., Urooj, U., Woods, W., & Ellis, A. W. (2011). The neural basis of the right visual field advantage in reading: An MEG analysis using virtual electrodes. *Brain Lang.*, Vol. 118, No. 3 (September 2011): pp. 53-71.

Berendse, H. W., Verbunt, J.P., Scheltens, P., van Dijk, B. W., & Jonkman, E. J. (2000). Magnetoencephalographic analysis of cortical activity in Alzheimer's disease: a pilot study. *Clinical Neurophysiology*, Vol. 111, No. 4 (2000): pp. 604-12.

Breier, J. I., Simos, P. G., Zouridakis, G., & Papanicolaou, A. C. (1998). Relative timing of neuronal activity in distinct temporal lobe areas during a recognition memory task for words. *J Clin Exp Neuropsychol.*, Vol. 20, No. 6 (December 1998): pp. 782-90.

Breier, J. I., Simos, P. G., Wheless, J.W., Constantinou, J. E., Baumgartner, J. E., Venkataraman, V., & Papanicolaou, A. C. (2001). Language dominance in children as determined by magnetic source imaging and the intracarotid amobarbital procedure: A comparison. *J Child Neurol.*, Vol. 16, No. 2 (February 2001): pp. 124-30.

Breier, J. I., Simos, P. G., Zouridakis, G., Wheless, J. W., Willmore, L. J., Constantinou, J. E., Maggio, W. W., & Papanicolaou, A. C. (1999). Language dominance determined by magnetic source imaging: a comparison with the Wada procedure. *Neurology*, Vol. 53, No. 5 (22 September 1999): pp. 938-45.

Buldú, J. M., Bajo, R., Maestú, F., Castellanos, N., Leyva, I., Gil, P., Sendiña-Nadal, I., Almendral, J. A., Nevado, A., Del-Pozo, F., & Boccaletti, S. (2011). Reorganization of functional networks in mild cognitive impairment. *PLoS One*, Vol. 6, No. 5 (2011): e19584. Epub 2011 May 23.

Campo, P., Maestú, F., Ortiz, T., Capilla, A., Fernández, S., & Fernández, A. (2005). Is medial temporal lobe activation specific for encoding long-term memories? *NeuroImage*, Vol. 25, No. 1 (March 2005): pp. 34-42.

Castro-Caldas, A., Nunes, M. V., Maestu, F., Ortiz, T., Simoes, R., Fernandes, R., de La Guia, E., Garcia, E., & Goncalves, M. (2009). Learning orthography in adulthood: A magnetoencephalographic study. *Journal of Neuropsychology*, Vol. 3 (2009): pp. 17-30.

Chan, A. M., Halgren, E., Marinkovic, K., & Cash, S. S. (2011). Decoding word and category-specific spatiotemporal representations from MEG and EEG. *Neuroimage*, Vol. 54, No. 4 (14 February 2011): pp. 3028-39.

Deeny, S. P., Poeppel, D., Zimmerman, J. B., Roth, S. M., Brandauer, J., Witkowski, S., Hearn, J. W., Ludlow, A. T., Contreras-Vidal, J. L., Brandt, J., & Hatfield, B. D. (2008). Exercise, APOE, and working memory: MEG and behavioral evidence for benefit of exercise in epsilon4 carriers. *Biol Psychol*, Vol. 78, No. 2 (May 2008): pp. 179-87.

Dixon R.A. e Nilsson L.G. (2004). Don´t fence us in: Probing the frontiers of cognitive aging (in *New frontiers in cognitive aging*, Eds. Dixon R.A., Backman L., Nilsson L.G. New York -Oxford University Press: pp 4-15

Dolan, R. J. (2008). Neuroimaging of cognition: Past, present, and future. *Neuron*, Vol. 60, No.3 (2008): pp. 496-502.

Donaldson, D. L. & Buckner, R. L. (2001). Effective paradigm design. In P.Jezzard, P. M. Matthews, & S. M. Smith (Eds.), *Functional MRI: An introduction to methods*. New York: Oxford University Press Inc.pp 177-195

Douw, L., Schoonheim, M. M., Landi, D., van der Meer, M. L., Geurts, J. J., Reijneveld, J. C., Klein, M., & Stam, C. J. (2011). Cognition is related to resting-state small-world network topology: A magnetoencephalographic study. *Neuroscience*, Vol. 175 (February 2011): pp. 169-77.

Fernández, A., Arrazola, J., Maestú, F., Amo, C., Gil-Gregorio, P., Wienbruch, C., & Ortiz, T. (2003). Correlations of hippocampal atrophy and focal low-frequency magnetic activity in Alzheimer's disease: Volumetric MR imaging-magnetoencephalographic study. *AJNR Am J Neuroradiol*, Vol. 24, No. 3 (March 2003): pp. 481-7.

Fernández, A., Hornero, R., Mayo, A., Poza, J., Gil-Gregorio, P., & Ortiz, T. (2006). MEG spectral profile in Alzheimer's disease and mild cognitive impairment. *Clinical Neurophysiology*, Vol. 117, No. 2 (2006): pp. 306-314.

Fernández, A., Maestú, F., Amo, C., Gil, P., Fehr, T., Wienbruch, C., Rockstroh, B., Elbert, T., & Ortiz, T. (2002). Focal temporoparietal slow activity in Alzheimer's disease revealed by magnetoencephalography. *Biol Psychiatry*, Vol. 52, No. 7 (1 October 2002): pp. 764-70.

Fernández, A., Turrero, A., Zuluaga, P., Gil, P., Maestú, F., Campo, P., & Ortiz, T. (2006). Magnetoencephalographic parietal dipole density in mild cognitive impairment: Preliminary results of a method to estimate the risk of developing Alzheimer's Disease. *Arch Neurol*, Vol. 63, No. 3 (March 2006): pp. 427-430.

Fisher, A. E., Furlong, P. L., Seri, S., Adjamian, P., Witton, C., Baldeweg, T., Phillips, S., Walsh, R.,Houghton, J. M., & Thai, N. J. (2008). Interhemispheric differences of spectral power in expressive language: A MEG study with clinical applications. *International Journal of Psychophysiology*, Vol. 68, No. 2 (2008): pp. 111-122.

Friston, K. J., & Dolan, R. J. (2010). Computational and dynamic models in neuroimaging. *Neuroimage*, Vol. 52, No. 3 (September 2010): pp. 752-65.

Frye, R. E., Rezaie, R., & Papanicolaou, A. C. (2009). Functional neuroimaging of language using magnetoencephalography. *Physics of Life Reviews*, Vol. 6, No. 1 (March 2009): pp. 1-10.

Gauthier, S., Reisberg, B., Zaudig, M., Petersen, R. C., Ritchie, K., Broich, K., Belleville, S., Brodaty, H., Bennett, D., Chertkow, H., Cummings, J. L., de Leon, M., Feldman, H., Ganguli, M., Hampel, H., Scheltens, P., Tierney, M. C., Whitehouse, P., & Winblad, B. (2006). International Psychogeriatric Association Expert Conference on mild cognitive impairment: Mild cognitive impairment. *Lancet*, Vol. 367, No. 9518 (15 April 2006): pp. 1262-70.

Grummicha, P., Nimskya, C., Paulic, E., Buchfeldera, M., & Ganslandta, M. (2006). Combining fMRI and MEG increases the reliability of presurgical language localization: A clinical study on the difference between and congruence of both modalities. *NeuroImage*, Vol. 32, No. 4.1 (October 2006): pp. 1793-1803.

Hämäläinen, M., & Hari, R. (2002). Magnetoencephalographic characterization of dynamic brain activation: Basic principles and methods of data collection and source analysis, In: *Brain Mapping: The Methods*, A. W. Toga & J. C. Mazziotta, Eds., Academic Press, Boston: pp. 227-253

Hari, R. (1993). Magnetoencephalography as a tool of clinical neurophysiology, In: *Electroencephalography: Basic principles, clinical applications, and related fields*, E. Niedermeyer & F. L. da Silva, Eds., pp. 1035-1061, Williams & Wilkins, Baltimore.

Hari, R., Levänen, S., & Raij, T. (2000). Timing of human cortical functions during cognition: Role of MEG. *Trends Cogn Sci*, Vol. 4, No. 12 (1 December 2000): pp. 455-462.

Hauk, O. (2004). Keep it simple: A case for using classical minimum norm estimation in the analysis of EEG and MEG data. *Neuroimage*, Vol. 21, No. 4 (April 2004): pp. 1612-21.

He, B., & Liu, Z. (2008). Multimodal functional neuroimaging: Integrating functional MRI and EEG/MEG. *IEEE reviews in biomedical engineering* (2008): pp. 23-40.

Hirschfeld, G., Zwitserlood, P., & Dobel, C. (2011). Effects of language comprehension on visual processing - MEG dissociates early perceptual and late N400 effects. *Brain Lang*, Vol. 116, No. 2 (2011): pp. 91-96.

Kaplan, A. Ya., Fingelkurts, A. A., Fingelkurts, A. A., Borisov, S. V., & Darkhovskye, B. S. (2005). Nonstationary nature of the brain activity as revealed by EEG/MEG: Methodological, practical and conceptual challenges. *Signal Processing*, Vol. 85, No. 11 (November 2005): pp. 2190-2212.

Kim, M. S., Kim, J. S., & Chung, C. K. (2008). Neural correlates of immediate and delayed word recognition memory: An MEG study. *Brain Res*, Vol. 1240 (November 2008): pp. 132-42.

Kober, H., Möller, M., Nimsky, C., Vieth, J., Fahlbusch, R., & Ganslandt, O. (2001). New approach to localize speech relevant brain areas and hemispheric dominance using spatially filtered magnetoencephalography. *Hum Brain Mapp*, Vol. 14, No. 4 (December 2001): pp. 236-50.

Lau, E., Almeida, D., Hines, P. C., & Poeppel, D. (2009). A lexical basis for N400 context effects:Evidence from MEG. *Brain Lang*, Vol. 111, No. 3 (December 2009): pp. 161-72.

Maestú, F., Baykova, E., Ruiz, J. M., Montejo, P., Montenegro, M., Llanero, M., Solesio, E., Gil, P., Yubero, R., Paul, N., Pozo, F., & Nevado, A. (2011). Increased biomagnetic activity in healthy elderly with subjective memory complaints. *Clin Neurophysiol*, Vol. 122, No. 3 (March 2011): pp. 499-505.

Maestú, F., Ortiz, T., Fernandez, A., Amo, C., Martin, P., Fernández, S., & Sola, R. G. (2002). Spanish language mapping using MEG: a validation study. *Neuroimage*, Vol. 17, No. 3 (November 2002): pp. 1579-86.

Maestú, F., Fernandez, A., Simos, P., Lopez-Ibor, M., Campo, P., Criado, J., Rodriguez-Palanca, A., Ferre, F., Amo, C., & Ortiz, T. (2004). Profiles of brain magnetic activity during a memory task in patients with Alzheimer's disease and in non-demented elderly subjects, with or without depression. *J Neurol Neurosurg Psychiatry*, Vol. 75, No. 8 (August 2004): pp. 1160–1162.

Maestú, F., Fernández, A., Simos, P. G., Gil-Gregorio, P., Amo, C., Rodriguez, R., Arrazola, J., & Ortiz, T. (2001). Spatio-temporal patterns of brain magnetic activity during a memory task in Alzheimer's disease. *Neuroreport*, Vol. 12, No. 18 (21 December 2001): pp. 3917-22.

Maestú, F., García-Segura, J., Ortiz, T., Montoya, J., Fernández, A., Gil-Gregorio, P., Campo, P., Fernández, S., Viaño, J., & Portera, A. (2005). Evidence of biochemical and biomagnetic interactions in Alzheimer's disease: An MEG and MR spectroscopy study. *Dement Geriatr Cogn Disord*, Vol. 20, No. 2-3 (2005): pp. 145-52.

Maestú, F., Arrazola, J., Fernández, A., Simos, P. G., Amo, C., Gil-Gregorio, P., Fernandez, A., Papanicolaou, A. C., & Ortiz, T. (2003). Do cognitive patterns of brain magnetic activity correlate with hippocampal atrophy in Alzheimer's disease? *J Neurol Neurosurg Psychiatry*, Vol. 74 (2003): pp. 208-12.

Maestú, F., Campo, P., Gil-Gregorio, P., Fernández, S., Fernández, A., & Ortiz, T. (2006). Medial temporal lobe neuromagnetic hypoactivation and risk for developing cognitive decline in elderly population: A 2-year follow-up study. *Neurobiol Aging*, Vol. 27, No. 1 (January 2006): pp. 32-37.

Maestú, F., Campo, P., Del Río, D., Moratti, S., Gil-Gregorio, P., Fernández, A., Capilla, A., & Ortiz, T. (2008). Increased biomagnetic activity in the ventral pathway in mild cognitive impairment. *Clinical Neurophysiology*, Vol. 85, No. 11 (2008): pp. 2190-2212.

Mirra, S. S., Heyman, A., McKeel, D., Sumi, S. M., Crain, B. J., Brownlee, L. M., Vogel, F. S., Hughes, J. P., van Belle, G., & Berg, L. (1991). The Consortium to Establish a Registry for Alzheimer's Disease (CERAD). Part II. Standardization of the neuropathologic assessment of Alzheimer's disease. *Neurology*, Vol. 41, No. 4 (April 1991): pp. 479-86.

Moran, R. J., Campo, P., Maestu, F., Reilly, R. B., Dolan, R. J., & Strange, B. A. (2010). Peak frequency in the theta and alpha bands correlates with human working memory capacity. *Front Hum Neurosci*, Vol. 11, No. 4 (November 2010): p. 200.

Osipovaa, D., Ahveninenb, J., Jensene, O., Ylikoskif, A., & Pekkonena, E. (2005). Altered generation of spontaneous oscillations in Alzheimer's disease. *NeuroImage*, Vol. 27, No. 4 (2005): pp. 835-41.

Osipovaa, D., Rantanend, K., Ahveninene, J., Ylikoskid, R., Häppöläd, O., Strandbergf, T., & Pekkonena, E. (2006). Source estimation of spontaneous MEG oscillations in mild cognitive impairment. *Neuroscience Letters*, Vol. 405, No. 1-2 (September 2006): pp. 57-61.

Osipovaa, D., Pekkonen, E., & Ahveninen, J. (2006). Enhanced magnetic auditory steady-state response in early Alzheimer's disease. *Clinical Neurophisiology*, Vol. 117, No. 9 (October 2006): pp. 1990-95.

Pang, E. W., Wang, F., Malone, M., Kadis, D. S., & Donner, E. J. (2011). Localization of Broca's area using verb generation tasks in the MEG: Validation against fMRI. *Neuroscience Letters*, Vol. 490, No. 3 (3 March 2011): pp. 215-19.

Papanicolaou, A. C. (1998). *Fundamentals of Functional Brain Imaging: A guide to the methods and their applications to psychology and behavioral neurosciences*. Swets & Zeitlinger, Netherlands.

Papanicolaou, A. C., Pazo-Alvarez, P., Castillo, E. M., Billingsley-Marshall, R. L., Breier, J. I., Swank, P. R., Buchanan, S., McManis, M., Clear, T., & Pássaro, A. D. (2006). Functional neuroimaging with MEG: Normative language profiles. *NeuroImage*, Vol. 33, No. 1 (October 2006): pp. 326-42.

Pasquale, F., Della Penna, S., Snyder, A. Z., Lewis, C., Mantini, D., Marzetti, L., Belardinelli, P., Ciancetta, L., Pizzella, V., Romani, G. L., & Corbetta, M. (2010). Temporal dynamics of spontaneous MEG activity in brain networks. *Proc Natl Acad Sci*, Vol. 107, No. 13 (30 March 2010): pp. 6040-45.

Petersen, R. C., Roberts, R. O., Knopman, D. S., Boeve, B. F., Geda, Y. E., Ivnik, R. J., Smith, G. E., Jack, C. R., Jr. (2009). Mild cognitive impairment: Ten years later. *Arch Neurol*, Vol. 66, No. 12 (December 2009): pp. 1447-55.

Petersen, R. C., Smith, G. E., Waring, S. C., Ivnik, R. J., Tangalos, E. G., & Kokmen, E. (1999). Mild cognitive impairment: Clinical characterization and outcome. *Arch Neurol*, Vol. 56, No. 3 (1999): pp. 303-8.

Poza, J., Hornero, R., Abásolo, D., Fernández, A., & García, M. (2007). Extraction of spectral based measures from MEG background oscillations in Alzheimer's disease. *Med Eng Phys*, Vol. 29, No. 10 (December 2007): pp. 1073-83.

Poza, J., Hornero, R., Abásolo, D., Fernández, A., & Mayo, A. (2008). Evaluation of spectral ratio measures from spontaneous MEG recordings in patients with Alzheimer's disease. *Computer Methods and Programs in Biomedicine*, Vol. 90, No. 2 (2008): pp. 137-47.

Puligheddu, M., de Munck, J. C., Stam, C. J., Verbunt, J., de Jongh, A., van Dijk, B. W., & Marrosu, F. (2005). Age distribution of MEG spontaneous theta activity in healthy subjects. *Brain Topogr.*, Vol. 17, No. 3 (Spring 2005): pp. 165-75.

Pulvermüller, F., Shtyrov, Y., & Ilmoniemi, R. (2003). Spatiotemporal dynamics of neural language processing: An MEG study using minimum-norm current estimates. *Neuroimage*, Vol. 20, No. 2 (October 2003): pp. 1020-5.

Püregger, E., Walla, P., Deecke, L., & Dal-Bianco, P. (2003). Magnetoencephalographic—features related to mild cognitive impairment. *Neuroimage*, Vol. 20, No. 4 (December 2003): pp. 2235-44.

Raichle, M. (19939 Functional Neuroimaging: A Historical and Physiological Perspective in Handbook of Functional Neuroimaging of Cognition: Cabeza R. & Kingstone A., Eds., pp. 3-26, MIT Press.

Robitaille, N., Marois, R., Todd, J., Grimault, S., Cheyne, D., & Jolicoeur, P. (2010). Distinguishing between lateralized and nonlateralized brain activity associated with visual short-term memory: fMRI, MEG, and EEG evidence from the same observers. *Neuroimage*, Vol. 53, No. 4 (December 2010): pp. 1334-45.

Rossini, P. M., Rossi, S., Babiloni, C., & Polich, J. (2007). Clinical neurophysiology of aging brain: From normal aging to neurodegeneration. *Progress in Neurobiology*, Vol. 83, No. 6 (December 2007): pp. 375-400.

Salmelin, R. (2007). Clinical neurophysiology of language: The MEG approach. *Clinical Neurophysiology*, Vol. 118, No. 2 (2007): pp. 237-54.

Silva Nunes, M. V., Castro-Caldas, A., Rio, D. D., Maestú, F., & Ortiz, T. (2009). The ex-illiterate brain: the critical period, the cognitive reserve and the HAROLD model. *Dement. Neuropsychol.*, Vol. 3, No. 3 (2009): pp. 222-27.

Simos, P. G., Breier, J. I., Zouridakis, G., & Papanicolaou, A. C. (1998). Identification of language-specific brain activity using magnetoencephalography. *J Clin Exp Neuropsychol.*, Vol. 20, No. 5 (October 1998): pp. 706-22.

Solomyak, O. & Marantz, A. (2009). Lexical Access in Early Stages of Visual Word Processing: A Single-Trial Correlational MEG Study of Heteronym Recognition. *Brain and Lang*, Vol. 108, No. 3 (March 2009): pp. 191-96.

Stam, C. J., Jones, B. F., Manshanden, I., van Cappellen van Walsum, A. M., Montez, T., Verbunt, J. P., de Munck, J. C., van Dijk, B. W., Berendse, H. W., & Scheltens, P. (2006). Magnetoencephalographic evaluation of resting-state functional connectivity in Alzheimer's disease. *NeuroImage*, Vol. 32, No. 3 (2006): pp. 1335-44.

Stam, C. J. (2010). Use of magnetoencephalography (MEG) to study functional brain networks in neurodegenerative disorders. *Journal of the Neurological Sciences*, Vol. 289, No. 15 (February 2010): pp. 128-34.

Stam, C. J. (2005). Nonlinear dynamical analysis of EEG and MEG: Review of an emerging field. *Clin Neurophysiol.*, Vol. 116, No. 10 (October 2005): pp. 2266-2301.

Stufflebeam, S. M., & Rosen, B. R. (2007). Mapping cognitive function. *Neuroimaging Clin N Am.*, Vol. 17, No. 4 (November 2007): pp. 469-84, viii-ix.

Tanaka, K., Kawakatsu, M., Fujiwara, K., Wang, G., & Yunokuchi, K. (2003). Tokyo Denki Effects on MEG coherence with working memory load. *The IEEE EMBS Asian-Pacific Conference on Biomedical Engineering 2003*, pp. 334-35.

Valaki, C. E., Maestu, F., Simos, P. G., Zhang, W., Fernandez, A., Amo, C. M., Ortiz, T., & Papanicolaou, A. C. (2004). Cortical organization for receptive language functions in Chinese, English, and Spanish: A cross-linguistic MEG study. *Neuropsychologia*, Vol. 42, No. 7 (2004): pp. 967-79.

Walla, P., Endl, W., Lindinger, G., Lalouschek, W., Deecke, L., & Lang, W. (1999). Early occipito-parietal activity in a word recognition task: an EEG and MEG study. *Clin Neurophysiol.*, Vol. 110, No. 8 (August 1999): pp. 1378-87.

Wehner, D. T., Ahlfors, S. P., & Mody, M. (2007). Effects of phonological contrast on auditory word discrimination in children with and without reading disability: A magnetoencephalography (MEG) study. *Neuropsychologia*, Vol. 45, No. 14 (November 2007): pp. 3251-62.

Zamrini, E., Maestu, F., Pekkonen, E., Funke, M., Makela, J., Riley, M., Bajo, R., Sudre, G., Fernandez, A., Castellanos, N., Del Pozo, F., Stam, C. J., van Dijk, B. W., Bagic, A., & Becker, J. T. (2011). Magnetoencephalography as a putative biomarker for Alzheimer's disease. *Int J Alzheimers Dis.* (10 April 2011): pp. 280-89.

3

Dynamic Imaging of Deep Brain Structures with MEG: Contributions to Understanding Human Memory

Sandra N. Moses[1,2,3], Faith M. Hanlon[4,5] and Jennifer D. Ryan[3,6,7]
[1]Department of Diagnostic Imaging, Hospital for Sick Children, Toronto,
[2]Department of Medical Imaging, University of Toronto, Toronto,
[3]Rotman Research Institute, Baycrest, Toronto,
[4]The Mind Research Network, Albuquerque, NM,
[5]Department of Psychology, University of New Mexico, Albuquerque, NM,
[6]Department of Psychology, University of Toronto, Toronto,
[7]Department of Psychiatry, University of Toronto, Toronto,
[1,2,3,6,7]Canada
[4,5]USA

1. Introduction

MEG is traditionally conceived of as a tool that provides excellent temporal and spatial resolution to characterize the dynamic time-course of brain responses originating within superficial cortex, such as basic primary sensory or motor responses. However, this dynamic imaging of brain activity within specific regions could also be very useful for expanding upon our knowledge of the neural underpinning of complex cognitive processes, such as memory. Although cognitive neuroscientists are now beginning to appreciate the utility of MEG imaging to illuminate the underlying mechanisms of human cognition, there has been a considerable debate regarding whether it is feasible to apply MEG to the study of memory. This chapter will briefly outline this debate, and provide a selective review of the literature that suggests that not only can MEG be a reliable tool with which to investigate memory in multiple populations, but that the insights gained by the application of MEG technology to the field of memory research are beyond those provided by other neuroimaging tools, such as functional magnetic resonance imaging (fMRI), positron emission tomography (PET) and electroencephalography (EEG). These insights come from the examination of the spatiotemporal dynamics of healthy brain function, as well as how these patterns are perturbed in pathological conditions such as in individuals with brain damage or psychiatric disorders. Ultimately, we suggest that recent findings from MEG have encouraged researchers to reconsider their conceptualizations of memory. For example, memory is often thought of as a modular cognitive process, distinct from other faculties such as perception. However, we will show new evidence from recent MEG studies that suggests a more distributed and interactive conceptualization of memory, and of cognition in general.

2. Detection of hippocampal signal using MEG

The difficulty surrounding the application of MEG to the study of human memory is that brain structures critical for memory are located deep within the brain. Neuropsychological and neuroimaging (MRI and PET) studies have implicated the hippocampus, a structure deep within the medial temporal lobe, as a crucial region supporting memory (e.g. for reviews see Cohen & Eichenbaum, 1993; Cohen et al., 1999; Cohen & Squire, 1980; Moses & Ryan, 2006). Specifically, bilateral damage to the hippocampus in humans leads to profound and pervasive amnesia in which the ability to remember or acquire particular classes of long-term memories is lost (Rosenbaum et al., 2008; Scoville & Milner, 1957; Tulving 1972). However, it has traditionally been assumed that reliable signal could not be obtained from deep sources such as the hippocampus, and as a result, MEG investigations have focused on recording from superficial cortices and have constrained the kinds of conceptual questions that were being investigated. Thus, in order to apply MEG technology to the study of human memory, thereby developing a new avenue of research in cognitive neuroscience, the validity of imaging hippocampal activation had to be demonstrated (for in depth discussions see Quraan et al., 2011; Riggs et al., 2009; Stephen et al., 2005).

The first challenge to hippocampal imaging with MEG lies with the structural property of the hippocampus itself. The spiral or spherical shape of the hippocampus could theoretically lead to cancellation of all signal, which would allow no detectable activation to pass outside of the hippocampus (Baumgartner et al., 2000, Mikuni et al., 1997). This type of complete cancellation would require perfect anatomical symmetry, as well as simultaneous activation of the dentate and cornu ammonis (CA) fields with equal signal intensity. However, this assumption of perfect symmetry is incongruent with studies that have demonstrated anatomical and electrophysiological asymmetries within the hippocampus (Duvernoy, 1988; Yeckel & Berger, 1990). Moreover, simultaneous recording from MEG and subdural electrodes demonstrates that strong epileptic discharges originating from within the hippocampus can, indeed, be detected using MEG (Mikuni et al., 1997). Additionally, simulation work demonstrates that MEG has the sensitivity to detect epileptic spike activity from the hippocampus and surrounding cortex (Stephen et al., 2005). Thus, cancellation of signal from the hippocampus is, at the very least, incomplete. Therefore, the imperfect symmetry of hippocampal anatomy and physiology permits activity from this structure to be detected by MEG sensors.

The second challenge to hippocampal imaging with MEG is that magnetic field strength decreases with increasing distance between neural sources and MEG sensors. Thus, there is concern that signal from deep sources, which are the furthest from the MEG sensor array, will be at least weaker than signal from superficial sources, and perhaps not detectable at all (Hillebrand and Barnes, 2002; Baumgartner et al., 2000; Hämäläinen et al., 1993). Simulation and empirical studies have been conducted to systematically investigate this issue regarding the strength of hippocampal and cortical sources (Mills et al., in review; Qurann et al., 2011). These studies have demonstrated that even weak stimulus-evoked hippocampal and cortical activity can be detected if care is taken in experimental design (i.e. appropriate behavioural and control tasks, sufficient numbers of trials) and selection of optimal analysis methods. In support of the conclusions from simulation work, an increasing body of empirical evidence demonstrates that although hippocampal activation may be more difficult to detect than superficial sources, it can be reliably detected with a range of experimental paradigms and analysis techniques (Breier, 1998, 1999; Hanlon et al., 2003, 2005, 2011; Hopf et al., 2010;

Ionnides et al., 1995; Kirsh et al., 2003; Leirer et al., 2010; Martin et al., 2006; Mikuni et al., 1997; Mills et al., in review; Moses et al., 2009, Nishitani et al., 1999; Papanicolaou et al., 2002; Stephen et al., 2005; Quraan et al., 2010; Riggs et al., 2009; Tesche, 1997; Tesche & Karhu, 1999, 2000; Tesche, Karhu & Tissari, 1996). Thus, using a well-designed paradigm and appropriate analysis techniques, stimulus-evoked hippocampal activation is detectable using MEG.

3. Insights into human memory gained from MEG

As stated above, MEG is an ideal tool to study human memory due to its excellent temporal and spatial resolution. Memory processes rely on the dynamic interaction among superficial sensory and association cortices with deep neural structures such as the hippocampus. Simulation studies and empirical findings demonstrate that MEG can reliably detect activation from the hippocampus, in addition to superficial cortical structures. The combination of this spatial resolution and high temporal resolution can elucidate at which particular stage of processing different brain regions contribute to the task, or cognitive operation, at hand, as well define the parameters (e.g. frequency) under which neural regions operate. In this capacity, MEG stands apart from other neuroimaging tools. FMRI is known for its high spatial resolution, but is not a direct measure of neuronal activity and has poor temporal resolution. EEG, like MEG, has superb temporal resolution. However, EEG is limited in its spatial resolution due to the brain, skull, and CSF smearing the electric potential patterns assessed from the scalp surface. In addition, EEG is recorded as a difference in potential between two electrode sites, with the pattern of electric potentials at the scalp surface contingent on the electrode site used as a reference for the sites of interest. Although MEG is not faced with these particular limitations of EEG, it is important to recognize that like EEG, MEG shares the uncertainties in source localization algorithms imposed by the "inverse problem". Confidence in the solutions however has been acquired through the use of simulation studies and empirical findings. Thus, overall, MEG can be used to compare the dynamics of healthy brain activation to that found in pathological conditions, such as in cases of brain damage or psychiatric disorders and as such, is well poised to provide new insights about human memory.

In this portion of the chapter, we will first discuss MEG studies that have characterized the dynamics of neural system activations involved in different types of memory processes in the healthy brain. We will then examine how facilitating the recruitment of one system over another may allow for compensation under pathological conditions. Subsequently, we will discuss studies that have used MEG to directly examine the neural basis of compensation in pathological conditions that arise due to brain lesions and schizophrenia. Lastly, we will report on applications of MEG to understanding the neural organization of memory during development.

3.1 How does the hippocampus contribute to memory?

Previous fMRI studies have documented the role of the hippocampus in the encoding and subsequent retrieval and recognition of newly learned information (e.g. Kirchhoff et al., 2000; Stark & Okado, 2003; Weis et al., 2004; Kapur et al., 1995; Schacter et al., 1995; Squire et al., 1992). However, these studies could not tell us the mechanisms (e.g., frequency, timing) by which the hippocampus supports such memory processes.

MEG studies have demonstrated that theta oscillations within the hippocampus are associated with memory processing. For instance, Guderian and Duzel (2005) required participants to study a series of faces superimposed on a background image. During a retrieval phase, faces were re-presented and participants were required to recollect the context (i.e., background image) with which the face had been paired. Recollection of the context in which a face had been learned was associated with an increase in the amplitude of theta oscillations. In a subsequent study, Guderian, Schott, Richardson-Klavehn and Duzel (2009) demonstrated that theta oscillations could be localized to the medial temporal lobes and that the amplitude of the theta oscillations observed prior to the onset of words were positively correlated with subsequent memory for the words. Using a working memory paradigm in which participants were required to maintain a series of integers in memory, Tesche and Karhu (2000) further localized theta oscillations to the hippocampus and additionally observed that such oscillations were stimulus-locked to the presentation of the memory set and that the duration of this stimulus-locked theta increased with increasing memory load. All together, these studies suggest that theta oscillations may mediate the dynamic interplay between the hippocampus and the cortex allowing for disparate cortical representations to be bound together and maintained in memory.

More recent evidence from MEG studies has suggested that via theta oscillations, the hippocampus supports memory through its dynamic interconnections with the cortex. For example, in Cashdollar et al., (2009), healthy participants and participants with bilateral hippocampal sclerosis (BHS) performed a delayed match-to-sample (DMS) task in which memory for the relations depicted within each scene stimulus had to be maintained in order for successful performance to occur. Specifically, in the non-relational condition, participants were presented with a single indoor or outdoor scene as the sample stimulus, and then were presented with the probe display in which the same exact scene was re-presented alongside a novel scene. In the relational condition, one of the scenes in the probe display was an exact repetition of the sample stimulus, and the other was again this same scene, but some relational change had occurred to the objects within the scene (e.g., an item had been added, deleted or moved in its spatial location). In healthy participants, an occipito-temporal theta synchrony was observed during the relational DMS task, whereas a frontal-parietal synchrony was observed for the non-relational DMS. Patients with left temporal lobe epilepsy (who had structurally intact hippocampi) showed similar effects to control participants; however, patients with BHS did not demonstrate the occipito-temporal theta synchrony in the relational DMS task and showed decreased accuracy on the task relative to the other participant groups, demonstrating that occipito-temporal theta synchrony critically supports relational memory.

A further specification regarding how the hippocampus supports memory concerns the timing by which the hippocampus contributes to processing. The cognitive implications of hippocampal responses that are earlier versus later in the processing stream are very different. For example, activation found later during the processing stream (e.g. 250+ ms following stimulus onset) would suggest that the hippocampus becomes involved only after the stimulus has already been perceived. This paints a modular and serial view of perception and memory processing -- first we perceive the stimulus, then we search our memory stores for a match.

In contrast, hippocampal activation found early in the processing (e.g. prior to 250 ms following stimulus onset) stream is suggestive of a role for this structure during perceptual processing. Such a finding may be interpreted as a contribution from memory in shaping and/or encoding our initial perception of a stimulus. This leads to a more distributed and interactive view of memory and perception. This integrated view of memory is expressed nicely by McIntosh (2007): "Memory is not the domain of particular systems in the brain, but of the brain as a whole.... The act of seeing, hearing and acting makes use of the brain's capacity for memory". Using MEG, serial modular versus distributed interactive views of the neural organization of cognitive functions such as perception and memory can be tested. Riggs et al. (2009) conducted a MEG investigation regarding the relative timing of the contribution of hippocampal responses to scene recognition. They examined hippocampal responses during the processing of novel and recently studied indoor and outdoor scenes. In support of the distributed interactive view of cognitive organization, they found very early hippocampal responses, during the first 200 ms following scene presentation, to both novel and previously studied scenes. This early latency is within the time window within which perception is thought to occur independently of the hippocampus (Tsivilis et al., 2001). Riggs et al. also found that this hippocampal activity consistently oscillated within the theta frequency band. They concluded that the hippocampus may be involved during early perceptual processing of old and new information, or at the very least, that memory processing begins rapidly and operates in conjunction with, or parallel to, visual processing when perception is thought to occur.

3.2 Perceptual plasticity: MEG studies of the effect of memory on perceptual processing

The idea of distributed interactive memory and perceptual processing was taken one step further by Ryan et al. (2008), with their discussion of *perceptual plasticity*. Their study built on fMRI work demonstrating that the information that has come to be associated with an object over time can change subsequent brain activation patterns that are invoked during processing when the object is subsequently presented in isolation (Nyberg, Habib, McIntosh & Tulving, 2000; Wheeler, Petersen & Buckner, 2000). For instance, visually presented words, when presented in isolation, do not elicit responses in auditory regions. However, following repeated pairings between the visually presented words and auditorily presented sounds, the presentation of a previously studied word elicits activation within auditory regions (Nyberg et al., 2000). Ryan et al. (2008) point out that although these fMRI studies can tell us that memory for associated information is related to the processing of sensory inputs, they cannot tell us precisely at what stage of processing activation is observed in these associated regions. Therefore, we do not know whether prior experience results in the activation of associated information that occurs following perceptual processing, or whether prior experience results in the activation of associated information during the time of perceptual processing itself. Hence, the dynamic description of brain systems obtained using MEG can inform our overall conceptualization of memory and perception, including the relationship between these faculties and whether they are, indeed, dissociable.

3.3 When does memory modulate primary sensory activity?

The unique combination of excellent temporal and spatial resolution of MEG allows for an investigation regarding the timing of primary sensory cortical modulations, and to infer whether the influence of prior experiences, or memory, can occur early enough to affect our perceptions. Moses et al. (2005) exposed participants to an auditory noise burst that was repeatedly paired with a visual presentation of a geometric figure. Initial presentation of the visual stimulus alone did not elicit activity within auditory regions. However, following training trials in which the noise and visual stimulus were presented together, the presentation of the geometric figure alone elicited a response within the auditory cortex. Interestingly, this response within the auditory cortex occurred early (approximately 50 ms) following the time when the presentation of the noise would have ordinarily been expected. This time interval of 50 ms coincides with the time at which sensory processing associated with tone perception occurs within the auditory cortex. In a further analysis, early responses were observed in the amygdala within 200 ms following the onset of the visual stimulus that had been previously paired with the noise compared to visual stimuli that had never been paired with the noise (Moses et al., 2007). These findings suggest that the experience of hearing a sound coincident with seeing a picture leads to changes in the way the brain processes that picture. In other words, the memory acquired by the participants within the laboratory altered their subsequent neural responses, and possibly, their perception of the items. These findings have also been replicated in the somatosensory domain (Moses et al., 2010).

3.4 Does memory alter primary perception?

Ryan et al. (2008) expanded on this question and asked whether pre-existing knowledge about an object changes the way the object is ''perceived''. Specifically, they asked whether the presence of memories about an object changes the way the brain responds at the time of initial perception, or whether the changes occur following initial perceptual processing at a time when memory processing is traditionally thought to occur. In contrast to Moses et al. (2005, 2007, 2010), in which memory acquisition occurred within the experimental session, Ryan et al. (2008) used a paradigm in which the ''previous learning episodes'' occurred in real life prior to the experiment, and in which the learned associated information was not presented at any time during the study and was not needed in order to complete the task given to the participants. Thus, they could ask whether early changes in neural activity actually represent a long-term change in perceptual processing, or whether they are merely a short-lived artificial change induced only in the laboratory as a result of the particular experimental procedures.

Ryan et al. (2008) gave participants visual presentations of famous and non-famous (novel) faces and, and auditory presentations of famous and non-famous names while neural responses were recorded with MEG. Interestingly, responses within the *auditory* cortex were larger for *visually* presented famous versus nonfamous faces. Likewise, activation within the *visual* cortex was larger for *auditorily* presented famous versus nonfamous names. These effects were found early during processing, within 150–250 ms, which is within the time window during which most perceptual processes are thought to occur, as opposed to a later time window (e.g 250-1000 ms) during which conceptual/semantic processes and/or the retrieval of associated information are largely purported to occur (e.g., Itier et al., 2006; Schweinberger et al., 2002; Donaldson & Rugg, 1998, 1999). These data suggested that, when a famous name is heard, there is obligatorily activation of a visual representation of the person's face; however, this visual representation is not present for non-famous names. Similarly, the presentation of a famous person's face obligatorily activated an auditory representation of the sound of their name. Thus, our memories, or knowledge about an individual, actually change how we initially perceive that individual during subsequent encounters. In a broader sense, Ryan et al. (2008) proposed that memories and prior experiences not only influence processing but that they may do so in an unconscious, obligatory manner. They contend that each encounter leads to a sort of "perceptual plasticity", meaning that subsequent processing of the same item is "ever-changing".

4. MEG studies of compensation for neural damage

Although the hippocampus plays a crucial role in memory, not all types of memory processing are mediated by the hippocampus. Hippocampal lesions in humans and non-human animals specifically lead to impairments in the ability to learn the relations among multiple items (Cohen & Eichenbaum, 1993; Sutherland & Rudy, 1989); an ability that is essential for acquiring episodic and autobiographical memory as well as semantic memories (Moses & Ryan, 2006; Eichenbaum & Cohen, 2001; Cohen & Eichenbaum, 1993). It is generally agreed upon that after a period of consolidation, semantic memories can be retrieved independently from the hippocampus, although there is currently still debate regarding whether the retrieval of episodic or autobiographical memories can ever occur independently from the hippocampus (Moscovitch, Rosenbaum, Gilboa et al., 2005). Other mnemonic functions such as skill learning and priming are considered procedural in nature, rather than relational, and can be mediated by extra-hippocampal structures (Cohen & Eichenbaum, 1993). Therefore, following hippocampal damage, extra-hippocampal structures can mediate the retrieval of semantic memory, as well as support procedural learning such as skill learning and priming (Cohen & Eichenbaum, 1993; Squire, 1992; Tulving, 1972). The recruitment of these extra-hippocampal regions during performance of a memory task may allow alternate cognitive strategies to support performance, thereby demonstrating a potential mechanism whereby one may circumvent a damaged hippocampal system. MEG can define the spatial distribution of distinct neural networks that can each support performance, and provide detail regarding when distinct networks are engaged.

4.1 Imaging the potential for compensation

Using MEG, Moses et al. (2010) investigated the conditions under which extra-hippocampal systems can facilitate performance on what has traditionally been shown to be a hippocampal-dependent relational memory task: transverse patterning. (e.g. Alvarado & Bachvallier, 2005; Astur & Constable, 2004; Driscoll et al., 2003; Hanlon et al., 2003, 2005, 2011; Meltzer et al., 2008, Moses, Ostreicher, Rosenbaum & Ryan, 2008; Moses et al., 2009; Rickard & Grafman, 1998; Rickard, Verfaellie & Grafman, 2006; Reed & Squire, 1996; Ostreicher, Ryan, Moses & Rosenbaum, 2010; Saksida et al., 2007).

The transverse patterning task is structurally analogous to the childhood game "rock-paper-scissors" (Rock crushes Scissors, Scissors cut Paper, Paper covers Rock), but uses novel stimuli (A, B, C) that have ambiguous meanings outside the context of their pairings (A beats B, B beats C, C beats A; or A+B-, B+C-, C+A-; Fig. 1A). Performance on the transverse patterning task is impaired following hippocampal damage, and is correlated with measures of hippocampal neuronal integrity (Driscoll et al., 2003). Transverse patterning deficits are also observed in conditions associated with impaired hippocampal functioning such as schizophrenia (Hanlon et al., 2005, 2011) and normal aging (Dricoll et al., 2003). Additionally, transverse patterning performance elicits hippocampal activation measured with fMRI (Astur & Constable, 2004: Melzer, Nigishi & Constable, 2008; Rowland et al., 2010) and MEG (Hanlon et al., 2003; 2005; 2011; Hopf et al., in reivew; Leirer et al., 2010; Mills et al., in review, Moses et al., 2009).

However, the transverse patterning task can be solved despite bilateral hippocampal damage if the stimuli involved are designed to tap previously acquired semantic memories (Moses et al., 2008), the retrieval of which is thought to be mediated by frontal and anterior temporal cortices (Cabeza & Nyberg, 2000). In Moses et al. (2008), amnesic patient K.C., whose damage includes the hippocampus bilaterally, was tested on four transverse patterning conditions that varied the extent to which the stimuli and relations among them were semantically meaningful, or known pre-experimentally: 1) abstract objects; 2) geometric shapes; 3) playing cards; 4) rock-paper-scissors (RPS). K.C. could solve the transverse patterning task using meaningful, but not arbitrary stimulus relations, suggesting that his successful performance was supported by an increased contribution from semantic memory (Moses et al., 2008).

In support of the notion that the transverse patterning task with meaningful stimulus relations can be solved by extra-hippocampal structures, an MEG study with neurologically intact participants revealed a bilateral decrease in hippocampal activation for the meaningful RPS condition compared to the other conditions (Moses et al., 2009). Hippocampal peaks were apparent as early as 120 ms, and maximum differentiation in hippocampal activation between the meaningful RPS and the other conditions occurred at approximately 300 ms in the right, and 550 ms in the left hippocampus. These time-course differences across conditions suggest that the meaningfulness of the stimuli affected later, conceptual, processing, rather than early perceptual processing.

Additionally, participants recruited left inferior frontal gyrus, as well as left perirhinal and anterior temporal cortices, to a greater extent for the meaningful RPS compared to the other stimulus conditions (Moses et al., 2009). Activation in left cortical regions has been shown to be involved in the processing of semantic information (Cabeza & Nyberg, 2000; Mummery et al., 2000; Taylor et al., 2006). Interestingly, the maximum differentiation between the meaningful RPS and the other conditions in these left cortical regions occurred at 500–550 ms, which coincides with the observed reduction in left hippocampal activation. This pattern of results suggests that a tradeoff can occur between two memory systems late in the processing stream; one memory system is mediated by the hippocampus and is involved in acquiring memory for novel relations and one memory system is mediated by left cortical regions and is involved in the use of semantic memory (Moses et al., 2009; Ryan and Cohen, 2003, 2004). The dynamic interplay between these two systems allows for semantic memory to be used to perform a relational memory task when stimulus relations are meaningful. Future work can investigate the extent to which alternate brain systems can be invoked to support new learning to allow for compensation in pathological conditions (e.g., Tse et al., 2007). However, such findings demonstrate that MEG can be used to examine the pattern of brain activation within specific regions or networks, such as the hippocampus and frontal cortex, as well as the latency of those activation patterns during the processing stream. This type of dynamic information regarding the temporal tradeoff between hippocampal and frontal brain networks has not been provided by other imaging modalities such as fMRI or EEG.

4.2 MEG provides direct evidence of compensation in pathological conditions

The previous work demonstrates that there is potential for dynamically interacting brain systems to allow for compensation in pathological conditions. As outlined below, numerous MEG studies have examined how neural dynamics are altered in the pathological brain, and how these changes affect cognition. Below, we focus the discussion on studies that have examined memory performance in individuals with compromised hippocampal function.

Using MEG, Hanlon and colleagues found evidence for compensation or functional plasticity in patients who have hippocampal damage or dysfunction (Hanlon et al. 2003).

During performance of the transverse patterning task using abstract pictures or "nonverbal" stimuli, neurologically intact control participants activate their right hippocampus. This is consistent with the idea that the right hippocampus is particularly implicated in nonverbal/visuo-spatial memory (Burgess et al., 2002; Smith and Milner, 1981, 1989) and left in verbal/narrative or episodic memory (Burgess et al., 2002; Frisk and Milner, 1990). Similarly, a patient with left hippocampal sclerosis also showed right hippocampal activation. In contrast, a patient with a right hippocampal lesion showed left hippocampal activation during performance of this nonverbal transverse patterning task (Hanlon et al. 2003). This increased left hippocampal activation found with right hippocampal damage may allow for behavioural compensation for an impaired right hippocampus.

The idea that the left hippocampus allowed for compensation for right hippocampal abnormalities is supported by the findings of Hanlon et al. (2005). They found that patients with schizophrenia were more likely than healthy control participants to show left or bilateral hippocampal activation during performance of a nonverbal transverse patterning task. Importantly, this increased left hippocampal activation in schizophrenia was correlated with higher performance accuracy on the transverse patterning task. In contrast, this relationship was not found in the control participants, who showed predominantly right hippocampal activation. Thus, the patients with schizophrenia who were the most successful at transverse patterning were most likely to show an atypical laterality pattern of hippocampal activation. These findings suggest that the additional recruitment of left hippocampal activation in patients with schizophrenia provided a compensatory mechanism for a dysfunctional right hippocampal system and led to improved behavioural performance.

In order to further investigate this compensation phenomenon, Hanlon and colleagues have recently developed a version of transverse patterning that uses visually presented novel verbal stimuli, or "non-words" (eg. "VULG", "COSE", "RINT") to compare to the novel nonverbal abstract pictures (Hanlon et al., 2011). In healthy control participants, this verbal transverse patterning task activates the left hippocampus to a greater extent than the right (Hanlon et al., 2011), in contrast to the nonverbal transverse patterning task, which, as noted above, activates the right hippocampus to a greater degree than the left (Hanlon et al., 2003, 2005, 2011; Leirer et al., 2010; Mills et al., in review; Moses et al., 2009). This reinforces the notion that the left and right hippocampi process different information modalities, and also allows for the non-invasive evaluation of the functioning of right and left hippocampus separately.

This lateralized hippocampal activation found in control participants was not seen in patients with schizophrenia, who instead showed more bilateral or left hippocampal activation for both the verbal and nonverbal transverse patterning tasks (Hanlon et al., 2011). This result was interpreted as the left hippocampus possibly trying to compensate for a right hippocampal deficit, using a verbal strategy, although inefficiently, and the right hippocampus unable to do the same for the left deficit. In addition to lateralized hippocampal activation, prefrontal cortex activation was observed, consistent with other neuroimaging studies using the transverse patterning task (Meltzer et al., 2008; Moses et al., 2009). This prefrontal cortex activation is not surprising given that the task not only relies on relational memory, but also on working memory for maintaining the distinct relationships. Interestingly, patients and controls showed a lateralized activation difference in the prefrontal cortex. Patients activated the left prefrontal cortex during both the verbal and nonverbal transverse patterning tasks, in contrast to controls who activated the right prefrontal cortex (Hanlon et al., 2011). Thus, patients showed hyperactivation of both prefrontal cortex and hippocampus and prefrontal cortex in the left hemisphere. Overall, this pattern of results suggests that the patients with schizophrenia were recruiting the hippocampus bilaterally in each condition in an attempt to compensate for hippocampal dysfunction.

4.3 MEG studies of the organization of memory development

The work of Hanlon et al. (2003, 2005, 2011) demonstrates that in adults with hippocampal dysfunction, recruitment of the hippocampus bilaterally may support performance for a task that typically elicits unilateral activation. However, it is unclear whether this effect may be found in developmental populations, since children show different laterality patterns than adults. In general, many cognitive operations that are lateralized to one hemisphere in adults have bilateral hemispheric representation in children. For example, the semantic processing of sentences recruits more bilateral activation in children, compared to left lateralized activation in adults (Brauer & Friederici, 2007), and increased activation of left middle temporal gyrus and inferior parietal lobule is found with increasing age throughout childhood (Chou et al., 2006). This suggests that the cortex becomes more lateralized and specialized with development. The neural organization and lateralization patterns of hippocampal-dependent memory in children has not been well characterized.

Recent work has investigated the differences in the organization of hippocampal dependent memory function in children and adults, and how they relate to behavioural performance (Hopf et al., in review). Hopf et al. (in review) discuss previous literature pointing to two different ways in which the relationship between lateralization of hippocampal activation and behaviour may be manifest in children. The first possibility comes from the previously discussed findings of compensatory activation in adults with hippocampal dysfunction (Hanlon et al., 2005). In this work, healthy participants typically showed right hippocampal activation on the nonverbal transverse patterning task, while participants with schizophrenia showed bilateral or left hippocampal activation associated with increases in behavioral performance. Therefore, in adults with hippocampal dysfunction, bilateral hippocampal recruitment may have a compensatory function. Similarly, children may not have a fully developed hippocampal system with unilaterally specialized hemispheres, and, consequently, may recruit the hippocampus bilaterally in order to achieve performance similar to that of adults. Thus, it may be reasonable to predict that, in children, the presence of more bilateral hippocampal activation during the nonverbal transverse patterning task would also lead to improvements in behavioral performance.

However, an alternative prediction is that more right lateralized hippocampal activation during a nonverbal relational memory task (e.g. transverse patterning using visual stimuli) will lead to more accurate performance, as this may be a sign of a more mature and efficient brain. For instance, previous work has shown that children who show more right hemisphere lateralization of activation during navigation show superior performance (Tsujii, Yamammoto, Masuda & Wantabe, 2009). Additionally, language lateralization studies demonstrate that areas of the brain become more specialized with increasing age (Chou et al., 2006; Holland et al., 2001; Ressel et al., 2008; Szaflarski et al., 2006), and that this is associated with superior behavioural performance (Everts et al, 2009; Lebel & Beaulieu, 2009). Therefore, it is also reasonable to predict that children who show a more adult-like pattern of right hippocampal lateralization would show superior performance on a nonverbal relational memory task. These opposing predictions suggest a difference in the manner by which behavioral performance is achieved on a nonverbal transverse patterning task: bilateral, or stronger left hippocampal responses associated with superior performance in children would reflect compensation, whereas right lateralized responses associated with superior performance would reflect neural maturation.

Hopf et al. (in review) investigated these two competing hypotheses regarding the neural correlates of behavioral performance between adults and children (aged 11-17). The findings of Hopf et al. supported the "maturation" account. Across participants of all ages, the presence of stronger right versus left hippocampal activation was correlated with superior nonverbal transverse patterning accuracy. This relationship was strongest later in the processing stream, particularly around 600 ms, suggesting that the difference was not related to perception but rather higher cognitive processes. This relationship between right lateralization and superior performance was the strongest within the youngest group of children, aged 11-14. That is, the more right lateralized the participant's hippocampal activation, the more accurate their performance; and this was particularly true for the younger children or the least mature participants. Importantly, this positive association between right hippocampal lateralization and accuracy (neural maturation) is opposite to that in adults with hippocampal dysfunction, who show a positive relationship between left hippocampal lateralization and accuracy (compensation) (Hanlon et al., 2005).

Thus, the findings of Hopf et al. (in review) lend support to the notion that typically developing children were not recruiting left hippocampus to compensate for an immature organization of the hippocampal system, or at the very least, this contralateral recruitment was ineffective at boosting performance. Rather, these results suggest that the more the activation pattern of a child's brain resembles that of an adult, the more accurate their behavioural performance will be. In other words, superior performance in typical developing children is associated with a more "mature" brain.

5. Conclusions and future directions

This chapter has shown that MEG can be used to examine memory in healthy adults and in special populations, such as individuals with amnesia, individuals with schizophrenia, and children. MEG investigations with healthy adults have provided insights that invite a re-conceptualization of the construct of memory and how it relates to other cognitive faculties. This work suggests that memory is organized in a distributed manner throughout the brain, and that memory interacts closely with other cognitive operations, such as perception. In particular, memory may influence the way we perceive the world around us. In fact, from a neurological standpoint, the cognitive operations of memory and perception may not even be dissociable, since the effects of both faculties are found in multiple distributed regions throughout the brain and are observed at similar points in the processing stream. MEG investigations with special populations reveal how these distributed networks are altered in the face of neural dysfunction, and at what stage of processing cognitive function differs from the norm.

All together, the MEG studies described throughout this chapter demonstrate the utility of this technique in providing mechanistic detail regarding memory processes, the nature of the impairment in disorders that include hippocampal dysfunction, and the nature of the developmental process. MEG provides comprehensive detail regarding the spatiotemporal dynamics of neural activity that cannot be gleaned from the use of any other neuroimaging technique on its own. As a consequence, MEG is a valuable tool for cognitive neuroscientists to understand the underlying mechanisms of human cognition.

6. Acknowledgements

The authors wish to thank Lily Riggs and Rosanna Olsen for commenting on this chapter.

7. References

Alvarado, M.C., Bachvalier, J., 2005a. Selective neurotoxic damage to the hippocampal formation impairs performance of the transverse patterning and location memory tasks in rhesus macaques. Hippocampus 15, 118-131.

Astur RS, Constable RT. (2004) Hippocampal dampening during a relational memory task. Behav Neurosci. 118, 667-75.

Baumgartner, C., Pataraia, E., Lindinger, G., Deecke, L. (2000). Neuromagnetic recordings in temporal lobe epilepsy. Journal of Clinical Neurophysiology, 17, 177-189.

Breier, J.I., Simos, P.G., Zouridakis, G., Papanicolaou, A.C. (1998). Relative timing of neuronal activity in distinct temporal lobe areas during a recognition memory task for words. Journal of Clinical and Experimental Neuropsychology 20, 782-790.

Breier, J.I., Simos, P.G., Zouridakis, G., Papanicolaou, A.C. (1999). Lateralization of cerebral activation in auditory verbal and non-verbal memory tasks using magnetoencephlography. Brain Topography 12, 89-97.

Brauer, J., Friederici, A.D. 2007. Functional neural networks of semantic and syntactic processes in the developing brain. J. Cogn. Neurosci. 19:1609-23.

Burgess N, Maguire EA, O'Keefe J. 2002. The human hippocampus and spatial episodic memory. Neuron 35, 625-41.

Cabeza, R., Nyberg, L., 2000. Imaging cognition II: An empirical review of 275 PET and fMRI studies. Journal of Cognitive Neuroscience 12, 1-47.

Cashdollar N, Malecki U, Rugg-Funn FJ, Duncan JS, Lavie N, Duzel E. (2009). Hippocampus-dependent and –independent theta-networks of active maintenance. PNAS, 106(48), 20493-20498.

Chou, T.-L., Booth, J.R., Bitan, T., Burman, D.D., Bigio, J.D., Cone, N.E., Cao, F. 2006. Developmental and skill effects on the neural correlates of semantic processing to visually presented words. Hum. Brain Mapp., 27:915-24.

Cohen NJ, Eichenbaum H. 1993. Memory, amnesia, and the hippocampal system. Massachusetts: MIT Press.

Cohen NJ, Squire LR. 1980. Preserved learning and retention of pattern-analyzing skill in amnesia: dissociation of knowing how and knowing that. Science 210, 207–210.

Cohen NJ, Ryan J, Hunt C, Romine L, Wszalek T, Nash C. 1999. Hippocampal system and declarative (relational) memory: summarizing the data from functional neuroimaging studies. Hippocampus 9, 83–98.

Donaldson DI, Rugg MD. (1998) Recognition memory for new associations: Electrophysiological evidence for the role of recollection. 36, 377-95.

Donaldson DI, Rugg MD. (1999) Event-related potential studies of associative recognition and recall: electrophysiological evidence for context dependent retrieval processes. Brain Res Cogn Brain Res. 8, 1-16.

Driscoll, I., Hamilton, D.A., Petropoulos, H., Yeo, R.A., Brooks, W.M., Baumgartner, R.N., Sutherland, R.J., 2003. The aging hippocampus: Cognitive, biochemical and structural findings. Cerebral Cortex 13, 1344–51.

Driscoll, I., Howard, S.R., Prusky, G.T., Rudy, J.W., Sutherland, R.J., 2005. Seahorse wins all races: Hippocampus participates in both linear and non-linear visual discrimination learning. Behavioral Brain Research 164, 29–35.

Duvernoy, H.M. (1988). The human hippocampus. An atlas of applied anatomy. JF Bergmann, Munich.

Everts R, Harvey AS, Lillywhite L, Wrennall J, Abbott DF, Gonzalez L, Kean M, Jackson GD, Aderson V. (2010) Epilepsia 51, 627-38.

Frisk V, Milner B. 1990. The role of the left hippocampus in the acquisition and retention of story content. Neuropsychologia 28, 349-59.

Guderian S, Duzel, E. (2005). Induced theta oscillations mediate large scale synchrony with mediotemporal areas during recollection in humans. Hippocampus, 15, 901-912.

Guderian S, Schott BH, Richardson-Klavehn A, Duzel E. (2009). Medial temporal theta state before an event predicts episodic encoding success in humans. PNAS, 106(13): 5365-5370.

Hämäläinen, M., Hari, R., Ilmoniemi, R.J., Knuutila, J., & Lounasmaa, O.V. (1993). Magnetoencephalography - Theory, instrumentation, and applications to noninvasive studies of the working human brain. Review, Modern Physician, 65, 413-496.

Hanlon, F.M., Weisend, M.P., Huang, M., Lee, R.R., Moses, S.N., Paulson, K.M., Thoma, R.J., Miller, G.A., Cañive, J.M., 2003. A non-invasive method for observing hippocampal function. Neuroreport 14, 1957-60.

Hanlon, F.M., Houck, J.M., Pyeatt, C.J., Lundy, S.L., Euler, M.J., Weisend, M.P., Thoma, R.J., Bustillo, J.R., Miller, G.A., Tesche, C.D. 2011. Bilateral hippocampal dysfunction in schizophrenia, NeuroImage, doi:10.1016/j.neuroimage.2011.06.091

Hanlon, F.M., Weisend, M.P., Yeo, R.A., Huang, M., Lee, R.R., Thoma, R.J., Moses, S.N., Paulson, K.M., Petropoulos, H., Miller, G.A., Cañive, J.M., 2005. A specific test of hippocampal deficit in schizophrenia. Behavioral Neuroscience 119, 863–75.

Hillebrand A, Barnes GR. (2002) A quantitative assessment of the sensitivity of whole-head MEG to activity in the adult human cortex. Neuroimage. 16, 638-50.

Holland, SK, Plante, E, Weber Byars, A, Strawsburg, RH, Schmithorst, VJ, Ball, W S. (2001). Normal fMRI brain activation patterns in children performing a verb generation task. NeuroImage, 14(4), 837-843.

Hopf L, Quraan M, Cheung M, Lalancette M, Farrari P, Taylor MJ, Moses SN. (in review) A magnetoencephelographic investigation of hippocampal lateralization and memory in children and adults.

Itier RJ, Latinus M, Taylor MJ. (2006) Face, eye and object early processing: what is the face specificity? Neuroimage. 29, 667-76.

Ioannides, A.A., Liu, M.J., Liu, L.C., Bamidis, P.D., Hellstrand, E., Stephan, K.M. (1995). Magnetic field tomography of cortical and deep processes: Examples of "real time mapping" of averaged and single trial MEG signals. International Journal of Psychophysiology 20, 161-175.

Kapur S, Craik FI, Jones C, Brown GM, Houle S, Tulving E. (1995) Functional role of the prefrontal cortex in retrieval of memories: a PET study. Neuroreport 6, 1880-4.

Kirsch, P., Achenbach, C., Kirsch, M., Heinzmann, M., Schienle, A., Vaitl, D. (2003). Cerebellar and hippocampal actiation during eyeblink conditioning depends on the experimental paradigm: A MEG study. Neural Plasticity 10, 291-301.

Kirchhoff BA, Wagner AD, Maril A, Stern CE. (2000) Prefrontal-temporal circuitry for episodic encoding and subsequent memory. J Neurosci. 20, 6173-80.

Lebel C, Beaulieu C. 2009. Lateralization of the arcuate faciculus fron childhood to adulthood and its relation to cognitive abilities in children. Human Brain Mapping 30, 3563-73.

Leirer VM, Wienbruch C, Paul-Jordanov I, Kolassa S, Elbert T, Kolassa I. (2010). Hippocampal activity during the transverse patterning task declines with cognitive competence but not with age. BMC Neuroscience 2010 11:113.

Martin, T., McDaniel, M.A., Guynn, M.J., Houck, J.M., Woodruff, C.C., Bish, J.P., Moses, S.N., Kicić, D., Tesche, C.D. (2007). Brain regions and their dynamics in prospective memory retrieval: a MEG study. International Journal of Psychophysiology 64, 247-258.

McIntosh AR. Coding and representation: The importance of mesoscale dynamics. In: Roediger HL, Yadin D, Fitzpatric SM, eds. Science of Memory: Concepts. New York: Oxford; 2007:59-64.

Meltzer, J.A., Negishi, M., Constable, R.T., 2008. Biphasic hemodynamic responses influence deactivation and may mask activation in block-design fMRI paradigms. Hum. Brain Mapp. 4, 385–399.

Mikuni, N., Nagamine, T., Ikeda, A., Terada, K., Taki, W., Kimura, J., Kikuchi, H., Shibasaki, H. (1997). Simultaneous recording of epileptiform discharges by MEG and subdural electrodes in temporal lobe epilepsy. NeuroImage, 5, 298-306.

Mill T, Lalancette M, Moses SN, Taylor MJ, Quraan MA. (In review) Techniques for detection and localization of weak hippocampal and frontal sources using beamformers in MEG.

Moscovitch, M., Rosenbaum, R.S., Gilboa, A., Addis, D.R., Westmacott, R., Grady, C., McAndrews, MP., Levine, B., Black S., Winocur, G., Nadel, L. (2005). Functional neuroanatomy of remote episodic, semantic and spatial memory: a unified account based on multiple trace theory. Journal of Anatomy, 207(1):35-66.

Moses, S.N., Bardouille, T., Brown, T.M., Ross, B., McIntosh, A.R. (2010) Learning related activation of somatosensory cortex by an auditory stimulus recorded with magnetoencephalography. NeuroImage 53, 275-82.

Moses, S.N., Houck, J.M., Martin, T., Hanlon, F.M., Ryan, J.D., Thoma, R.J., Weisend, M.P., Jackson, E.M., Pekkonen, E., Tesche, C.D. (2007) Dynamic human neural activity recorded from amygdala using magnetoencephalography. Brain Research Bulletin. 7, 452-60.

Moses, S.N., Martin, T., Houck, J.M., Ilmoniemi, R., Tesche, C.D. (2005) The C50m response: conditioned magnetocerebral activity recorded from the human brain. NeuroImage 27, 778-88.

Moses, S.N., Ostreicher, M.L., Rosenbaum, R.S., Ryan, J.D., 2008. Successful transverse patterning in amnesia using semantic knowledge. Hippocampus 18, 121-4.

Moses, S.N., Ryan, J.D. 2006. A comparison and evaluation of the predictions of relational and conjunctive accounts of hippocampal function. Hippocampus 16, 43-65.

Moses, S.N., Ryan, J.D., Bardouille, T., Kovacevic, N., Hanlon, F.M., McIntosh, A.R., 2009. Semantic information alters neural activation during transverse patterning performance. NeuroImage 46, 863–873.

Mummery, C.J., Patterson, K., Price, C.J., Ashburner, J., Frackowiak, R.S., Hodges, J.R. (2000). A voxel-based morphometry study of semantic dementia: Relationship between temporal lobe atrophy and semantic memory. Annuls of Neurology 47, 36-45.

Ostreicher, M.L., Moses, S.N., Rosenbaum, R.S., Ryan, J.D. (2010) Remediation of age-related deficits in relational memory. Journal of Gerontology: Psychological Sciences. 65B, 32-41.

Nishitani, N., Ikeda, A., Nagamine, T., Honda, M., Mikuni, N., Taki, W., Kimura, J., Shibasaki, H. (1999). The role of the hippocampus in auditory processing studied by event-related electric potentials and magnetic fields in epilepsy patients before and after temporal lobectomy. Brain 122, 687-707.

Nyberg, L., Habib, R., McIntosh, A. R., & Tulving, E. (2000). Reactivation of encoding-related brain activity during memory retrieval. Proceedings of the National Academy of Sciences, 97, 1120–1124.

Papanicolaou AC, Simos PG, Castillo EM, Breier JI, Katz JS, Wright AA. (2002) The hippocampus and memory of verbal and pictorial material. Learn Mem 9, 99-104.

Quraan MA, Moses SN, Hung Y, Mills T, Taylor MJ. (2011) Detection and localization of hippocampal activity using beamformers with MEG: a detailed investigation using simulations and empirical data. Hum Brain Mapp, 32, 812-27.

Reed, J.M., Squire, L.R., 1996. Impaired transverse patterning in human amnesia is a special case of impaired memory for two-choice discrimination tasks. Behavioral Neuroscience 113, 3-9.

Ressel V, Wilke M, Lidzba K, Lutzenberger W, Krägeloh-Mann I. (2008) Increases in language lateralization in normal children as observed using magnetoencephalography. Brain Lang. 106, 167-76.

Rickard, T.C., Grafman, J., 1998. Losing their configural mind: Amnesic patients fail on transverse patterning. Journal of Cognitive Neuroscience 10, 509–16.

Rickard, T.C., Verfaellie, M., Grafman, J., 2006. Transverse patterning and human amnesia. Journal of Cognitive Neuroscience 18, 1723–33.

Riggs, L., Moses, S.N., Bardouille, T., Herdman, A.T., Ross, B., Ryan, J.D., 2008. A complementary analytic approach to examining medial temporal lobe sources using magnetoencephalography. NeuroImage 45, 627-42.

Rosenbaum RS, Moscovitch M, Foster JK, Schnyer DM, Gao F, Kovacevic N, Verfaellie M, Black SE, Levine B. 2008. Patterns of autobiographical memory loss in medial-temporal lobe amnesic patients. J Cogn Neurosci. 20, 1490-506.

Rowland LM, Griego JA, Spieker EA, Cortes CR, Holcomb HH. (2010) Neural changes associated with relational learning in schizophrenia. Schizophr Bull. 36, 496-503.

Ryan, J.D., Cohen, N.J., 2003. The contribution of long-term memory and the role of frontal-lobe systems in on-line processing. Behavioral and Brain Sciences 26, 756.

Ryan, J.D., Cohen, N.J., 2004. The nature of change detection and on-line representations of scenes. Journal of Experimental Psychology: Human Perception and Performance 30, 988-1015.

Ryan, J.D., Moses, S.N., Ostreicher, M.L., Bardouille, T., Herdman, A.T., Riggs, L., Tulving, E. (2008) Seeing sounds and hearing sights: The influence of prior learning on current perception. Journal of Cognitive Neuroscience. 20, 1030-42.

Saksida, L.M., Busey, T.J., Buckmaster, C.A., Murray, E.A., 2007. Impairment and facilitation of transverse patterning after lesions of the perirhinal cortex and hippocampus, respectively. Cerebral Cortex 17, 108-15.

Schacter DL, Reiman E, Uecker A, Polster MR, Yun LS, Cooper LA. (1995) Brain regions associated with retrieval of structurally coherent visual information. Nature. 376, 587-90.

Schweinberger SR, Pickering EC, Jentzsch I, Burton AM, Kaufmann JM. (2002) Event-related brain potential evidence for a response of inferior temporal cortex to familiar face repetitions. Brain Res Cogn Brain Res. 14, 398-409.

Scoville WB, Milner B. 1957. Loss of recent memory after bilateral hippocampal lesions. J. Neurol. Neurosurg. Psychiat. 20, 11-21.

Squire LR. (1992) Memory and the hippocampus: a synthesis from findings with rats, monkeys, and humans. Psychol Rev. 99, 195-231.

Stark CE, Okado Y. (2003) Making memories without trying: medial temporal lobe activity associated with incidental memory formation during recognition. J Neurosci. 23, 6748-53.

Stephen, J.M., Ranken, D.M., Aine, C.J., Weisend, M.P., Shih, J.J. (2005) Differentiability of simulated MEG hippocampal, medial temporal and neocortical temporal epileptic spike activity. Journal of Clinical Neurophysiology 22, 388-401.

Rudy JW, Sutherland RJ. (1989) The hippocampal formation is necessary for rats to learn and remember configural discriminations. Behav Brain Res 34, 97-109.

Szaflarski, JP, Holland, SK, Schmithorst, VJ, Byars, AW. (2006), fMRI study of language lateralization in children and adults. Human Brain Mapping, 27: 202–212.

Taylor, K.I., Moss, H.E., Stamatakis, E.A., Tyler, L.K., 2006. Binding crossmodal object features in perirhinal cortex. Proceeding of the National Academy of Sciences U.S.A. 21, 8239-44.

Tesche, C.D. (1997). Non-invasive detection of ongoing neuronal population in normal human hippocampus. Brain Research, 749, 53-60.

Tesche, C.D., & Karhu, J. (1999). Interactive processing of sensory input and motor input in the human hippocampus. Journal of Cognitive Neuroscience 11, 424-436.

Tesche, C.D., & Karhu, J. (2000). Theta oscillations index human hippocampal activation during a working memory task. Proceedings of the National Academy of Sciences, U.S.A. 97, 919-924.

Tesche, C.D., Karhu, J., Tissari, S.O. (1996). Non-invasive detection of neuronal population activity in human hippocampus. Cognitive brain research 4, 39-47.

Tse D , Langston RF, Kakeyama M, Bethus I, Spooner PA, Wood ER. (2007). Schemas and memory consolidation. Science, 316, 76 – 82.

Tsujii T, Yamamto E, Masuda S, Watanabe S. 2009. Longitudinal study of spatial working memory development in young children. NeuroReport 20, 759-63.

Tulving E. 1972. Episodic and semantic memory. In: Tulving E, Donaldson W, editors. Organization of memory. San Diego, CA: Academic Press. p. 381–403.

Weis S, Specht K, Klaver P, Tendolkar I, Willmes K, Ruhlmann J, Elger CE, Fernández G. (2004) Process dissociation between contextual retrieval and item recognition. Neuroreport 15, 2729-33.

Wheeler ME, Petersen SE, & Buckner RL. (2000). Memory's echo: Vivid remembering reactivates sensory-specific cortex. Proceedings of the National Academy of Sciences, 97, 1125–1129.

Yeckel, M.F., Berger, T.W. (1990). Feedforward excitation of the hippocampus by afferents from the entorhinal cortex: redefinition of the role of the trisynaptic pathway. Proceedings of the National Academy of Sciences, U.S.A., 87, 5832-5836.

Part 2

Current State of the Art: Addressing the Inverse Problem

4

Characterization of Brain Dynamics Using Beamformer Techniques: Advantages and Limitations

Maher A. Quraan
Krembil Neuroscience Centre & Toronto Western Research Institute, University Health Network, Toronto, Ontario Canada

1. Introduction

The objective of biomagnetic neuroimaging is to characterize the spatiotemporal distribution of electrical activity within the human brain by measuring the magnetic field outside the head. Magnetoencephalography (MEG) provides such a tool where measurements are performed non-invasively at numerous locations surrounding the head. The high sensitivity of Superconducting Quantum Interference Devices (SQUID) utilized by current MEG systems combined with advanced hardware and software noise cancellation techniques allow the detection of minute magnetic fields generated by electrical neural activity with good accuracy. The ability to directly observe the neuronal fields allows MEG to have millisecond time resolution, orders of magnitude higher than the time resolution of fMRI and PET. While the electrical signals measured by electroencephalography (EEG) are strongly influenced by inhomogeneities in the head, the magnetic fields measured by MEG are produced mainly by current flow in the relatively homogenous intracranial space, permitting more accurate spatial localization (Hamalainen et al. 1993).

Although electromagnetic fields are fully described by Maxwell's equations, the problem of obtaining the spatiotemporal distributions of the neural current generators from MEG data (referred to as the inverse problem) poses a challenge since it is inherently ill-defined (Hamalainen et al., 1993). Since the neural current generators lie within the human head, a conducting medium, it is not possible to develop a mathematical model that provides a unique solution. Instead, several methods with different assumptions have been developed, each of which has its own advantages and limitations (Pascarella et al., 2010; Sekihara and Nagarajan, 2008; Wipf and Nagarajan, 2009).

Generally, inverse models in MEG can be separated into two classes: parametric models and imaging models. Parametric models are global solutions that attempt to account for the measured fields in their entirety in terms of a small number of sources. The most popular model in this class is the equivalent current dipole model (ECD), where non-linear least-square fits are used to estimate the parameters of the current dipoles requiring the number of sources to be known *a priori*, and are not easily able to reconstruct spatially distributed or extended sources. More advanced techniques have been developed in this class such as multipole models that allow for modeling extended sources (Jerbi et al., 2002), as well as techniques that allow better estimates of source parameters such as those that employ simulated annealing and genetic algorithms (Uutela et al., 1998).

The most popular imaging models are local linear estimators (Greenblatt et al., 2005) that estimate the source activity at points of interest, treating each point as being independent of any other location, as opposed to finding a global solution. This class of solutions attempts to minimize contributions from all other source locations to estimates of source activity at the point of interest, and hence is often referred to as a spatial filter. Spatial filtering approaches can also be used to produce volumetric images of brain activity by choosing a region of interest divided uniformly into voxels often spanning the entire brain. A source is assumed at each voxel and a spatial filter is used to estimate its strength. Two classes of spatial filters are typically used: adaptive and non-adaptive. Non-adaptive spatial filters rely on the forward solution in their formulation of the inverse problem in a manner completely independent of the measurement, while adaptive spatial filters rely on both the forward solution and the field measurements. The popular minimum-norm solution (Hamalainen et al., 1993) as well as the more recent sLORETA (Pascual-Marqui, 2002) can be formulated as a non-adaptive spatial filter, and are therefore examples of this class (Sekihara, 2008).

In this chapter we will focus on one localization modality, the adaptive spatial filter or beamformer. Beamformers come in various forms, each with its own set of advantages and disadvantages in terms of location bias and resolution. The most widely used, the minimum-variance (MV) beamformer, was originally developed in the field of sonar and radar signal processing (Borgiotti and Kaplan, 1979) and later adapted to the bioelectromagnetic inverse problem (Robinson and Rose, 1992; Van Veen et al., 1997). The unit-gain constrained MV beamformer has been shown to be biased with artefacts near the center, while the lead-field constrained and the unit-noise-gain constrained MV beamformer have been shown to be unbiased even in the presence of random noise (Greenblatt et al., 2005; Sekihara et al., 2005). In addition, MV adaptive spatial filters generally attain much higher resolution than non-adaptive spatial filters, with the unit-noise-gain MV beamformer having the highest resolution. In this chapter we will present the formalism for these different kinds of beamformers in their scalar form, then develop the formalism for a vector beamformer (Sekihara et al., 2001, Quraan and Cheyne 2010) and an eigenstate-projected vector beamformer (Sekihara et al., 2001). We will discuss the advantage of the vector beamformer and present a comparison of the scalar and vector beamformers.

Despite their advantages in terms of spatial resolution and localization accuracy, the performance of beamformers is seriously degraded in the presence of sources with high temporal correlations. This has been demonstrated for neural sources that are known to be highly correlated, such as bilateral activation of the temporal lobes during steady-state auditory stimulation (Brookes et al., 2007; Dalal et al., 2006; Popescu et al., 2008; Quraan and Cheyne, 2008; Quraan and Cheyne, 2010), and for primary visual sources (Quraan and Cheyne, 2008; Quraan and Cheyne, 2010), and is likely the case for many other sources as most brain modules are organized with bilateral symmetry. The beamformer's susceptibility to temporally correlated sources limits the beamformer's ability to accurately localize such sources, and results in significant attenuation of the source magnitude and, hence, a poor reconstruction of the time courses. In addition, interactions between correlated sources can result in spurious activation patterns. For example, it has been shown that auditory sources result in broad activation patterns in the mid sagittal plane (Van Veen, 1997; Quraan and Cheyne, 2008; Quraan and Cheyne, 2010).

Another major limitation of beamforming algorithms is their inability to spatially filter out strong sources from outside the region of interest, a phenomenon often referred to as *leakage* (Reddy 1987). This presents a major challenge when attempting to detect and accurately localize weak sources in the presence of dominant sources, hindering the ability to study higher order cognitive processes. For example, activations related to memory and inhibition and originating in the hippocampi and frontal lobes are often activated by primary sensory inputs which evoke brain activity that is often an order of magnitude higher than the secondary cognitive processes.

2. Theory

2.1 The scalar beamformer

Beamformers are based on the concept of spatial filtering, where the aim is to pass the signal from the location of interest while blocking signals from all other locations. To achieve this, a weight vector, $w(r)$, is applied to the measurement vector to create a weighted sum representing an estimate of source activity from the desired location, $\boldsymbol{r}$. A functional image, therefore, requires N such weight vectors, where N is the number of brain locations (voxels) in the image. For a brain location of interest, $\boldsymbol{r}$, the source activity at time t is the output of the spatial filter and is given by

$$s(\boldsymbol{r},t) = \boldsymbol{w}^T(\boldsymbol{r})\boldsymbol{b}(t), \tag{1}$$

where $\boldsymbol{b}(t)$ is the measurement vector given by

$$\boldsymbol{b}(t) = \left[b_1(t), b_2(t), b_3(t), \ldots, b_M(t)\right]^T \tag{2}$$

for an MEG system with M sensors. Here we follow the convention that plain italics indicate scalars, boldface lower-case letters represent vectors, while boldface upper-case letters represent matrices.

Defining a lead field vector, $\boldsymbol{l}(\boldsymbol{r})$, as the output of the sensor array corresponding to a source of unit moment at location $\boldsymbol{r}$, the desired effect of passing signals from location $\boldsymbol{r}_p$ while blocking signals from other locations requires that

$$\boldsymbol{w}^T(\boldsymbol{r}_p)\boldsymbol{l}(\boldsymbol{r}_q) = 0, \tag{3}$$

where $\boldsymbol{r}_\text{p}$ and $\boldsymbol{r}_\text{q}$ represent any two distinct locations, and where for simplicity we assume that a fixed source direction at each location has been determined. We return to this topic below where we discuss source orientation.

In reality it is impossible to satisfy (3) and fully attenuate all sources outside the spatial location of interest. The exercise of designing an optimum spatial filter, therefore, amounts to minimizing the contribution from sources outside the location of interest. This is achieved either through a MV or least-mean-squares technique, and in all cases the solution to this problem takes the form (Reddy, et al. 1987)

$$w_{opt}(r) = \gamma R^{-1} l(r), \quad (4)$$

where γ is a scalar whose value depends on the details of the method used, and $\boldsymbol{R}$ is the second-order moment matrix about the mean (often referred to as the covariance matrix) given by

$$R = \left\langle b(t) b^T(t) \right\rangle, \quad (5)$$

where $\langle * \rangle$ indicates the expectation value.

2.1.1 Beamformer constraints

The MV based beamformers find a set of weights, *w(r)*, which minimize the variance at the filter output,

$$\min_w w^T(r) R w(r), \quad (6)$$

subject to a constraint; the choice of this constraint determines the beamformer properties in terms of location bias, resolution, and the presence of artefacts. One popular choice is the unit-gain (UG) constraint, where the signal from the location of interest, r_p, is required to satisfy

$$w_{UG}^T(r_p) l(r_p) = 1, \quad (7)$$

in order to preserve the source magnitude. While this choice yields a good image resolution, it can be shown to be biased, and can result in strong artefacts near the centre. The constraint

$$w_{LF}^T(r_p) l(r_p) = \| l(r) \|, \quad (8)$$

on the other hand, results in the same high resolution and can be shown to be unbiased with no artefacts near the centre (Sekihara, et al. 2005), although it applies a variable gain to the source amplitude depending on its location. This type of beamformer is often referred to as a lead-field (LF) constrained or array-gain constrained. A third type of beamformer, the unit-noise-gain (UNG) beamformer imposes a constraint on the gain such that the weights satisfy

$$w_{UNG}^T(r_p) w_{UNG}(r_p) = 1, \quad (9)$$

and results in no localization bias, and significantly higher resolution than the other two constraints above.

The bias of the unit-gain constrained beamformer has been corrected in the literature by dividing the source power by the noise power (Van Veen, et al. 1997), resulting in a quantity described in units of pseudo-z scores (Robinson and Vrba 1999). In the presence of uncorrelated random noise that is identical across all channels this modification is equivalent to normalizing the weights so that

$$w_{PZ} = \frac{w_x}{\sigma_N \left[w_x^T w_x \right]^{1/2}}, \quad (10)$$

where σ_N^2 is the noise variance, and w_x represents either w_{UG}, w_{LF}, or w_{UNG}. It is worth noting that this normalization makes the unit-gain beamformer or the lead-field normalized beamformer equivalent to the unit-gain-noise constrained beamformer in terms of resolution and localization accuracy since

$$\boldsymbol{w}_{UNG} = \frac{\boldsymbol{w}_x}{\left[\boldsymbol{w}_x^T \boldsymbol{w}_x\right]^{1/2}}. \tag{11}$$

In terms of constraints, this means that the normalization in (11) effectively removes the constraint in (7) (or (8)) and replaces it with the condition in (9). The performance of any adaptive spatial filter also depends on the parameters affecting the accuracy of the covariance matrix such as the frequency bandwidth and the integration time. For a detailed assessment of these parameters on the beamformer performance we refer the interested reader to the recent publication by Brookes et al. (2008).
The solution to the optimization problem in (6) can be achieved using the method of Lagrange multipliers which determines γ in (4) to be

$$\gamma_{UG} = \left[\boldsymbol{l}^T(\boldsymbol{r})\boldsymbol{R}^{-1}\boldsymbol{l}(\boldsymbol{r})\right]^{-1}, \tag{12}$$

For the unit-gain constrained beamformer. The solution with the lead-field constrained beamformer has the same format with $\boldsymbol{l}(\boldsymbol{r})$ replaced by $\boldsymbol{l}'(\boldsymbol{r})$ in (4), where

$$\boldsymbol{l}'(\boldsymbol{r}) = \frac{\boldsymbol{l}(\boldsymbol{r})}{\left\|\boldsymbol{l}(\boldsymbol{r})\right\|}. \tag{13}$$

The unit-noise-gain constrained beamformer gives

$$\gamma_{UNG} = \left[\boldsymbol{l}^T(\boldsymbol{r})\boldsymbol{R}^{-2}\boldsymbol{l}(\boldsymbol{r})\right]^{-1/2}. \tag{14}$$

2.2 The vector beamformer

The formalism presented so far assumes the source direction to be known, and hence applies to a scalar beamformer for which the source direction is determined by a separate procedure. The techniques usually employed to calculate the source direction, however, integrate over a wide time range often involving hundreds of milliseconds. Since sources are typically active over a short range, this results in averaging over significant amounts of noise (instrumental noise, brain noise, leakage) which may or may not be isotropic. This issue becomes particularly significant for small SNR sources. In addition, by integrating over a wide time range one assumes that only one source with a constant orientation is active at a given voxel over the entire time range. Using a vector beamformer one can avoid such assumptions and biases by calculating the three components of the weight vector in order to track the three components of the source activity vector. However, since radial components of source activity inside a conducting sphere are not detectable outside the sphere, in cases where the head model is assumed to be spherical, one can switch to spherical coordinates and track the tangential (θ and ϕ) components only. In this case the weights, source activity, and forward solution are given by

$$\boldsymbol{W}(\boldsymbol{r}) = \left[\boldsymbol{w}_{\vartheta}(\boldsymbol{r}), \boldsymbol{w}_{\varphi}(\boldsymbol{r}) \right], \tag{15}$$

$$s(\boldsymbol{r},t) = \left[s_{\vartheta}(\boldsymbol{r},t), s_{\varphi}(\boldsymbol{r},t) \right], \tag{16}$$

and

$$\boldsymbol{L}(\boldsymbol{r}) = \left[\boldsymbol{l}_{\vartheta}(\boldsymbol{r}), \boldsymbol{l}_{\varphi}(\boldsymbol{r}) \right], \tag{17}$$

respectively. The minimization in (6) and its constraint (7) now become

$$\min_{\boldsymbol{w}_{\vartheta}} \boldsymbol{w}_{\vartheta}^{T}(\boldsymbol{r}) \boldsymbol{R} \boldsymbol{w}_{\vartheta}(\boldsymbol{r}) \text{ subject to: } \boldsymbol{w}_{\vartheta}^{T}(\boldsymbol{r}) \boldsymbol{l}_{\vartheta}(\boldsymbol{r}) = 1 \;\&\; \boldsymbol{w}_{\vartheta}^{T}(\boldsymbol{r}) \boldsymbol{l}_{\varphi}(\boldsymbol{r}) = 0, \tag{18}$$

and

$$\min_{\boldsymbol{w}_{\varphi}} \boldsymbol{w}_{\varphi}^{T}(\boldsymbol{r}) \boldsymbol{R} \boldsymbol{w}_{\varphi}(\boldsymbol{r}) \text{ subject to: } \boldsymbol{w}_{\varphi}^{T}(\boldsymbol{r}) \boldsymbol{l}_{\varphi}(\boldsymbol{r}) = 1 \;\&\; \boldsymbol{w}_{\varphi}^{T}(\boldsymbol{r}) \boldsymbol{l}_{\vartheta}(\boldsymbol{r}) = 0, \tag{19}$$

yielding the solution

$$\boldsymbol{W}(\boldsymbol{r}) = \boldsymbol{R}^{-1} \boldsymbol{L}(\boldsymbol{r}) \left[\boldsymbol{L}^{T}(\boldsymbol{r}) \boldsymbol{R}^{-1} \boldsymbol{L}(\boldsymbol{r}) \right]^{-1}. \tag{20}$$

Following the approach of Sekihara et al. (2001) the metric

$$s(\boldsymbol{r},t) = \sqrt{s_{\vartheta}^{2}(\boldsymbol{r},t) + s_{\varphi}^{2}(\boldsymbol{r},t)} \tag{21}$$

can be used to construct the functional images.

2.3 The spatiotemporal (event-related) beamformer

For a spatiotemporal or "event-related" beamformer (Sekihara 2001, Robinson 2004) the source activity at a given instant in time can be calculated using (1) for each of the two orthogonal directions, where $\boldsymbol{b}(t)$ is the trial-averaged MEG data. The covariance matrix (eq. 5) on the other hand can be computed by either summing over the single trial data, or by averaging the data first (i.e. b(t) in (5) would correspond to the epoch averaged data). However, since data averaging reduces random noise, some of the eigenvalues of the covariance matrix may approach zero, resulting in an ill-conditioned matrix. In situations where the data are very clean (e.g., a large number of epochs are averaged), the number of non-zero eigenvalues of the covariance matrix can become lower than the matrix dimension (i.e, the number of sensors) and this matrix becomes singular and, hence, non-invertible. A common remedy for this is to apply a method known in signal processing theory as diagonal loading, which amounts to adding $\varepsilon\boldsymbol{I}$ to the covariance matrix $\boldsymbol{R}$, where ε is the loading factor, and $\boldsymbol{I}$ is the identity matrix (Carlson, 1988). This technique is also referred to as Tikhonov regularization in linear algebra (Tikhonov, 1963), and is used to improve the condition of an ill-conditioned matrix. Intuitively, diagonal loading amounts to adding random Gaussian noise to the original data, which when forming the covariance matrix appears as a constant value added to the diagonal elements. As such, covariance matrix regularization mainly impacts spatial resolution. Gaussian noise with a standard deviation of 3 to 5 ft/√Hz is typically sufficient to remedy this problem without having a significant impact on spatial resolution.

2.4 Computation of source orientation

Scalar beamformers rely on a determination of the source orientation to construct the component of source activity in what it deems to be the optimal direction. The source orientation is typically determined either through a grid-search aimed at maximizing source power in each voxel (Robinson and Vrba 1999), or through an eigendecompositon of the source power, where the largest eigenvalue is identified as the one corresponding to the source originating from that voxel (Sekihara, et al. 2001). The eigendecomposition method is essentially equivalent to the grid-search method, but achieves the purpose in a more computationally efficient fashion. In both methods, however, the power is calculated over a wide time range, typically spanning hundreds of milliseconds. Furthermore, the assumption is made that all activity determined by the beamformer to originate from a given voxel is indeed generated by brain sources originating at that location. For cases where the source of interest is weak and in the presence of other strong sources that result in strong leakage into the region of interest, this assumption fails. In other words, in such cases, most of the activity in the region of interest over a long time range results from leakage from strong sources outside the region of interest, and hence, the determination of the source orientation using either of these methods is subject to significant errors. The scalar beamformer, therefore, ends up constructing the component of the source activity in a direction different from that of the source of interest and dismissing what might be a significant component of the source of interest. The vector beamformer, on the other hand, constructs the source activity in the two tangential directions, dismissing only the radial component which is typically small. In many applications of the scalar beamformer, however, the source of interest is the dominant one, and the effect of leakage is small (in the absence of strong external noise artefacts). In this case an accurate determination of the source angle can be achieved, and the construction of the source activity component in only this direction is justified. However, constructing source activity of both tangential components even in such cases guards against dismissing unexpected components, and provides verification that the source orientation was properly computed.

Figure 1 shows a performance comparison of the scalar and vector beamformers in localizing simulated hippocampal sources folded in with real visual data (Quraan et al. 2010c, Quraan et al. 2011). For the vector beamformer, the averaged localization error increases from ~15 mm at 40 nAm to ~18 mm at 20 nAm, while the scalar beamformer results in an averaged localization error of ~18 mm at 40 nAm, increasing to ~27 mm at 20 nAm. Figure 1 (right) shows the number of failures for both the vector and scalar beamformers as a function of simulated source strength, where a failure is defined to be a case where the localization error exceeds 20 mm. At 40 nAm the vector beamformer fails 20% of the time, while the scalar fails 40% of the time. While the failure rate of the vector beamformer remains relatively unchanged as the simulated source strength is reduced to 20 nAm (~20%), the scalar beamformer fails 47% of the time at 30 nAm and 60% of the time at 20 nAm. As the source strength is further reduced, the signal strength drops well below the background noise level, and both beamformers fail equally at identifying and properly localizing the sources.

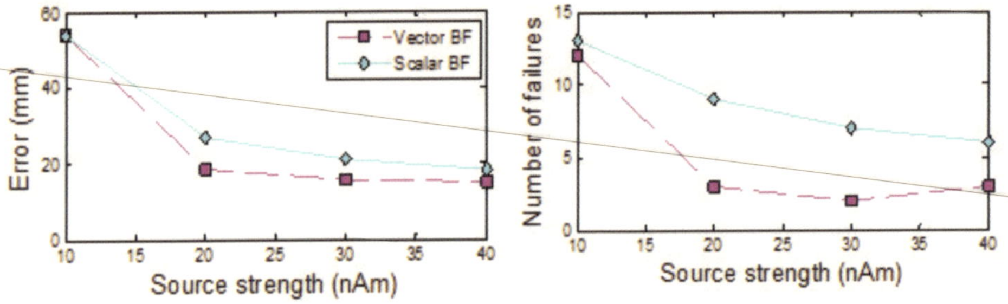

Fig. 1. (left) Beamformer localization error averaged over 15 subjects for hippocampal sources simulated at various source strengths (as indicated on the figure) then added to individual-subject VEF data at a latency far from the active region (800 ms – 830 ms). Scalar and vector beamformers were used to perform the localization as indicated on the plot. (right) Number of localization failures for the same where a localization failure is defined as a distance error exceeding 20 mm

2.5 Computation of head model

The magnetic fields measured by MEG are produced mainly by current flow in the relatively homogenous intracranial space, and are not significantly affected by the poor conductivity of the scalp. The performance of the inverse solution, however, depends on assumptions regarding the head shape. For example, when a spherical approximation of the head shape is used, a radial source component relative to this sphere will yield a null value outside the head (Sarvas 1988). Since the human head deviates significantly from a sphere, in reality, spherical approximations present a source of error, the magnitude of which is highly dependent on the source location and orientation. The use of boundary element models (BEM) and finite element models (FEM) provides a significant improvement. In such cases a 3D vector beamformer can be used instead of the 2D beamformer discussed above.

3. Temporal correlations

3.1 Effects of temporal correlations on the performance of the beamformer

To demonstrate the effect of temporal correlations on the performance of the beamformer, we simulate two sources in the auditory cortex, one in the right and one in the left temporal lobe. Figure 2a shows the images resulting from this analysis when the sources are uncorrelated, superimposed on a subject's MRI. The simulated positions of both sources were recovered to within the scanning resolution (0.25 cm) of the beamformer. Also shown in Figure 2a are slices in the xy-plane at the position of the sources (z=4.5). The sources were then made fully correlated and the simulation was repeated with the same parameters. In this case the beamformer finds no peaks, and a z-slice at the position of the two sources looks completely flat with pseudo-z values corresponding to the noise level as shown in Figure 2b. In this case the two correlated sources fully attenuated each other.

The simulation was then repeated with the same parameters as above but this time random Gaussian noise was added at values corresponding roughly to those of a typical MEG system. For the case when the two sources are uncorrelated, they were localized to their simulated position to within the scanning resolution of the beamformer, as shown in Figure

3a. The lower resolution is a result of using much higher noise values compared to the previous simulation. When the sources were made fully correlated, localization revealed three sources instead of two, the source with the highest strength being a broad source in the mid-sagittal plane, as shown in Figure 3b. The next two sources were in the right and left temporal lobes but were poorly localized, appearing ~2 cm away from the simulated position, closer to the skull.

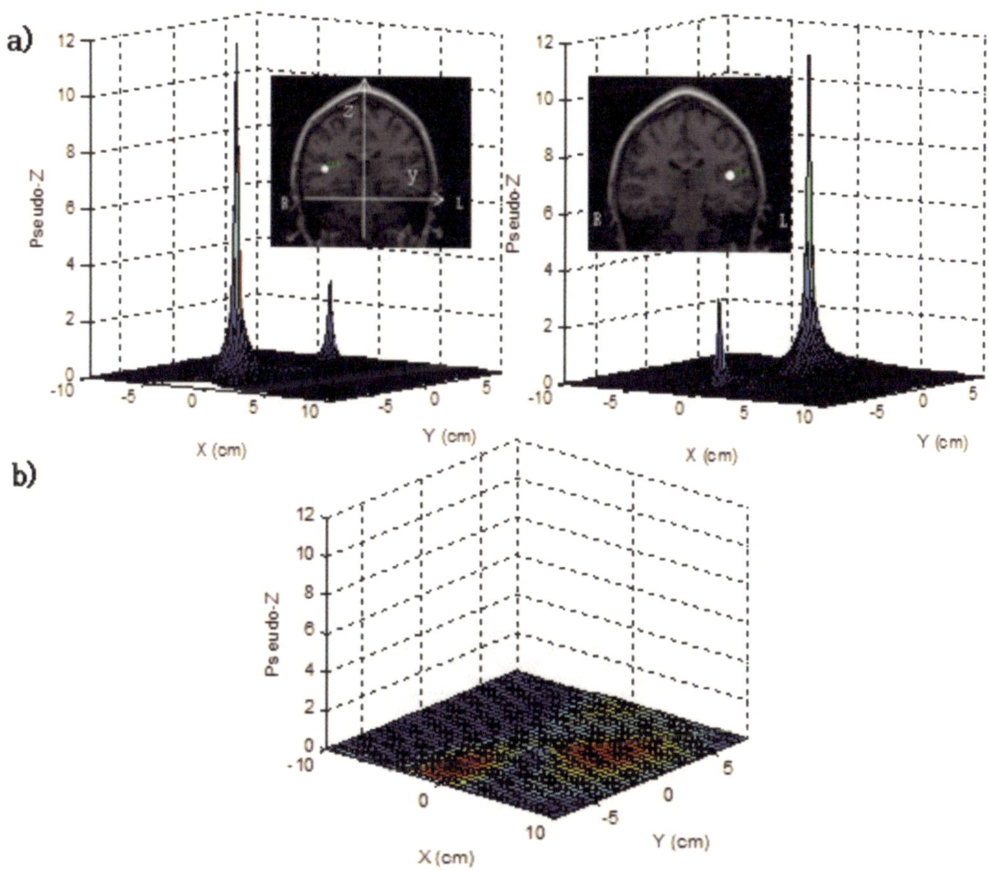

Fig. 2. Localization of bilateral sources simulated with random Gaussian noise added to each channel. (a) Images of the right and left source reconstructions when 20 nAm uncorrelated sources are placed in the right and left temporal lobes, superimposed on a coronal MRI slice intersecting the position of the source along the x direction of a right-handed coordinate system, with the y and z directions indicated by the white arrows. The random noise level was chosen to be 10 times smaller than that of a typical MEG system. The location of the peaks of the left and right reconstructed source images are indicated by white dots. The mesh plots show the spatial distribution of the reconstructed source strength in the xy-plane at the z-position of the peaks. (b) Same as (a) but the sources are fully correlated showing no peaks exceeding the noise level

Figure 4 shows another simulation were the two sources were brought closer together so that they are only separated by 3 cm. For the case when the two sources were made uncorrelated, they were localized to their simulated position to within the beamformer scanning resolution, as shown in Figure 4a. When the two sources were made correlated, instead of observing two distinct sources, the beamformer shows only one broad source half way between the other two sources as shown in Figure 4b.

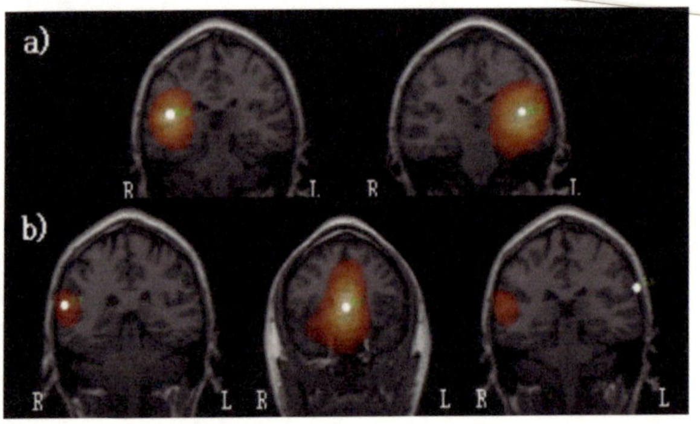

Fig. 3. (a) Same as Figure 2a but noise is added at typical MEG levels (5ft/√hz). (b) Same as (a) but the sources are fully correlated

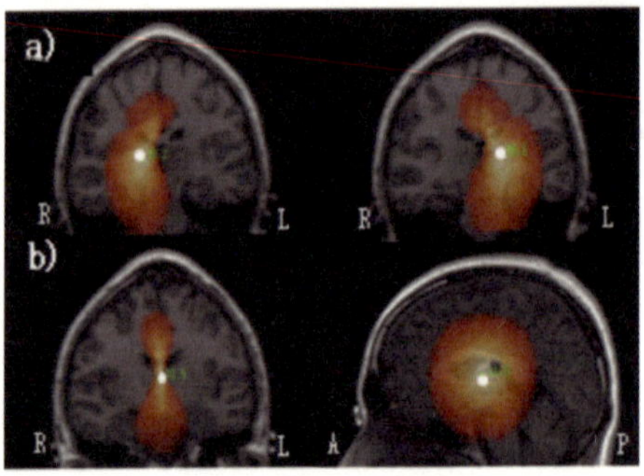

Fig. 4. Same as Figure 3 but the sources are placed at close proximity (3 cm apart) and given a strength of 40 nAm. When (a) uncorrelated the peaks are localized to a position consistent with their simulated location; when (b) correlated the two sources merge together resulting in a single activation in the mid-sagittal plane

3.2 Correcting for temporal correlations

Few techniques have been recently developed to correct for the adverse effects of temporal correlations on the performance of the beamformer. In this section we discuss and compare four of these techniques.

3.2.1 Higher order covariance matrix

Huang et al. (2007) suggested that the use of a higher order covariance matrix improves the performance of the beamformer in the presence of temporally correlated sources. In particular, a third-order covariance matrix was suggested for optimal performance. This method was applied to the simulations described in the previous section using a third order covariance matrix to calculate the beamformer weights. For uncorrelated sources the result (Figure 5a) was similar to Figure 3a, but the pseudo-z scores were a few percent higher, while the resolution was noticeably lower. The result for the case of correlated sources is shown in Figure 5b. We observe that the highest peak belongs to a spurious broad source in the mid-sagittal plane analogous to that of Figure 3b, except that the source here is stronger and broader. While the other two sources are found in the left and right temporal lobes, the localization error is greater than 2 cm, similar to that obtained from the use of a first order covariance matrix. We therefore conclude that this model fails at correcting for correlation effects in beamformer localization.

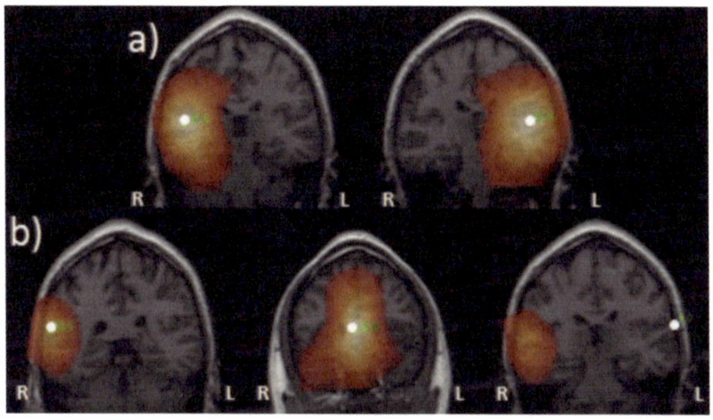

Fig. 5. (a) Localization of the same correlated simulated sources as in Figure 3 except that a 3rd order covariance was used as in the model by Huang et al. with the two sources uncorrelated (a) and correlated (b)

3.2.2 The dual lead-field approach

Another method proposed by Brookes et al. (2007) relies on calculating a dual lead field based on the two interfering sources

$$l_{dual} = \frac{1}{2} l_1(r_1, \xi_1) + \frac{1}{2} l_2(r_2, \xi_2), \tag{22}$$

where l_1 and l_2 are the lead fields from the correlated sources located at positions r_1 and r_2 and pointing in directions ξ_1 and ξ_2, respectively. The weight vector is then calculated using l_{dual} and hence acts to pass the field from the locations of the two sources while attenuating sources originating from other spatial locations, resulting in the sum of the strength of the two sources. Although this method can successfully recover correlated sources, it presents some practical limitations. First, in order to calculate the lead field of the interfering source, its location must be known. Since the source location is not usually known *a priori*, one can use another technique to uncover the source location, or perform a grid search. One might attempt to use the beamformer first in normal mode to get an estimate of the source location; however, as we have seen in the previous section, the beamformer localization accuracy may be significantly compromised when correlated sources are present, thus requiring the use of a grid search in such a case. Second, the orientation of the sources is not usually known, and in the context of the scalar beamformer employed by the authors, a very computationally intensive 2-dimensional search over the directions of the two sources would be required. Third, the spatial resolution gets progressively worse as the correlation between the two sources decreases and the correct source strength cannot be recovered, to the point where it may fail to reveal an uncorrelated source. Fourth, the assumption in (22) is that the two sources have equal magnitude and are therefore weighted equally. In reality, since bilateral sources are often of different magnitude, one would have to allow for more flexibility. To do so Brookes et al. re-write (22) as

$$\boldsymbol{l}_{dual} = a\boldsymbol{l}_1(\boldsymbol{r}_1,\xi_1)+(1-a)\boldsymbol{l}_2(\boldsymbol{r}_2,\xi_2), \tag{23}$$

adding yet another parameter, a, to be determined by optimizing the pseudo-z statistic.

3.2.3 Selecting a subset of sensors

Another approach that has been used as an alternative to implementing explicit corrections in the algorithms for reducing correlation effects in beamformer localization is to use only the sensors from the left side of the MEG array to analyze left-hemisphere sources and, conversely, right-hemisphere sensors to analyze right-hemisphere sources (Herdman et al., 2003). This approach is mainly applicable to auditory cortex sources with widely separated field patterns. However, a recent publication (Popescu et al., 2008) has shown that such a technique can result in significant localization errors due to incomplete removal of the signal from the contralateral source, in agreement with our own results (Quraan, unpublished).

3.2.4 The coherent source suppression model (CSSM)

A more general model has been proposed by Dalal et al. (2006) which relies on specifying additional constraints in deriving the beamformer weights. As shown in eq. 3, the condition to block signals from outside the location of interest is not explicitly specified, but rather one relies on the minimization in (18) and (19) to achieve it. Since this is not achieved in the presence of correlated sources, one can explicitly add constraints to demand it be achieved. In particular, the constraints

$$\begin{aligned} \boldsymbol{w}_\vartheta^T(\boldsymbol{r})\boldsymbol{l}_\vartheta(\boldsymbol{r}_i)=0 \\ \boldsymbol{w}_\vartheta^T(\boldsymbol{r})\boldsymbol{l}_\varphi(\boldsymbol{r}_i)=0 \end{aligned} \tag{24}$$

and

$$\begin{aligned} \boldsymbol{w}_\varphi^T(\boldsymbol{r})\boldsymbol{l}_\varphi(\boldsymbol{r}_i)=0 \\ \boldsymbol{w}_\varphi^T(\boldsymbol{r})\boldsymbol{l}_\vartheta(\boldsymbol{r}_i)=0 \end{aligned} \tag{25}$$

are added to equations (18) and (19), respectively, where $\boldsymbol{r}_i$ is the location of the interfering source. The solution to this constrained minimization problem takes the form (Sekihara, 2008)

$$\boldsymbol{W}(\boldsymbol{r})=\left[\boldsymbol{C}^T(\boldsymbol{r})\boldsymbol{R}^{-1}\boldsymbol{C}(\boldsymbol{r})\right]^{-1}\boldsymbol{R}^{-1}\boldsymbol{C}(\boldsymbol{r})\boldsymbol{c}, \tag{26}$$

where

$$\boldsymbol{c}=[1,0,0,...,0]^T, \tag{27}$$

and $\boldsymbol{C}$ is the composite lead-field matrix given by

$$\boldsymbol{C}(\boldsymbol{r})=\left[\boldsymbol{l}_\vartheta(\boldsymbol{r}),\boldsymbol{l}_\varphi(\boldsymbol{r}),\boldsymbol{l}_\vartheta(\boldsymbol{r}_i),\boldsymbol{l}_\varphi(\boldsymbol{r}_i)\right]^T. \tag{28}$$

Implementations of this model can therefore allow the user to specify the location of the suspected correlated source to be suppressed, or suppression point, $\boldsymbol{r}_i$. The algorithm can then calculate the lead fields for the location of interest, as well as the location of the suppression point, to formulate the composite matrix (eq. (28)) which in turn is used to calculate the weights (eq. (26)). When the precise location of the interfering source is not known *a priori*, or the source is expected to have a large spatial extent, a suppression region (i.e. a collection of adjacent suppression points), $\{ \boldsymbol{r}_i \}$, can be specified. In this case constraints similar to those of equations (24) and (25) are added to correspond to the locations to be suppressed, and the composite lead field (eq. (28)) would have 2 additional columns per extra suppression point. As more suppression points are added, however, the number of degrees of freedom in the minimization is quickly reduced, hence, impacting the performance of the model.

Figure 6 shows the beamformer localization of the two simulated correlated auditory sources discussed above when applying CSSM to correct for temporal correlations. First, we note that the mid-sagittal source has now disappeared verifying that it is an artefact of the interference effect between the two sources. Second, the strength of the reconstructed sources in the simulated dataset have increased by ~90% and ~130%, since the attenuation effects due to correlations are reduced. Third, both sources were localized to their simulated positions to within the beamformer scanning resolution.

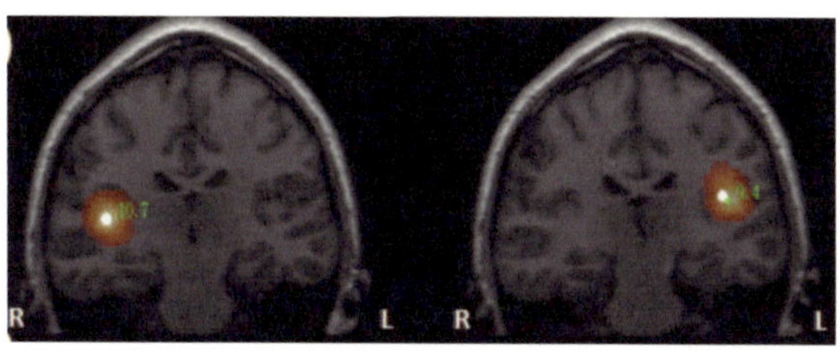

Fig. 6. (a) Localization of the same correlated simulated sources as above when CSSM was used to correct for correlation effects. The suppression region was chosen to surround the right source when the left source was localized and vice versa resulting in the left and right figures, respectively

3.2.4.1 Systematic effects of CSSM

To consider the effect of distance between source and suppression point on beamformer source reconstruction, a single source was simulated in the right temporal lobe and random Gaussian noise was added to the simulation at levels typical in an MEG system. The beamformer was then used to localize the source first with no suppression points, then a suppression point was added at a position 9 cm away from the source and the localization procedure was repeated. This was repeated with the suppression point brought closer to the source as illustrated in Figure 7b. Figure 7a shows the percentage reconstructed source strength (i.e. reconstructed source strength with suppression relative to no suppression) with the suppression point at various distances along this line. The figure shows that even when the suppression point was more than a few centimetres away from the interfering source, a large portion of this source was still suppressed. While the amount of suppression applies to the simulation at hand (i.e. the actual amount depends on the number of sources and their locations, the orientation of the sources, the amount of noise, and the parameters used in the suppression model, etc), the general effect holds; namely the suppression point has a long range effect, and the amount of suppression will increase with decreasing distance. This indicates that this method is effective even if we do not have precise information regarding the location of the correlated (interfering) source. However, this has a negative consequence as well; we saw that in this example even when the suppression point was 7 cm away from a source of interest, that source was suppressed by ~20%. This issue becomes more problematic when the interferer and source of interest are close together. In this example, when the correlated bilateral sources were a distance of 3 cm apart, and the suppression point was placed at the location of one of the two sources, the source of interest was suppressed by ~50%. In such cases one can achieve a better outcome by choosing a suppression point not to coincide with the interferer, but rather some distance away in a direction opposite to that of the source of interest. In this example, if one chooses a suppression point 1 cm away from the interferer (4 cm away from the source of interest), the interferer will be suppressed by ~80% while the source of interest will only be suppressed by ~30%. This long range effect of suppression points poses a serious limitation to this model with respect to general applications (such as grid search algorithms), but allows its application to specific cases where the suppression point(s) are carefully chosen for the case at hand. It should be noted however, that spatial localization of the source, regardless of distance from the suppression point, remained within the scanning resolution (0.25 cm) of the beamformer in these simulations in all cases except when the attenuation exceeded 80% (i.e. when the suppression point was within 1 cm from the source to be localized).

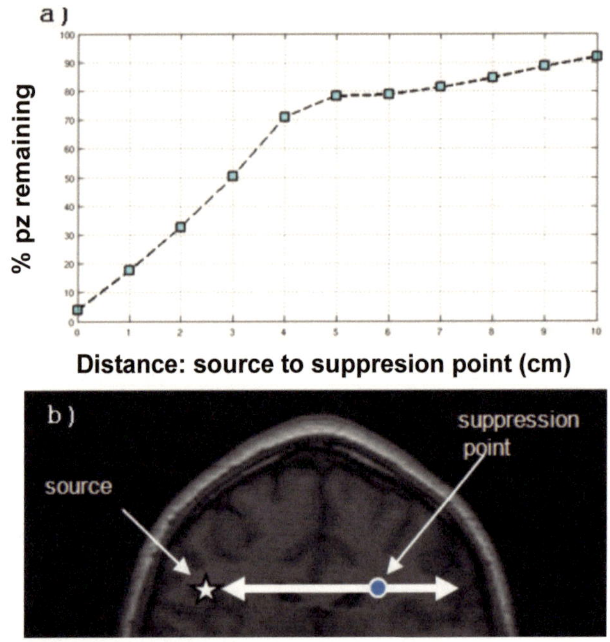

Fig. 7. (a) Percentage pseudo-z remaining (pseudo-z with suppression relative to pseudo-z without suppression) after a suppression point was introduced at various distances from a point source along a line joining the left and right temporal lobes as illustrated in Figure (b). The source was simulated with a strength of 40 nAm and random Gaussian noise at levels typical in an MEG system was added to the simulation

Other systematic effects of the CSSM model were also considered and evaluated in Quraan and Cheyne (2010), including the effect of distance between suppression point and interferer, the effect of the size of the suppression region, the effect of reducing the suppression region using singular value decomposition and the effect of resolution of the suppression region.

3.2.4.2 Example from Auditory data

Table 1 shows the results from datasets acquired from eight subjects listening to a tone, analyzed with and without correlation suppression. Significant mid-sagittal artefacts are seen in seven out of the eight datasets, with the mid-sagittal spurious sources peaking higher than one of the two auditory sources in three out of the eight datasets. Significant increases in source amplitude are observed when correlation suppression is used in all cases, ranging from 17% to 189%. We also note the uneven suppression of left and right sources, and the absence of one of the bilateral sources in one subject as a result of correlations. We also note the uneven suppression of bilateral sources which is highly significant as laterality indices are often used to assess cognitive function and is sometimes used to aid presurgical mapping. Changes in source localization of up to 1.1 cm are also observed.

Figure 8 shows the group averaged functional images from all 13 subjects that participated in the same tone perception task study as well as in a vowel-speak condition (Beal et al. 2010). We note that the reconstructed sources were localized to the auditory cortex with a high degree of symmetry consistent with other neuroimging studies of M100. We also note that the time courses of the left and right auditory sources are highly correlated and peak at ~100 ms, as expected.

Amplitude change (%)		**Location change (cm)**		**Spurious source amplitude (%)**
Left	**Right**	**Left**	**Right**	
81	39	0.5	0.0	56
64	78	0.6	0.8	86
69	34	0.8	0.4	86
189	52	0.6	0.3	126
69	36	0.8	0.0	130
38	122	0.5	1.1	116
n/a	17	n/a	0.5	n/a
54	26	0.4	0.4	0

Table 1. Effects of correlation suppression on datasets acquired from eight subjects showing the percentage increase in amplitude and the change in localization for the left and right auditory (M100) sources when correlations are corrected for. Also shown is the relative strength of mid-sagittal spurious sources when no correlation correction is used, calculated as a percentage of the strength of the weaker of the two auditory sources. The left auditory source was not observed in one subject (row 7)

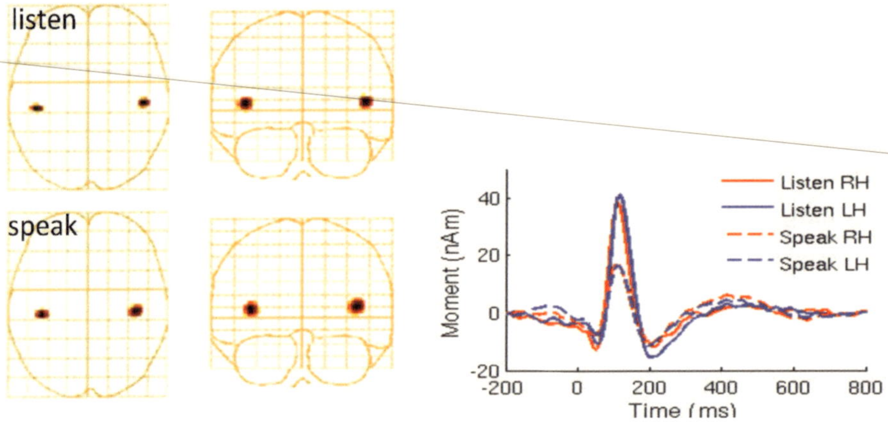

Fig. 8. (left) Group averaged functional images from 13 healthy subjects that participated in a tone perception task study as well as in a vowel-speak study. (right) Group averaged time courses obtained from the auditory sources localized on the left (Beal et al. 2010)

4. Leakage

4.1 Effects of leakage on the performance of the beamformer

The purpose of a beamformer is to block signals from outside the voxel for which the source magnitude is being determined; in the presence of noise or other strong signals, however, beamformers can only partially attenuate such signals. Strong sources from other locations may make significant contributions to the source activity, thereby limiting the localization accuracy or even obscuring a weak source. Reddy et al. (1987) derived an expression for the power output of two fully uncorrelated point sources and showed that in the presence of noise, the complete blocking of signals from outside the location of interest may not be achieved. Leakage presents a serious challenge for the beamformer when the source of interest is a weak source and other strong sources are present, a case that is typical in cognitive paradigms that rely on sensory inputs to evoke much weaker activations in structures such as the hippocampus, and the amygdala. Figure 9 shows beamformer localization of two uncorrelated simulated point sources (indicated by the red dots) where random Gaussian noise is added at typical MEG noise levels. While the peak activity is detected within the beamformer scanning resolution (5 mm), broad bands of activity are observed surrounding the actual point sources confirming the beamformer's inability to block the strong auditory sources from leaking into the surrounding volume. In cases where the source of interest is a weak source lying in the vicinity of these leakage patterns, the detection and accurate localization of such source will be compromised.

Figure 10a shows a group-averaged glass-brain plot of source activity in the Talairach coordinate system for sources simulated at 40, 30, 20, and 10 nAm, where the simulated signals were folded in with visual data. The group averages include datasets from 15-subjects with 150 trials/dataset. As can be seen from this figure, the 40 nAm hippocampal activation was detected as the strongest activation, but at 30 nAm the primary visual activation was the strongest. Although hippocampal activation is still visible, a leakage pattern resulting from the activation of the visual cortices and extending all the way to the hippocampus is also visible. At 20 and 10 nAm the hippocampal signal is no longer visible due to leakage from the primary visual sources. Since most hippocampal signals are below the 30 nAm range, the ability to properly detect and localize small signals is crucial (Quraan et al. 2011).

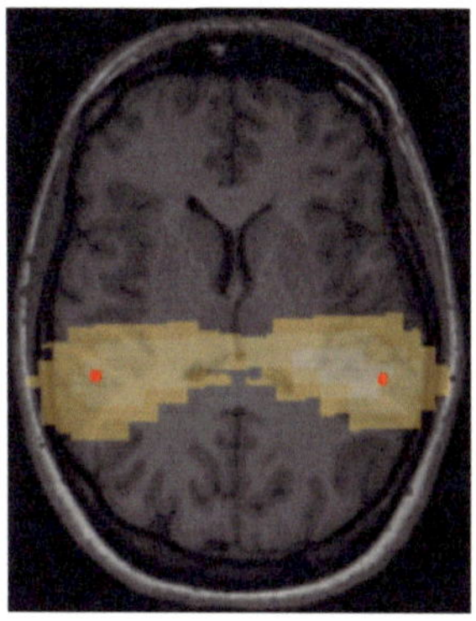

Fig. 9. Beamformer localization of two point sources simulated at the positions indicated by the red dots. The broad activation patterns result from leakage of activation into neighbouring voxels

4.2 Reducing the impact of leakage on the performance of the beamformer

An approach that is highly effective in reducing the effect of leakage from the dominant sensory sources when higher cognitive processes are of interest is achieved by designing experiments that include appropriate control conditions. We have used this approach (Quraan et al. 2010b, Quraan et al. 2010c, Quraan et al. 2011, Mills et al., submitted) to investigate hippocampal activations. In such experiments the condition of interest (which we will call the *experimental* condition) involves a task that is expected to activate the hippocampus while the control condition (which we will call *control*) involves a task that is not expected to involve the hippocampal system to the same extent. For example, for experiments that use visual presentations as stimuli, both the experimental condition and the control condition would include the visual activation. One can then construct *experimental* images and *control* images and subtract them. Since both images include the visual activation as well as its leakage patterns, ideally, subtracting the two would also subtract leakage from the primary visual sources that hinder the detection and localization of the hippocampal sources. Realistically, efficient subtraction of such sources relies on the way these control conditions are constructed and the number of trials used. One would expect the best subtraction of such leakage patterns to occur if the control trials were interleaved with the experimental trials, to ensure that the subject is responding to the visual stimuli similarly in both cases. In addition, interleaving ensures the capture of noise variations almost simultaneously for both conditions, as well as any head movement variations. However, it is not always possible to interleave conditions since achieving the experimental condition may require separation from the control condition. In this case one would have to subtract images constructed from individual runs (one run for the experimental and one run for the control), and while optimal leakage subtraction efficiency is not achieved, a reasonable subtraction efficiency can still be obtained as we demonstrate on both simulations and real data.

Figure 10b shows the *experimental-control* group averaged images for the same experimental condition as in Figure 10a. As is the case with no control condition, hippocampal activation is successfully detected for the 40-20 nAm range. Furthermore, while at 10 nAm a reminant of the primary visual activation is still present, its leakage patterns are effectively reduced, allowing the detection of the hippocampal signal. For such signals, however, the localization bias becomes fairly strong, as a result of the strong leakage and brain noise relative to the hippocampal signal, and the group averaged image shows hippocampal activation shifted laterally by 15 mm. As we have seen, this bias arises from the localization algorithm in the presence of noise and the subtraction of *experimental-control* images does not eliminate this bias.

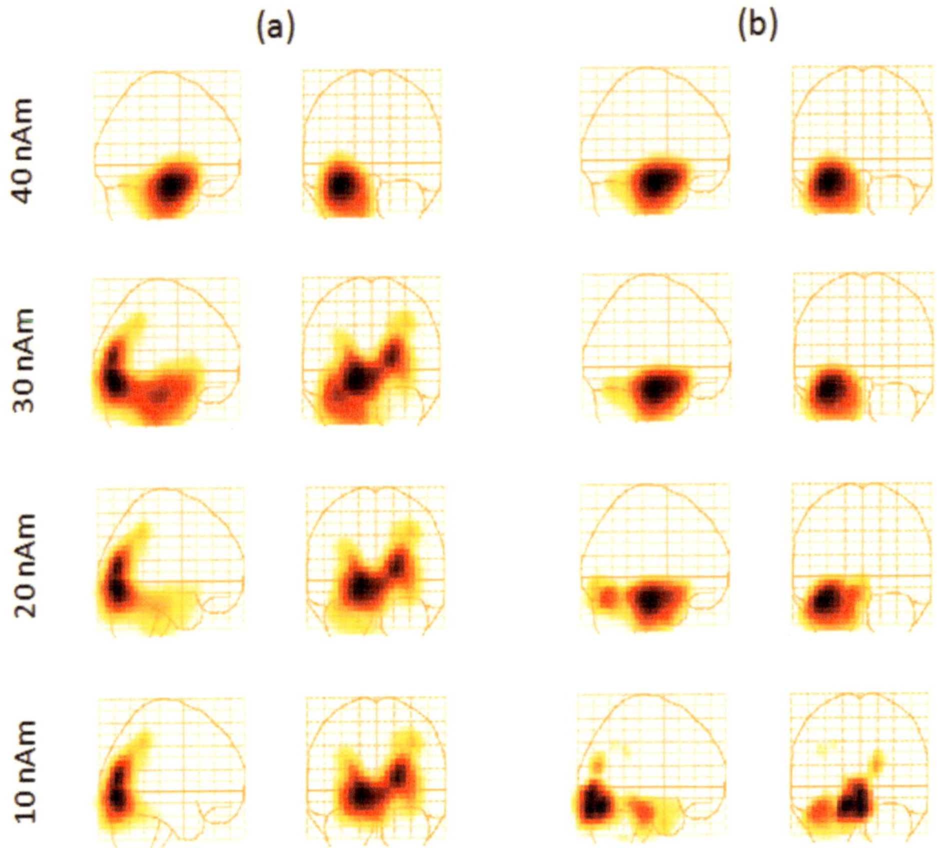

Fig. 10. (a) Group averaged functional images of VEF data obtained from 15 subjects. Simulated hippocampal source with various strengths (as indicated on the figure) were added to each dataset at a latency within the active region (200 ms – 230 ms). (b) The same as in (a) but the images obtained from the control condition were subtracted from the experimental condition for each subject prior to averaging

4.2.1 Data subtraction techniques

In the discussion above we demonstrated that subtracting source images reconstructed from *experimental* and *control* conditions, which we will refer to as image subtraction (IS), enhances our ability to localize weak sources. We now compare IS to two other subtraction techniques, the first based on the subtraction of epoch-averaged sensor data (SAD), and the second based on the subtraction of unaveraged sensor data (SUD). We note that IS differs from SAD and SUD in that the subtraction occurs post source localization only in the former. When localizing weak sources, the advantage of subtraction prior to localization is that the dominant sources are largely removed, allowing the beamformer to achieve a better minimization and reducing possible interferences and biases.

We compared the performance of these three subtraction techniques by simulating hippocampal and medial prefrontal sources of various strengths (Mills et al., submitted). The simulated sources were embedded in real visual data obtained from 22 subjects at a latency of 300 ms, where the brain noise background from the visual activity has largely subsided, and at 100 ms, where the visual activity is at its peak. Three assessment measures were used in this comparison: the strength of the weakest source detected by each technique, the relative strength of signal and noise and the localization accuracy. Figure 12 shows the results for the low (top) and high (bottom) brain noise background conditions, respectively.

For the low brain noise region we were able to detect both the medial prefrontal and the hippocampal source to below ~5 nAm with all techniques. However, IS yielded the least accurate localization of all three techniques, particularly for the hippocampal source. For example, for a source with a strength of 10 nAm the error exceeded 20 mm for the IS technique, SUD gave a localization error of ~13 mm, and SAD ~8 mm. For the hippocampal source, the SAD and SUD techniques were more effective at localizing the deep hippocampal source than the IS technique in the low brain noise condition.

For the more challenging high brain noise condition, the post-localization subtraction techniques outperformed IS for detection of the medial prefrontal source. This simulated source was only detected down to ~12 nAm with the IS technique, while both the SUD and SAD techniques were able to detect the source with a strength below 5 nAm. Similarly, the intersection of the signal and noise curves and localization error showed IS to be the least accurate. In the case of the hippocampal signal under the high brain noise condition, the difference between the techniques was substantial when considering the intersection of the signal and noise curves. For IS the intersection occurred at ~18 nAm, compared to ~7 nAm for SAD and ~2 nAm for SUD. For the localization error, IS showed the least accuracy, while SUD and SAD were comparable.

4.2.2 Emperical data example

The SUD and SAD techniques can be combined to capture their advantages by averaging the control block first then subtracting this average from every trial in the experimental condition. We applied this analysis technique to real data obtained with a transverse patterning paradigm, which requires memory for relations among stimuli and has been shown to depend upon the integrity of the hippocampal system (Driscoll et al., 2005; Rickard et al., 2006). A control task corresponding to this paradigm is known as an elemental task, and can be solved by learning about the individual elements rather than the relations among them, and may not rely on the hippocampal system to the same extent (Hanlon et al. 2003, 2005; Moses et al., 2009). For this task group averages across 16 adult datasets were constructed. Images from the individual subjects were averaged over 40 ms time ranges with a 20 ms sliding window covering the range of 80 to 720 ms, resulting in 32 group averages (Figure 12).

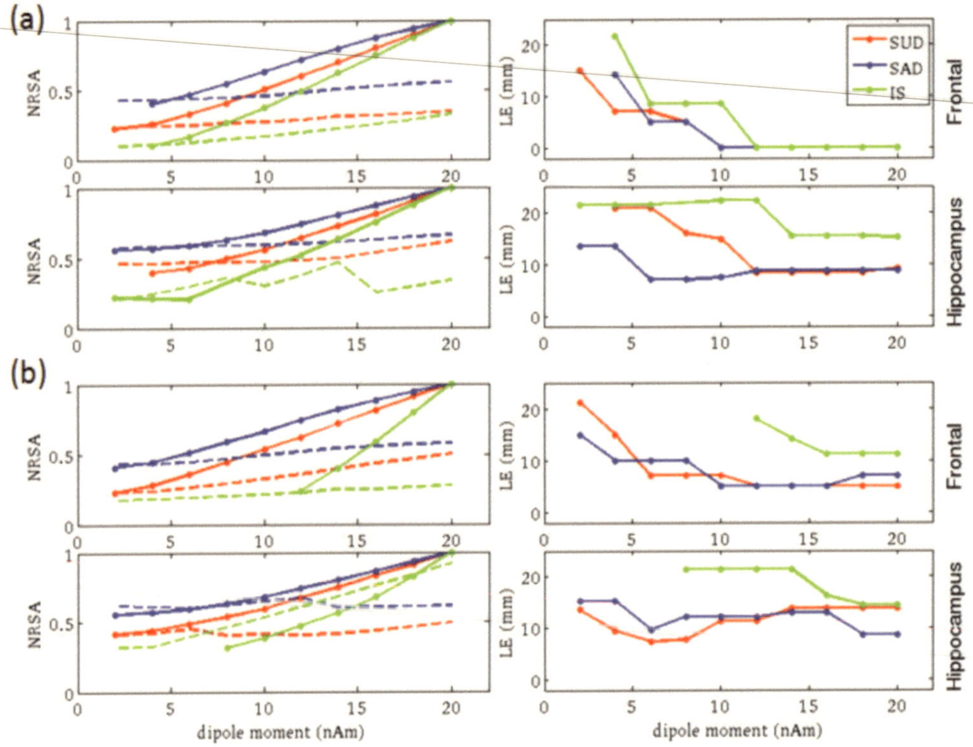

Fig. 11. Beamformer localization results at a latency of (a) 300 ms and (b) 100 ms for a group average of 22 subjects participating in a visual experiment, where a simulated medial prefrontal or hippocampal source was added to the visual data, peaking at 300 ms and 100 ms in figures (a) and (b), respectively. Left panel: Reconstructed source activity normalized to the maximum of the signal curve as a function of simulated source strength for the largest peak in the signal category (solid lines) and the largest peak in the noise category (dashed lines) using the three analysis techniques: IS, SAD and SUD, as labelled on the figure. Right panel: Localization error for the same sources as in the left panel

4.3 Caveats and systematic effects

4.3.1 Experimental design

It is important to note that these analysis techniques depend on compatible experimental and control paradigms, where the two paradigms are as equivalent as possible except in the experimental paradigm's ability to evoke the weak activation of interest. This includes the background activations that both paradigms evoke, as well as the timing of these activations. Nonetheless, this does not require that the resulting brain activity from the two conditions differs only by one feature. In fact, the main purpose is to subtract the dominant sensory sources that result in most of the leakage. If several weak sources still exist, the beamformer will be able to localize them more accurately than in the presence of the dominant sources. Even if the dominant source is not fully subtracted out, a significant reduction of its magnitude is advantageous as the leakage from a source increases with

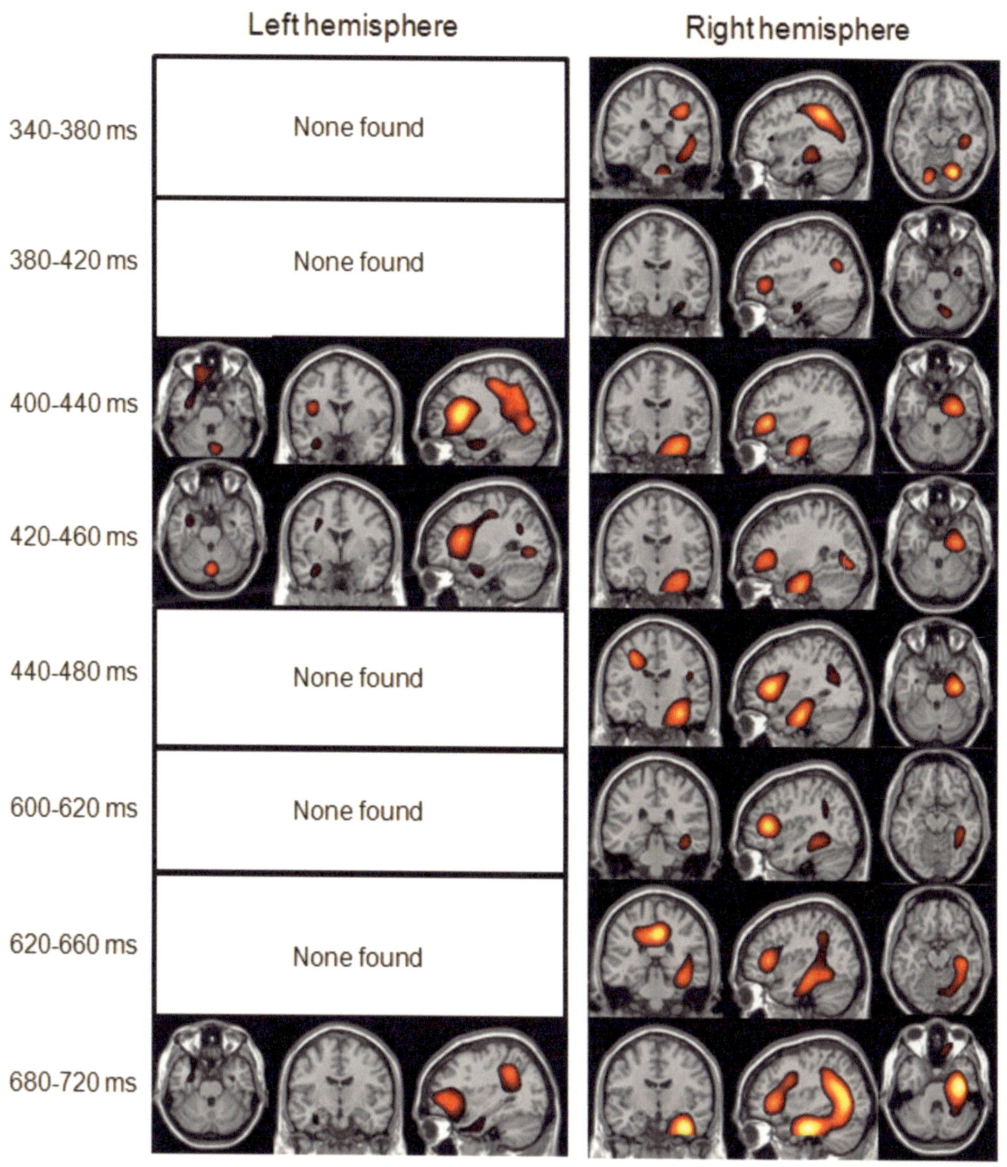

Fig. 12. Localization of hippocampal and frontal sources from a transverse patterning task using pre-localization data subtraction for a group average of 16 subjects. The functional images are averaged over time samples in the latency range labeled on the left side of each figure. The images were normalized to the maximum intensity and thresholded at 80%, and reveal robust hippocampal activation that is largely right dominant

source strength. Generally, differences between experimental and control conditions may arise from changes in the basic sensory processes rather than the higher cognitive process of interest. This emphasizes the need for careful paradigm design and multi-modality validations as different imaging methods are subject to different systematic effects. When differences between experimental and control paradigms are observed at the sensor level, it is not possible to differentiate between these two cases as the sources responsible for these differences are unknown. However, when these differences are localized (i.e. in source space), we are able to tell whether the intended outcome of the paradigm (e.g. increased hippocampal involvement) has been achieved. For the case above, for example, we were able to localize hippocampal and frontal activations in both the n-back and the transverse patterning paradigms.

4.3.2 Head motion

Differences in head position relative to the sensors between the experimental and control conditions represent a source of error for the pre-localization subtraction techniques as data subtraction occurs prior to MRI-MEG co-registration. However, the use of head motion correction techniques, which has been demonstrated to have an accuracy below 2 mm (Taulu et al., 2005; Wilson et al., 2007), will alleviate such shortcomings. The same algorithms can also be used to reference the head position relative to the sensors from multiple datasets to the same frame, allowing multiple datasets to be added or subtracted with high precision. This allows referencing the experimental and control blocks to the same frame, allowing the use of pre-localization data subtraction with improved accuracy. While specialized hardware and software for head motion correction is available for head-tracking, most MEG systems currently in use do not have this capability. In cases where the experimental and control condition can be interleaved, however, this issue would no longer be a concern. Furthermore, in protocols where multiple trials are averaged, the smearing in source position that results from head position differences among trials, not only increases the localization error, but also reduces the ability to detect weak sources.

4.3.3 Leakage from other sources of noise

Strong sources of noise other than brain noise can also result in significant leakage and hinder the detection and localization accuracy of weaker sources. Signals resulting from eye movement and eye blinks typically result in signals much larger than brain signals. Similarly, artefacts resulting from braces and fillings result in large signals. Independent component analysis (ICA) techniques can help remove some noise components. Open source packages such as EEGlab can be used to remove such artefacts prior to applying a beamformer solution, although regularization will be needed as the removal of components results in a reduction of the covariance matrix rank.

5. Conclusions

We conclude that in the absence of robust inverse models that are able to accurately localize sources with good precision and high resolution, and yet be robust to interference from other sources be they correlated or uncorrelated, the analysis of MEG data requires careful validations. In this respect, many of the inverse models typically employed are complementary, often requiring the use of multiple techniques in order to arrive at proper conclusions. Whenever ambiguities are present such as in the case of weak or deep sources, or when using imaging techniques that are known to suffer from spatial biases and low resolution, or in the presence of correlations when beamformers are used, it is prudent to carry out the necessary corroboration procedures. Realistic simulations are a necessary tool to quantify the performance of the various inverse models and analysis techniques, including what brain activity can and cannot be detected. It can also shed light on the experimental parameters needed to optimize the experimental design.

While beamformer techniques have been gaining popularity in the MEG field due to their ease of use, their limitations and drawbacks have often been largely ignored leading to inappropriate use of these modalities. Beamformer susceptibility to correlation effects has strong consequences on the ability to properly reconstruct brain activity as it results in significant attenuation of temporally correlated signals, false positives, and localization inaccuracies. The often uneven attenuation of correlated bilateral sources leads to unreliable laterality information (e.g. laterality index). In addition, this attenuation (which varies depending on signal to noise ratio as we have shown here), results in altering the source time course and any measure derived from it such as frequency spectra and functional connectivity measures.

Similarly, leakage effects which result in broad reconstructed activation patterns as a result of the beamformer's inability to block signals from outside the voxel for which the source strength is estimated often lead to misinterpreted results. In fact, one of the most commonly cited advantages of spatial filtering techniques is their ability to reconstruct spatially distributed sources, as opposed to dipole fits which assume a point source. In reality, in the presence of typical MEG instrumental noise (as well as background brain noise) resolution limitations (e.g. as a result of leakage) result in a wide source spread obscuring the spatial spread of actual brain sources. In addition, leakage from the strong sensory activations, which, as we have seen in this chapter in the context of auditory and visual activations, span a large volume surrounding the sources of interest hindering the detection of weaker sources such as memory activations originating in the hippocampus.

Spatial filters of the adaptive and non adaptive type are local linear estimators that estimate source activity at a given location, completely independently of any other location. In this respect, no attempt is made to account for the measured fields in their entirety. If the magnetic fields at the sensors are to be calculated from the beamformer solution from every voxel, the calculated field will exceed the measured field by a large amount due to resolution/leakage effects. In this respect no acceptable χ^2 (or goodness of fit) measure can be achieved making it difficult to differentiate between acceptable and unacceptable solutions based on their ability to reproduce the measured fields. Acknowledging this fact, in this chapter (and other publications) we relied on extensive realistic simulations to verify beamformer solutions. Such simulations are a necessity for verifying the outcome of any mathematical model, and not least a model where no quality assurance metric is employed.

While we have shown in this chapter that models and analysis techniques are available to work around these difficulties, in closing we emphasize that none of these techniques provide a robust solution. Appropriate validations based on the use of multiple inverse models and simulations are necessary to validate experimental outcomes.

6. Acknowledgements

The author would like to acknowledge Dr. Margot Taylor, Dr. Sandra Moses and Dr. Deryk Beal for providing the data and for many interesting discussions; Mr. Travis Mills and Mr. Marc Lalancette for many interesting discussions and for help with data analysis.

7. References

Borgiotti, G., Kaplan, L.J., 1979. Superresolution of uncorrelated intereference sources by using adaptive array technique. IEEE Transactions on Antenna and Propagation 27, 842-845.

Beal DS, Cheyne DO, Gracco VL, Quraan MA, Taylor MJ, De Nil F. 2010. Auditory evoked fields to vocalization during passive listening and active generation in adults who stutter. Neuroimage 52(4):

Brookes, M.J., Stevenson, C.M., Barnes, G.R., Hillebrand, A., Simpson, M., Francis, S.T., Morris, P.G., 2007. Beamformer reconstruction of correlated sources using a modified source model. Neuroimage 34, 1454-1465.

Brookes, M.J., Vrba, J., Robinson, S.E., Stevenson, C.M., Peters, A.M., Barnes, G.R., Hillebrand, A., Morris, P.G., 2008. Optimising experimental design for MEG beamformer imaging. Neuroimage 39, 1788-1802.

Carlson BD. 1988. Covariance matrix estimation errors and diagonal loading in adaptive arrays. IEEE Trans. Aerospace and Electronic Systems 24:397-401.

Greenblatt, R.E., Ossadtchi, A., Pflieger, M.E., 2005. Local linear estimators for the bioelectromagnetic inverse problem. IEEE Trans. Signal Process. vol. 53, 3403-3412.

Hamalainen, M., Hari, R., Ilmoniemi, R.J., Knuutila, J.L., Olli V., 1993. Magnetoencephelography - theory, instrumentation, and applications to noninvasive studies of the working human brain. Reviews of Modern Physics 65, 413-497.

Hanlon FM, Weisend MP, Huang M, Lee RR, Moses SN, Paulson KM, Thoma RJ, Miller GA, Canive JM. 2003. A non-invasive method for observing hippocampal function. Neuroreport 14(15):1957-60.

Hanlon FM, Weisend MP, Yeo RA, Huang M, Lee RR, Thoma RJ, Moses SN, Paulson KM, Miller GA, Canive JM. 2005. A specific test of hippocampal deficit in schizophrenia. Behav Neurosci 119(4):863-75.

Herdman, A.T., Wollbrink, A., Chau, W., Ishii, R., Ross, B., Pantev, C., 2003. Determination of activation areas in the human auditory cortex by means of synthetic aperture magnetometry. Neuroimage 20, 995-1005.

Huang, M.X., Shih, J.J., Lee, R.R., Harrington, D.L., Thoma, R.J., Weisend, M.P., Hanlon, F., Paulson, K.M., Li, T., Martin, K., Millers, G.A., Canive, J.M., 2004. Commonalities and differences among vectorized beamformers in electromagnetic source imaging. Brain Topogr 16, 139-158.

Jerbi, K., Mosher, J.C., Baillet, S., Leahy, R.M., 2002. On MEG forward modelling using multipolar expansions. Phys Med Biol 47, 523-555.

Mills T, Lalancette M, Moses SN, Taylor MJ, Quraan MA. Techniques for detection and localization of weak sources using MEG, submitted.

Moses SN, Ryan JD, Bardouille T, Kovacevic N, Hanlon FM, McIntosh AR. 2009. Semantic information alters neural activation during transverse patterning performance. Neuroimage 46(3):863-73.

Pascarella A., Sorrentino A., Campi C. and Piana M., Particle filtering, beamforming and multiple signal classication for the analysis of magnetoencephalography time series: a comparison of algorithms". Inverse Problems and Imaging (in press).

Pascual-Marqui, R.D., 2002. Standardized low-resolution brain electromagnetic tomography (sLORETA): technical details. Methods Find Exp Clin Pharmacol 24 Suppl D, 5-12.

Popescu, M., Popescu, E., Chan, T., Blunt, S.D., Lewine, J.D., 2008. Spatio-Temporal Reconstruction of Bilateral Auditory Steady-State Responses Using MEG Beamformers. IEEE Transactions on Biomedical Engineering 55, 1092-1102.

Quraan MA, Cheyne D. 2008. Correcting for correlations in beamformer localization. 15th International Conference on Biomagnetism.

Quraan MA, Cheyne D. 2010. Reconstruction of correlated brain activity with adaptive spatial filters in MEG. Neuroimage 49, 2387-2400.

Quraan MA, Moses SN, Hung Y, Mills T, Taylor MJ. 2011. Detection and localization of hippocampal activity using beamformers with MEG: A detailed investigation using simulations and empirical data. Human Brain Mapping 32 (5):812-827.

Quraan MA, Hopf L, Mills T, Marc Lalancette M and Moses SN (2010) Localization of Hippocampal & Frontal Activity Using Beamformers in MEG. 16th Annual Meeting of the Organization of Human Brain Mapping.

Quraan MA, Moses SN, Hung Y, Mill T and Taylor MJ (2010). Detection and Localization of Hippocampal Activity Using Beamformers in MEG. 16th International Conference on Biomagnetism.

Reddy, V.U., Paulraj, A., Kailath, T., 1987. Performance analysis of the optimum beamformer in the presence of correlated sources and its behavior under spatial smoothing. IEEE Transactions on Acoustics and Speech Signal Processing ASSP-35, 927-936.

Robinson, S.E., 2004. Localization of event-related activity by SAM(erf). Neurol Clin Neurophysiol 2004, 109.

Robinson, S.E., Rose, D.F., 1992. Current source imaging estimation by spatially filtered MEG. Biomagnetism: Clinical Aspects, 761-765.

Robinson, S.E., Vrba, J., 1999. Recent Advances in Biomagnetism. In: Yoshimoto, T., Kotani, M., Kuriki, S., Karibe, S., Nakasato, N. (Eds.), Functional neuroimaging by synthetic aperature magnetometry (SAM). Tohoku University Press, Sendai, Japan, 302-305.

Sekihara, K., 2008. Adaptive spatial filters for electromagnetic brain imaging, 1st ed. Springer, New York.

Sekihara, K., Nagarajan, S.S., Poeppel, D., Marantz, A., 2002a. Performance of an MEG adaptive-beamformer technique in the presence of correlated neural activities: effects on signal intensity and time-course estimates. IEEE Trans Biomed Eng 49, 1534-1546.

Sekihara, K., Nagarajan, S.S., Poeppel, D., Marantz, A., Miyashita, Y., 2001. Reconstructing spatio-temporal activities of neural sources using an MEG vector beamformer technique. IEEE Trans Biomed Eng 48, 760-771.

Sekihara, K., Nagarajan, S.S., Poeppel, D., Marantz, A., Miyashita, Y., 2002b. Application of an MEG eigenspace beamformer to reconstructing spatio-temporal activities of neural sources. Hum Brain Mapp 15, 199-215.

Sekihara, K., Sahani, M., Nagarajan, S.S., 2005. Localization bias and spatial resolution of adaptive and non-adaptive spatial filters for MEG source reconstruction. Neuroimage 25, 1056-1067.

Shan, T., Kailath, T., 1985. Adaptive Beamforming for Coherent Signals and Interference. IEEE Transactions on Acoustics, Speech, and Signal Processing ASSP-33, 527-536.

Taulu S, Simola J. 2006. Spatiotemporal signal space separation method for rejecting nearby interference in MEG measurements. Phys Med Biol 51(7):1759-68.

Tikhonov AN. 1963. Solution of incorrectly formulated problems and the regularization method. Soviet Mathematics Doklady 4:1035-1038.

Uutela, K., Hamalainen, M., Salmelin, R., 1998. Global optimization in the localization of neuromagnetic sources. IEEE Trans Biomed Eng 45, 716-723.

Van Veen, B.D., van Drongelen, W., Yuchtman, M., Suzuki, A., 1997. Localization of brain electrical activity via linearly constrained minimum variance spatial filtering. IEEE Trans Biomed Eng 44, 867-880.

Wilson H, Moiseev A, Podin S, Quraan M. 2007. Continuous head localization and data correction in MEG. Proceedings of the 15th International Conference in Biomagnetism:623-626.

Wipf D, Nagarajan S. 2009. A unified Bayesian framework for MEG/EEG source imaging. Neuroimage 44(3):947-66.

5

Statistical Approaches to the Inverse Problem

A. Pascarella[1] and A. Sorrentino[2]
[1]*Dipartimento di Neuroscienze, Universitá di Parma*
[2]*Department of Statistics, University of Warwick*
[1]*Italy*
[2]*United Kingdom*

1. Introduction

Magnetoencephalography (MEG) can be considered as one of the most powerful instruments for non-invasive investigation of the brain functions (Hämäläinen et al., 1993). Its good temporal resolution (sampling frequency can reach several thousands of Hertz), only comparable to the sampling frequency of electroencephalography (EEG), allows following the neural dynamics on a millisecond time scale. This implies that, with respect to other functional imaging modalities, MEG provides an enormous amount of information about the brain activity. On the other hand, localization of brain activity from MEG data requires to solve a highly ill-posed inverse problem (Sarvas, 1987): exact reconstruction of the neural current is not possible even with noise-free data, and the debate about the actual spatial resolution of MEG is still open. Despite this drawback, the appeal of MEG data is such that a large number of methods have been developed for localizing brain activity from MEG recordings. Starting from the middle Eighties, when the first Minimum Norm Estimate (Hämäläinen & Ilmoniemi, 1984) appeared, to the recent developments in spatio temporal regularization (Ou et al., 2009), state space models (Long et al., 2006; Sorrentino et al., 2009) and Markov Chain Monte Carlo (Jun et al., 2005), the attempts to insert enough a priori information to actually provide stable and reliable solutions have been rising rather than diminishing. The goal and the scope are clear: automatic and reliable source localization can be of practical use in several fields, possibly including clinical applications (pre-surgical evaluation, foci localization in epilepsy), new technology development (e.g. brain computer interfaces), and scientific research (e.g. for analysis of large datasets).

Despite having been presented in rather different frameworks and with largely different names and techniques, most methods appeared so far in the MEG inverse literature can be described rather straightforwardly in a statistical setting, which helps unifying and clarifying the assumptions and the limitations of the methods. In this chapter, we attempt a brief review of the most largely known methods, as well as of some of the most recently appeared ones, highlighting the statistical features. We first provide a brief description of the statistical approach to inverse problems in Section 2; then we describe the main features of the MEG inverse problem in Section 3; in Section 4 and 5 we review methods developed by other authors, while in Section 6 we discuss our work on Bayesian filtering for MEG.

2. Statistics and inverse problems

2.1 Inverse problems

In applied mathematics the term inverse problem denotes a class of problems, often originating from physics equations, where the unknown is an unobserved quantity which has to be recovered from indirect measurements. Rather often, there is a causal relationship between the unknown and the data, and the inverse problem involves moving backwards from a measured effect to an unknown cause. An excellent source of inverse problems is the field of medical imaging, where one tries to recover information about quantities within the body from external measurements.

Inverse problems are usually represented in functional form as

$$g = A(f) \tag{1}$$

where $g \in H_2$, $f \in H_1$, and $A : H_1 \to H_2$ is an operator between the two possibly distinct functional spaces (e.g. Banach spaces, Hilbert spaces, etc.) H_1 and H_2. From a mathematical viewpoint, the inverse problem consists in finding the function f given the function g and the operator A. In most cases of practical interest, however, the solution of the inverse problem cannot be found exactly, because the operator A is pathological: either its kernel is non-empty - leading to non-uniqueness of the inverse solution - or the range of A is not the whole H_2 - leading to non-existence problems - or the inverse operator, when it exists, is not continuous - leading to stability problems. In applied mathematics, the typical solution to these pathologies is provided in the celebrated regularization framework for linear inverse problems (Bertero & Boccacci, 1998), where the ill-posed problem is replaced by a one-parameter family of well-posed ones. The most common regularization algorithm, Tichonov method, consists in finding the minimizer $\hat{f}$ of

$$||g - A \cdot f||^2_{H_2} + \bullet\, ||f||^2_{H_1} \tag{2}$$

which is rather straightforwardly

$$\hat{f} = (A^*A + \bullet\, I)^{-1}A^*g \tag{3}$$

where A^* is the adjoint of A and $\bullet$ is the regularization parameter, which tunes the balance between stability of the solution and its capability to explain the measured data. More in general, the recipe of any regularization algorithm is to minimize a functional which combines the misfit - the difference between the actual data and the model - with some type of norm of the solution - implicitely encouraging some stability property for the solution. The choice of this norm, together with a criterion for choosing the value of the regularization parameter, are key ingredients which highly depend on the specific problem.

2.2 Statistics for inverse problems

Given the stochastic nature of noise affecting the data, it is natural to view inverse problems as statistical inference problems. The core of this approach is to model the data as a Random Variable (RV). Then, there exist two main frameworks for dealing with the inverse problem: in the Maximum Likelihood (ML) framework, the unknown is viewed as a set of parameters which characterize the probability distribution of the data, and the inverse problem is re-phrased as a parameter estimation problem; in the Bayesian framework, the unknown is viewed as a Random quantity as well, and the inverse problem is re-phrased as the problem of calculating the posterior distribution of the unknown, given the data.

More specifically, let y be the realization of the Random Variable Y, representing the measured data. In the ML framework, x represents the unknown parameters; the distribution of the data $L(y|x)$ is called likelihood function and contains both the physical model - the operator A mapping the unknown onto the data - and the assumptions on the statistical distribution of noise. Typically one wants to find the x which maximizes L for the observed noisy data y; such

$$\hat{x} = \arg\max(L(y|x)) \tag{4}$$

is naturally called Maximum Likelihood estimate of x.
In the Bayesian framework, on the other hand, x is viewed as the realization of the Random Variable X rather than as a parameter, and it is given a prior distribution; this prior is then combined with the likelihood through Bayes theorem to produce the so called posterior distribution, i.e. the probability distribution for the unknown, conditioned on the realization of the data. The solution of the inverse problem is here defined to be the posterior distribution of the unknown, which can then be used to compute point estimates and bounds. More specifically, let $p(x)$ be the prior probability distribution for the unknown, emboding all the information which is known a priori, before the data are collected; let $L(y|x)$ be the likelihood function, the same function which is used in the ML framework; the posterior distribution is given by Bayes theorem as

$$p(x|y) = \frac{L(y|x)p(x)}{p(y)} \tag{5}$$

where $p(y)$ is the normalizing constant and is given as $p(y) = \int L(y|x)p(x)dx$.

2.3 The linear Gaussian case

Let us briefly consider a linear inverse problem with additive zero-mean Gaussian noise N, with standard deviation $\bullet$; in the ML framework, the model equation is

$$Y = Ax + N \tag{6}$$

and the likelihood function is

$$L(y|x) = \frac{1}{\sqrt{2\bullet}\,\bullet} \exp\left(-\frac{||y - Ax||^2}{2\bullet^2}\right). \tag{7}$$

The ML estimate in this example is the solution of the least squares problem.

In Bayesian terms, the model equation becomes

$$Y = AX + N \tag{8}$$

and the posterior distribution under zero-mean Gaussian prior for the unknown turns out to be:

$$p(x|y) \propto \exp\left(-\frac{||y - Ax||^2}{2\bullet^2}\right) \exp\left(-\frac{||x||^2}{2\bullet^2}\right) \tag{9}$$

where $\bullet$ is the standard deviation of the prior. Comparison of equations (9) and (2) suggests that the minimizer of the Tichonov functional is the mode of the posterior distribution, provided that the regularization parameter is identified with the ratio between the noise variance and the variance of the prior distribution.

As this simple example suggests, in the statistical framework regularization is interpreted as providing a priori information to solve the ill-posed problem. Furthermor, the statistical framework is an elegant and unifying framework where linear as well as non-linear problems can be formally described. Rather than providing computational recipes, this framework provides a theoretical background which is general enough for different kinds of problems, for different kinds of distributions of the noise, and always provides a meaningful interpretation of the variables and parameters in the game.

3. Basic facts about the MEG inverse problem

3.1 Ill posedeness

The magnetic field $\mathbf{b}$ produced by a given electrical current distribution $\mathbf{j}(\mathbf{r})$ inside a volume V and measured at a point $\mathbf{r} \notin V$ is given by the Biot-Savart equation

$$\mathbf{b}(\mathbf{r}) = \frac{\bullet_0}{4\bullet} \int_V \mathbf{j}(\mathbf{r}') \times \frac{\mathbf{r}-\mathbf{r}'}{|\mathbf{r}-\mathbf{r}'|^3} d\mathbf{r}' \quad . \tag{10}$$

It has been known for 150 years that the problem of estimating the electrical current from measurements of the magnetic field is an ill posed problem. Recently a few rigorous proofs have appeared in the literature, which are summarized in the following.

Let $\mathcal{B}_1 : (C(V))^3 \to (C(D))^3$ be the operator described by (10), mapping the electrical current distribution, belonging to the space $(C(V))^3$ of continuous function within the brain volume V, onto the magnetic field, belonging to the space $(C(D))^3$ of continuous functions on a surface D which contains the boundary of V. In Kress et al. (2002) it has been proved that the kernel of $\mathcal{B}_1$ contains the linear subspace

$$M = \{\mathbf{j} | \mathbf{j} = \Delta m, m \in (C_0^2(V))^3\}. \tag{11}$$

This implies that the inverse problem has no unique solution; in particular, given a solution $\mathbf{j}^*$ of the inverse problem (10), any current distribution of the form $\tilde{\mathbf{j}} = \mathbf{j}^* + \bullet \mathbf{j}'$, with $\mathbf{j}' \in M$ and $\bullet \in \mathbb{R}$ is also a solution of the problem.

Let $\mathcal{B}_2 : (L^2(V))^3 \to (L^2(V))^3$ be the operator described by (10), mapping the electrical current distribution in the volume V onto the magnetic field within the same volume V. In this case, all three components of both the electrical current and the magnetic field are assumed to be L^2 functions. In Cantarella et al. (2001), it has been proved that $\mathcal{B}_2$ is a compact operator. This result implies that the generalized inverse is not a continuous operator.

3.2 The inverse model

The Biot Savart equation (10) is only a partial description of the MEG inverse problem: there are two main issues which need to be discussed in order to provide computational solutions to the inverse problem. The first issue, only mentioned here because it is not relevant in the rest of the Chapter, concerns the geometrical and physical model used to approximate the head; it is usually referred to as the forward problem, because it amounts to accurate calculations of the magnetic field produced by a known neural current distribution. Due to the non-zero conductivity of the tissues inside the head, the electrical currents elicited by brain activity are only a portion of the electrical currents flowing in the brain; this means that $\mathbf{j}(\mathbf{r})$ in (10) contains both neural activity and passively flowing currents, which are generated by the neural activity itself and contribute to the measured field as well. The forward problem accounts for the mechanisms by which the neural currents generate the passive currents, and how these passive currents flow in the brain. In the simplest model, available since the Eighties, the head is modelled as a homogeneous spherical conductor, and the effect of the passive currents can be calculated analytically (Sarvas, 1987). A more realistic model, nowadays largely used, takes into account the actual shape of the brain, while maintaining a piecewise homogeneous conductivity, and is solved with numerical integration techniques known as Boundary Element Methods (Gramfort et al., 2011). More recently the use of Finite Element Methods (Pursiainen et al., 2011), far more computationally demanding, allows implementation of completely non-homogeneous and even anisotropic conductivity models.

The second relevant point is the discretization of equation (10). The standard approach comprises discretization of the brain volume with a finite set of $\mathcal{N}_{points}$ points, possibly distributed along the cortical surface. The neural current is then represented as a vector field on these support points. The single current element, with support in a single point of the brain, is usually referred to as *current dipole*. It is characterized by a location $\mathbf{r}$ and a dipole moment $\mathbf{q}$; mathematically speaking it is an applied vector, while from the physical viewpoint it represents the first order approximation of any current distribution. The whole neural current is then viewed as the superposition of thousands of current dipoles:

$$\mathbf{j}(\mathbf{r}) = \sum_{k=1}^{\mathcal{N}_{points}} \mathbf{q}^k \bullet (\mathbf{r} - \mathbf{r}^k) \tag{12}$$

where $\mathbf{q}^k$ is the dipole moment of the current dipole at location $\mathbf{r}^k$ and $\bullet(\cdot)$ is the Dirac delta. The Biot-Savart operator is discretized in a matrix $\mathbf{G} = [\mathbf{G}(\mathbf{r}^1), \ldots, \mathbf{G}(\mathbf{r}^{\mathcal{N}_{points}})]$ of size $\mathcal{N}_{sensors} \times 3\mathcal{N}_{points}$ where each column of the matrix $\mathbf{G}(\mathbf{r}^k)$ represents the magnetic field produced by a unit current dipole at a given position and oriented according to one of the three orthogonal directions; this matrix is usually referred to as the leadfield matrix. The discretized mathematical model becomes here

$$\mathbf{b} = \mathbf{G} \cdot \mathbf{j} \tag{13}$$

where the vector $\mathbf{b}$ is $\mathcal{N}_{sensors} \times 1$ and contains the collection of data measured by all the sensors, while the vector $\mathbf{j} = [\mathbf{j}^1, \ldots, \mathbf{j}^{\mathcal{N}_{points}}]^T$ is $3\mathcal{N}_{points} \times 1$ and contains the dipole moments of the current dipoles located at the fixed locations contained in the leadfield $\mathbf{G}$. In the remainder of the Chapter we will denote by $\mathbf{b}_t$ and $\mathbf{j}_t$ the measured data and the neural current at time t; the leadfield matrix is usually assumed to be not time dependent.

3.3 Classification of inverse methods

Equation (13) is the main equation of practical interest for the solution of the inverse problem. It reflects the fact that the inverse problem is linear, in the sense that the measured data are the linear superpositions of the contributions of individual current dipoles. The physical and geometrical model discussed in the previous section is embodied in the matrix $\mathbf{G}$, which is assumed to be known when solving the inverse problem. However, talking about *the* MEG inverse problem may be misleading for the following reason. While in the general case one will model the neural current as a vector field with support in the whole brain, and the inverse problem amounts to inversion of the (non-invertible) matrix $\mathbf{G}$, in an alternative approach one can assume that the brain activity is highly localized in few brain regions; if these regions

are small compared to their distance from the sensors, each region can be approximated as a single current dipole; in this case, the inverse problem consists in estimating the number of sources, their location, orientation and strength. The mathematical properties of the two inverse problems are rather different. In the former case, one will face a linear equation resulting in a highly under-determined problem due to the ratio between the typical number of sensors ($\simeq$ 100) and the typical number of points ($\simeq 10,000$). In the following, we will call *imaging methods* the methods based on a continuous current distribution model. In the second case, one will want to estimate the intensity, the orientation, as well as the number and the locations of the point sources; the dependence of the magnetic field on the two latter parameters is highly non-linear, thus resulting in a genuinely non-linear problem. In the following, we will call *parametric methods* the methods based on a point source model.
The classification of inverse methods in imaging and parametric methods is rather common practice in many reviews and dates back at least to Hämäläinen et al. (1993), where dipole methods are separated from regularization methods. In this chapter, we introduce a new - to the best of our knowledge - classification of inverse methods, which accounts for a recent trend in the MEG inverse problem community. We will call *static methods* the inverse methods which do not give a priori information on the temporal behaviour of the neural sources, and *dynamic methods* those which do provide a prior on it. The recent appearance of dynamic methods is indeed a consequence of the increased availability of cheap computational power. Dynamic methods are far more computationally demanding for the simple reason that they perform regularization in a much higher-dimensional space. At the same time, prior information in the temporal domain can really help in stabilizing the solution of this highly ill-posed problem.

4. Imaging methods

Imaging methods solve the linear inverse problem defined by

$$\mathbf{B}_t = \mathbf{G}\mathbf{J}_t + \mathbf{N}_t \tag{14}$$

where: $\mathbf{B}_t \in \mathbb{R}^{\mathcal{N}_{sensors}}$ is the Random Vector representing the measured data at time t; $\mathbf{G}$ is the leadfield matrix as in (13); $\mathbf{J}_t \in \mathbb{R}^{3\mathcal{N}_{points}}$ is the Random Vector representing the neural current distribution at time t; $\mathbf{N}_t \in \mathbb{R}^{\mathcal{N}_{sensors}}$ explicitely accounts for the presence of noise in the data. The output of an imaging method is an estimate of $\mathbf{J}_t$ for every t; as such, it is a sequence of current distributions which can be visualized as a dynamic intensity map representing the flow of brain activity.
From a statistical perspective, all the imaging methods we will describe can be interpreted as Bayesian estimation methods; this is due to the ill-posedeness of the inverse problem which requires rather strong regularization algorithms, i.e. a priori information, to get stable solutions. Due to the fact that most of these methods have been first described in a regularization/ optimization framework, the estimate they provide is always easily interpreted as the MAP of the posterior distribution. All methods share basically the same likelihood function: since noise is assumed to have a zero-mean Gaussian distribution and to be uncorrelated with the sources, the likelihood function is:

$$\bullet\,(\mathbf{b}_t|\mathbf{j}_t) = \frac{1}{\sqrt{(2\bullet)^M|\mathbf{\Sigma}|}} \exp\left(-(\mathbf{b}_t - \mathbf{G}\mathbf{j}_t)^T \mathbf{\Sigma}^{-1} (\mathbf{b}_t - \mathbf{G}\mathbf{j}_t)\right) \tag{15}$$

where $\mathbf{b}_t$, $\mathbf{j}_t$ are realizations of the data and the unknown RV, $\mathbf{\Sigma}$ is the noise covariance matrix and $M = \mathcal{N}_{sensors}$.

What really makes each method unique is the specific choice of the prior distribution for the spatio/ temporal distribution of the neural current.

4.1 Static imaging methods - Minimum Norm Estimate

Minimum Norm Estimate (MNE) is perhaps the most popular method for solving the MEG inverse problem. It has been introduced almost thirty years ago and is the straightforward implementation of the Tichonov algorithm. As seen in Section 2, this choice corresponds to a Gaussian prior distribution

$$\bullet\,(\mathbf{j}_t) = \frac{1}{\sqrt{2\bullet\,\bullet}} \exp\left(-\frac{||\mathbf{j}_t||^2}{2\bullet\,^2}\right). \qquad (16)$$

The explicit form of the MNE solution, i.e. the MAP of the posterior distribution under the given prior, is given by

$$\hat{\mathbf{j}}_t = (\mathbf{G}^T\boldsymbol{\Sigma}^{-1}\mathbf{G} + \bullet\,\mathbf{I})^{-1}\mathbf{G}^T\boldsymbol{\Sigma}^{-1}\mathbf{b}_t \qquad (17)$$

where the regularization parameter is $\bullet \propto \frac{1}{\bullet^2}$. Due to the Gaussian spatial prior, solutions provided by MNE tend to be rather smooth, a feature that makes MNE less suitable than other methods for estimating focal activity. Furthermore, another limitation of MNE is that the zero-mean Gaussian prior gives an implicit preference to superficial sources, which need lower intensity to produce the meaured field. This results in an estimation bias which is stronger for deeper sources. Despite these drawbacks, MNE is a very attractive method thanks to its simplicity and to the very low computational cost.

4.2 Static imaging methods - weighted MNE, LORETA and LCMV beamformer

The class of weighted minimum norm solutions has been developed with the aim of overcoming the depth bias introduced by the simple prior used by MNE. The main difference with respect to standard MNE is that the prior is still Gaussian but the source covariance matrix is no longer proportional to the identity matrix; instead, the source covariance matrix contains a weighting factor for each source, aimed at removing the bias towards superficial solutions. In Lin et al. (2006), for instance, the $3\mathcal{N}_{points} \times 3\mathcal{N}_{points}$ source covariance matrix $\mathbf{R}$ is diagonal with

$$\mathbf{R}_{j,j} = ||\mathbf{G}(\mathbf{r}^k)||^{-p}, j = 3k-2, 3k-1, 3k, \;\; k = 1, \ldots, \mathcal{N}_{points} \qquad (18)$$

where $\mathbf{G}(\mathbf{r}^k)$ is the lead field corresponding to the k-th source point, $||\cdot||$ is the euclidean norm and p is the depth weighting parameter. With this choice, deeper sources have a Gaussian prior with larger variance with respect to shallower sources. The final solution of WMNE is given by the two following equivalent formulations

$$\begin{aligned}\hat{\mathbf{j}}_t = &\quad \mathbf{R}\mathbf{G}^T(\mathbf{G}\mathbf{R}\mathbf{G}^T + \boldsymbol{\Sigma})^{-1}\mathbf{b}_t = \\ = &\; (\mathbf{G}^T\boldsymbol{\Sigma}^{-1}\mathbf{G} + \mathbf{R}^{-1})^{-1}\mathbf{G}^T\boldsymbol{\Sigma}^{-1}\mathbf{b}_t.\end{aligned} \qquad (19)$$

Low Resolution Electromagnetic Tomography (LORETA) (Pascual-Marqui et al., 1994) is a WMNE with the further addition of a Laplacian operator. The prior for LORETA is given by

$$\bullet\,(\mathbf{j}_t) \propto \exp\left(-\mathbf{j}_t^T\mathbf{R}^T\mathbf{L}^T\mathbf{L}\mathbf{R}\mathbf{j}_t\right) \qquad (20)$$

where $\mathbf{R}$ is as in (18) and $\mathbf{L}$ is the discrete spatial laplacian operator (Pascual-Marqui, 1999). Such operator $\mathbf{L}$ produces a smoother estimate of the current distribution since the inverse matrix $\mathbf{L}^{-1}$ implements a discrete spatial smoothing operator. LORETA has been shown to provide accurate localization even for deep sources.

The term *beamformer* encompasses a broad range of algorithms which have become popular in the last fifteen years. In one way or the other, most or all of them can be proved to be particular choices of WMNE (Mosher et al., 2003). Here we only consider the Linearly Constrained Minimum Variance Beamformer (Van Veen et al., 1997). The derivation of this method is made in an engineering framework and is based on a constrained minimization. The idea behind beamforming is that of constructing a spatial filter which isolates the activity produced in a selected location, blocking the activity originated elsewhere. The main working assumption of the method described in (Van Veen et al., 1997) is that all the sources are uncorrelated. The result of the constrained minimization turns out to be

$$\hat{\mathbf{j}}_t^k = \left[(\mathbf{G}(\mathbf{r}^k))^T \mathbf{R}_b^{-1} \mathbf{G}(\mathbf{r}^k)\right]^{-1} (\mathbf{G}(\mathbf{r}^k))^T (\mathbf{G}\mathbf{R}\mathbf{G}^T + \boldsymbol{\Sigma})^{-1} \mathbf{b}(t) \tag{21}$$

where $\mathbf{R}_b$ is the data covariance matrix and $\hat{\mathbf{j}}_t^k$ is the estimated current density at k-th location. We remark that this solution corresponds to the WMNE solution (19) if the source covariance matrix $\mathbf{R}$ is a block diagonal matrix, composed by the 3×3 matrices:

$$\mathbf{R}(\mathbf{r}^k) = \left[(\mathbf{G}(\mathbf{r}^k))^T \mathbf{R}_b^{-1} \mathbf{G}(\mathbf{r}^k)\right]^{-1} \tag{22}$$

and zero elsewhere. Importantly, the assumption that the neural sources are not correlated in time is a strong assumption, often not verified in experimental data. As a consequence of this assumption, however, beamformers face severe difficulties when the data actually contain signals produced by correlated sources. An improved version of the beamforming technique has been proposed, which tries to overcome this limitation (Sekihara et al., 2002).

4.3 Static imaging methods - dSPM and SLORETA

Dynamic Statistical Parametric Mapping (dSPM) and Standardized LORETA (sLORETA) combine Bayesian inference for the electrical current with noise normalization. The ouput of these methods is no longer an estimate of the neural current distribution, but rather a statistical measure of brain activity.

Instead of imaging the estimated electrical current intensity, dSPM (Dale et al., 2000) produces maps of the following neural activity index

$$z_t^k = \frac{||\hat{\mathbf{j}}_t^k||_2^2}{||(\mathbf{W}(\mathbf{r}^k))^T \boldsymbol{\Sigma} \mathbf{W}(\mathbf{r}^k)||_F^2} \tag{23}$$

where $\mathbf{W}(\mathbf{r}^k)$ is the regularized inverse operator in (19)

$$\mathbf{W}(\mathbf{r}^k) = (\mathbf{G}\mathbf{R}\mathbf{G}^T + \boldsymbol{\Sigma})^{-1} \mathbf{G}(\mathbf{r}^k) \mathbf{R}(\mathbf{r}^k) \tag{24}$$

$\boldsymbol{\Sigma}$ is the noise covariance matrix, and $||\cdot||_F$ is the Frobenius norm; in practice, the output of a weighted MNE $\hat{\mathbf{j}}_t$ at the k-th location is divided by an estimate of the portion of the source variance, at the same location, which is due to the noise in the data. Under the null hypothesis of zero brain activity, the resulting quantity z_t has a Student's t distribution.

sLORETA (Pascual-Marqui, 2002) consists in a similar approach, but the standardization is obtained considering the variance of the estimated sources (19), instead of using just the variance due to the noise component. SLORETA produces maps of the quantity

$$z_t^k = \frac{||\hat{\mathbf{j}}_t^k||_2^2}{||(\mathbf{W}(\mathbf{r}^k))^T(\mathbf{G}R\mathbf{G}^T + \mathbf{\Sigma})^{-1}\mathbf{W}(\mathbf{r}^k)||_F^2}. \tag{25}$$

The claim of the authors is that this method produces unbiased, zero-error localization of point sources. sLORETA is largely used in EEG source analysis, where source localization is made particularly difficult by the strongest impact of the passive currents on the measured data.

4.4 Static imaging methods - minimum current estimate

The MCE algorithm (Uutela et al. (1999)) is substantially different from all the imaging methods presented so far in that it does not use a Gaussian prior for the current distribution, but an exponential prior instead:

$$\bullet\,(\mathbf{j}_t) = \exp(-||\mathbf{j}_t||_1) \tag{26}$$

where $||\mathbf{j}_t||_1 = \sum_{k=1}^{3N_{points}} \left|\mathbf{j}_t^k\right|$.

This is usually phrased in the regularization framework as using an L^1 prior, and the main consequence of this choice is that sparsity of the solution is promoted, so that estimates provided by MCE are typically highly focused.

In contrast to the MNE, MCE is therefore well suited for estimating focal activity. As a drawback, it has been suggested that MCE is in fact not capable to recover smooth current distributions, always shrinking to few points the estimated active area. From a computational viewpoint, the minimization with the L1 norm cannot be expressed any more in a closed form. Linear programming algorithms can be used to solve the minimum problem, but the computational cost is remarkably higher compared to that of methods based on a Gaussian prior.

4.5 Dynamic imaging methods - L1L2 regularization

From the conceptual point of view, the L1L2 approach (Ou et al., 2009) consists in replacing the time-varying Random Vectors in equation (14) with the full random matrices containing the whole spatio-temporal pattern of the data and of the brain activity:

$$\mathbf{B} = \mathbf{G}\mathbf{J} + \mathbf{N} \tag{27}$$

where $\mathbf{B} = [\mathbf{B}_1, \ldots, \mathbf{B}_T]$, $\mathbf{J} = [\mathbf{J}_1, \ldots, \mathbf{J}_T]$ and $\mathbf{N} = [\mathbf{N}_1, \ldots, \mathbf{N}_T]$; the functional to be minimized is now

$$||\mathbf{B} - \mathbf{G}\mathbf{J}||_F^2 + ||\mathbf{J}||_2^1 \tag{28}$$

with

$$||\mathbf{J}||_2^1 = \sum_{k=1}^{3N_{points}} \sqrt{\sum_{t=1}^{T} (\mathbf{J}_t^k)^2}. \tag{29}$$

In Bayesian terms, this can be viewed as using a Gaussian prior distribution in time and a Laplacian prior distribution in space. This type of regularization promotes both sparsity in the spatial domain, in order to produce good estimates of focal sources, and smoothness in the temporal domain. From the computational viewpoint, this method is realized by means of a projection of the data and of the source space onto a subset of basis functions, to reduce the dimensionality; a gradient method is used to minimize the functional, i.e. to calculate the approximate MAP of the posterior distribution.

4.6 Dynamic imaging methods - Kalman filter

In Kalman filtering, one explicitely models the neural currents and the measurements as two stochastic processes, $\{\mathbf{J}_1, \ldots, \mathbf{J}_T\}$, $\{\mathbf{B}_1, \ldots, \mathbf{B}_T\}$. Under Markovian assumptions for these processes, the posterior distribution $\bullet\ (\mathbf{j}_t|\mathbf{b}_{1:t})$ can be computed at any time-point t applying sequentially the following two equations:

$$\bullet\ (\mathbf{j}_t|\mathbf{b}_{1:t-1}) = \int \bullet\ (\mathbf{j}_t|\mathbf{j}_{t-1}) \bullet\ (\mathbf{j}_{t-1}|\mathbf{b}_{1:t-1}) d\mathbf{j}_{t-1} \tag{30}$$

$$\bullet\ (\mathbf{j}_t|\mathbf{b}_{1:t}) = \frac{\bullet\ (\mathbf{b}_t|\mathbf{j}_t) \bullet\ (\mathbf{j}_t|\mathbf{b}_{1:t-1})}{\bullet\ (\mathbf{b}_t|\mathbf{b}_{1:t-1})} \tag{31}$$

where $\{\mathbf{b}_{1:t}\}$ denotes the set of measurements up to time t and $\bullet\ (\mathbf{j}_t|\mathbf{j}_{t-1})$ is the transition kernel wich describes the evolution of the neural currents in time. Under Gaussian noise, Gaussian prior assumptions, the posterior distribution remains Gaussian at any time point, and these two equations have closed form solution through the so-called Kalman filter: at every time point, the mean and the covariance matrix of the Gaussian distribution are updated. The main difference between this approach and all the previously described approaches is that here the data are analyzed in sequence. The solution at time t depends on all the past history of observations; the prior density in the Kalman filter is time dependent and is given by

$$\bullet\ (\mathbf{j}_{1:t}) = \bullet\ (\mathbf{j}_0) \prod_{n=0}^{t} \bullet\ (\mathbf{j}_{n+1}|\mathbf{j}_n). \tag{32}$$

The main practical issue in the application of a Kalman filter to the MEG inverse problem is that the Kalman filter requires to invert the source covariance matrix at each time step. In MEG, this covariance matrix is typically very large, being $3\mathcal{N}_{points} \times 3\mathcal{N}_{points}$. In Galka et al. (2004), the very high dimensional problem is decomposed in a collection of low dimensional problems, exploiting the local nature of the covariance matrix; in Long et al. (2006), a network of computers is instead used to solve the full problem.

5. Parametric methods

Parametric methods solve the non-linear inverse problem defined by

$$\mathbf{B}_t = \sum_{i=1}^{\mathcal{N}_{dipoles}} \mathbf{G}(\mathbf{R}_t^i)\mathbf{Q}_t^i + \mathbf{N}_t \tag{33}$$

where $\mathcal{N}_{dipoles}$ is the unknown number of active dipoles at time t, $\mathbf{R}_t^i$ and $\mathbf{Q}_t^i$ are the Random Vectors representing the location and the dipole moment of the i-th source at time t, respectively, and $\mathbf{G}(\mathbf{r})$ is the lead field of a unit dipole at location $\mathbf{r}$. Remarkably, the number of active dipoles is not expected to be higher than, say, ten; this implies that the number of unknowns in the parametric approach is considerably lower than the number of unknowns in the imaging approach. However, as already observed, the data depend now non-linearly on the parameters, namely, on the number of sources and on the source locations. This non-linearity causes in fact several problems if one attempts to solve the full problem. For this reason, several methods for dipole estimation work under two important assumptions: first that the number of sources is constant in time, and second that the source locations are fixed. Only recently, Bayesian methods have appeared which try to overcome these artificial constraints. The authors have personally developed one of these methods, namely particle filtering; to this method is devoted Section 6. In the present Section, we give a brief overview of the other main parametric methods.

5.1 Static parametric methods - dipole fitting

Dipole fitting is one of the oldest and most largely used methods for solving the MEG inverse problem. In dipole fitting, current dipoles are estimated one at a time, at fixed time points; the user typically chooses the best time point, the one at which the data exhibit a dipolar field pattern, and then starts a non-linear optimization algorithm - typically a Levemberg-Marquardt algorithm - which maximizes the likelihood for a single current dipole at that particular time point

$$\exp\left(-(\mathbf{b}_t - \mathbf{G}(\mathbf{r})\cdot\mathbf{q})^T\mathbf{\Sigma}^{-1}(\mathbf{b}_t - \mathbf{G}(\mathbf{r})\cdot\mathbf{q})\right) \tag{34}$$

$\mathbf{r}$ and $\mathbf{q}$ being the location and dipole moment of one single source. The single dipole fitting procedure is typically iterated, usually at different time points, until a satisfactory set of different dipoles is found. To produce an estimate of the temporal behaviour of the estimated sources, a multiple dipole model is constructed by combining the estimated dipole locations and - possibly - orientations; the dipole strengths are then estimated linearly from the data, by optimization of the likelihood

$$\exp\left[-\left(\mathbf{b}-\sum_{i=1}^{\mathcal{N}_{dipoles}}\mathbf{G}(\mathbf{r}^i)\cdot\mathbf{q}^i\right)^T\mathbf{\Sigma}^{-1}\left(\mathbf{b}-\sum_{i=1}^{\mathcal{N}_{dipoles}}\mathbf{G}(\mathbf{r}^i)\cdot\mathbf{q}^i\right)\right] \tag{35}$$

A key problem with dipole fitting is that it strongly relies on the personal experience of the person who performs the analysis; in some sense then, despite it never formally makes use of a prior density, it may be considered as a Bayesian method due to the strong prior embodied in the human experience. A second relevant problem of dipole fitting is that, involving decision making from the user, it is usually quite time consuming.

5.2 Static parametric methods - MUSIC and RAP-MUSIC

The Recursively Applied and Projected MUltiple SIgnal Classification (RAP MUSIC) algorithm is perhaps the most largely known method for automatic estimation of current dipoles from MEG data. It was first introduced in Mosher et al. (1992) and further developed in order to deal efficiently with correlated sources (Mosher & Leahy, 1999).

MUSIC is based on a simplified version of the model described in equation (33), as it assumes that the number of dipoles and their locations are fixed in time; thus the model becomes now

$$\mathbf{B}_t = \sum_{i=1}^{\mathcal{N}_{dipoles}}\mathbf{G}(\mathbf{R}^i)\mathbf{U}^i\cdot S_t^i + \mathbf{N}_t = \mathbf{A}\cdot\mathbf{S}_t + \mathbf{N}_t \tag{36}$$

where $\mathbf{A} = [\mathbf{G}(\mathbf{R}^1)\mathbf{U}^1, \ldots, \mathbf{G}(\mathbf{R}^{\mathcal{N}_{dipoles}})\mathbf{U}^{\mathcal{N}_{dipoles}}]$ is the field generated by $\mathcal{N}_{dipoles}$ dipoles with locations $\{\mathbf{R}^i\}$ and orientations$\{\mathbf{U}^i\}$; S_t^i is the strength of the i-th dipole and $\mathbf{S}_t = [S_t^1, \ldots, S_t^{\mathcal{N}_{dipoles}}]$ the amplitudes vector; the dipole moment is therefore $\mathbf{Q}^i = \mathbf{U}^i \cdot S^i$.
If one further assumes that the neural sources are not correlated, simple calculations yield for the data covariance matrix $\mathbf{R}_b$

$$\mathbf{R}_b = \mathbf{A}^T \mathbf{R}_s \mathbf{A} + \bullet^2_{noise} \mathbf{I} \tag{37}$$

where $\mathbf{R}_s$ is the covariance matrix of the sources. Due to the assumption of uncorrelated sources, the source covariance matrix has full rank, and the data covariance matrix contains $\hat{\mathcal{N}}_{dipoles}$ eigenvalues considerably larger than the others; this number represents an estimate of the number of dipoles.
Furthermore the corresponding eigenvectors span the so called signal subspace $\hat{\bullet}_s$ and an estimate of the unknown parameters $\{\mathbf{r}^i, \mathbf{u}^i\}$ is obtained by maximizing the subspace correlation (Golub & Loan, 1984) between the dipole field and the signal subspace:

$$subcorr(\mathbf{G}(\mathbf{r})\mathbf{u}, \hat{\bullet}_s). \tag{38}$$

Once the locations and orientations are estimated, the source amplitudes are found by a least square approach. A recursive procedure deals with the problem of local minima.
From a statistic view point it can be shown that the estimated parameters represent a Maximum Likelihood estimate of the Random Vector in the model (33) (Stoica & Nehorai, 1989).

5.3 Dynamic parametric methods - MCMC of current dipoles

A more recently proposed strategy for solving the parametric MEG problem is that of using Bayesian inference for approximating the posterior density in the parameter space (Jun et al., 2005). In these studies, the authors assume a fixed but unknown number of spatially stationary dipolar sources; the modeling parameters are then the Random Variable of the number of sources $\mathcal{N}_{dipoles}$ and the Random Vectors of the source locations $\mathbf{R} \in \mathbb{R}^{3\mathcal{N}_{dipoles}}$, of the source time courses $\mathbf{S} \in \mathbb{R}^{\mathcal{N}_{dipoles} \times T}$ and of the dipole orientations $\mathbf{U} \in \mathbb{R}^{3\mathcal{N}_{dipoles}}$. The authors seek an approximation of the posterior density through Bayes theorem (5):

$$\begin{aligned} \bullet\,(n_{dipoles}, \mathbf{r}, \mathbf{s}, \mathbf{u}|\mathbf{b}) = \\ \bullet\,(\mathbf{b}|n_{dipoles}, \mathbf{r}, \mathbf{s}, \mathbf{u})\bullet\,(\mathbf{u}|\mathbf{r}, n_{dipoles}) \times \\ \times \bullet\,(\mathbf{s}|n_{dipoles})\bullet\,(\mathbf{r}|n_{dipoles})\bullet\,(n_{dipoles}) \quad , \end{aligned} \tag{39}$$

where the probability distributions for the source parameters are (necessarily) conditioned on the number of sources. Uniform distributions are used for $\mathcal{N}_{dipoles}$, $\mathbf{U}$ and $\mathbf{R}$, while a Gaussian distribution is assumed for $\mathbf{S}$. In order to explore the high-dimensional posterior density, they resort to reversible jump Markov Chain Monte Carlo techniques after marginalization of the posterior density with respect to the noise covariance matrix and the source time courses. In Jun et al. (2006), the multi-dipole model is refined by introducing a source-dependent temporal activity window: in other words, each dipole is active only for a finite time interval, and is totally silent for the rest of the sequence, thus avoiding possible cross-talk phenomena. The implementation is again performed with a Reversible Jump Markov Chain Monte Carlo algorithm.

6. Highly Automated Dipole EStimation

In this section we present the formulation of the multi-dipole particle filter we have been developing in collaboration with our colleagues, and which we have published as an online open source code under the name of HADES (Highly Automated Dipole EStimation). The idea behind the method is that of using the Bayesian filtering equations (43)-(44) in a multi-dipole setting rather than in the imaging framework. In practice, the algorithm tracks in time the probability distribution of the dipole parameters; the main difficulties here are related to the non-linear dependence of the data on the dipole parameters, and on the necessity of estimating the number of dipoles as well. The particle filtering approach has been first proposed in a methodological paper, (Somersalo et al., 2003). In a subsequent set of publications, with our colleagues we have investigated the use of particle filtering for estimation of current dipoles from experimental MEG data (Sorrentino, 2010; Sorrentino et al., 2009), and compared particle filtering with other source estimation methods in Pascarella et al. (2010). Particle filtering has also been used to solve the EEG inverse problem in Antelis & Minguez (2010) and Mohseni et al. (2008); however, in these studies a simpler setting was used where the number of dipoles is fixed a priori.
The main advantages of the approach outlined below are that (i) it is a very general approach to multiple dipole modeling, as it explicitely allows the number of dipoles to be time varying and provides dynamically a posterior probability for the number of sources; (ii) it can be used online in real time, at least in principle, because data are processed in sequence and not as a whole.
In the following, we first describe the mechanism of the most basic particle filter; we then consider the practical modeling of multiple dipole with Random Finite Sets; we outline briefly the use of semi-analytic techniques, and eventually describe the open source software with Graphical User Interface for use of particle filtering.

6.1 Particle filtering

Bayesian filtering relies on Markovian assumptions for the data and the unkown processes: if $\mathbf{J}_t$ and $\mathbf{B}_t$ represent the neural current and the measured data at time t, respectively, these assumptions can be formulated in terms of conditional distributions, and amount to

$$\bullet\,(\mathbf{b}_t|\mathbf{j}_t, \mathbf{j}_{t-1}, \mathbf{j}_{t-2}, ..., \mathbf{j}_1) = \bullet\,(\mathbf{b}_t|\mathbf{j}_t) \tag{40}$$

$$\bullet\,(\mathbf{j}_t|\mathbf{j}_{t-1}, \mathbf{b}_{t-1}, ..., \mathbf{b}_1) = \bullet\,(\mathbf{j}_t|\mathbf{j}_{t-1}) \tag{41}$$

$$\bullet\,(\mathbf{j}_t|\mathbf{j}_{t-1}, ..., \mathbf{j}_1) = \bullet\,(\mathbf{j}_t|\mathbf{j}_{t-1}) \ . \tag{42}$$

Given these premises, and assuming knowledge of the two conditional distributions at the right hand side of (40)-(42), the posterior distribution at time t can be obtained from the posterior distribution at time $t-1$ with the two following equations

$$\bullet\,(\mathbf{j}_t|\mathbf{b}_{1:t-1}) = \int \bullet\,(\mathbf{j}_t|\mathbf{j}_{t-1}) \bullet\,(\mathbf{j}_{t-1}|\mathbf{b}_{1:t-1}) d\mathbf{j}_{t-1} \tag{43}$$

$$\bullet\,(\mathbf{j}_t|\mathbf{b}_{1:t}) = \frac{\bullet\,(\mathbf{b}_t|\mathbf{j}_t) \bullet\,(\mathbf{j}_t|\mathbf{b}_{1:t-1})}{\bullet\,(\mathbf{b}_t|\mathbf{b}_{1:t-1})} \ . \tag{44}$$

in (43) a prior density at time t is obtained by convolution of the posterior density at time $t-1$ with the transition kernel; in (44), the posterior density at time t is obtained by combining the prior with the likelihood in the standard Bayes theorem. In addition to the two conditional

distributions mentioned above, the density $\bullet\,(\mathbf{j}_0|\mathbf{b}_0) = \bullet\,(\mathbf{j}_0)$ at time $t = 0$ is needed for initialization.
Exact computation of these two equations is possible under rather restrictive assumptions, such as the ones leading to Kalman filtering and described in Section 4. For more general cases, such as the one considered here which involves a non-linear relationship between the data and the unkonwns, numerical techniques have to be used to get reasonable approximations of the posterior densities. Particle filters are one of the most used numerical techniques for solving this type of problems. They are basically a sequential Monte Carlo sampling technique. In their simplest form, the SIR (Sampling Importance Resampling) particle filter, they amount to sequential application of an importance sampling - resampling mechanism.
The main steps of the SIR particle filter are:

0 [initialization] draw $\mathcal{N}_{particles}$ sample points $\{\tilde{\mathbf{j}}_0^i\}_{i=1,\ldots,\mathcal{N}_{particles}}$ distributed according to $\bullet\,(\mathbf{j}_0|\mathbf{b}_0)$; the sampled points represent therefore an approximation of the initializing density:

$$\bullet\,(\mathbf{j}_0) \simeq \sum_{i=1}^{\mathcal{N}_{particles}} \frac{1}{\mathcal{N}_{particles}} \bullet (\mathbf{j}_0 - \tilde{\mathbf{j}}_0^i) \quad ; \tag{45}$$

1 [Evolution] for $t \geq 0$, let $\{\tilde{\mathbf{j}}_t^i\}_{i=1,\ldots,\mathcal{N}_{particles}}$ be a sample distributed according to $\bullet\,(\mathbf{j}_t|\mathbf{b}_{1:t})$; then exploiting the Chapman-Kolmogorov equation we may approximate the next prior probability density function as follows:

$$\bullet\,(\mathbf{j}_{t+1}|\mathbf{b}_{1:t}) = \int \bullet\,(\mathbf{j}_{t+1}|\mathbf{j}_t) \bullet\,(\mathbf{j}_t|\mathbf{b}_{1:t}) d\mathbf{j}_t \simeq$$

$$= \frac{1}{\mathcal{N}_{particles}} \sum_{i=1}^{\mathcal{N}_{particles}} \bullet\,(\mathbf{j}_{t+1}|\tilde{\mathbf{j}}_t^i) \quad ; \tag{46}$$

sample the so obtained prior density, by drawing a single particle $\mathbf{j}_{t+1}^i$ from $\bullet\,(\mathbf{j}_{t+1}|\tilde{\mathbf{j}}_t^i)$ for each i; we have now an approximation of the prior at time $t+1$:

$$\bullet\,(\mathbf{j}_{t+1}|\mathbf{b}_{1:t}) \simeq \sum_{i=1}^{\mathcal{N}_{particles}} \frac{1}{\mathcal{N}_{particles}} \bullet (\mathbf{j}_{t+1} - \mathbf{j}_{t+1}^i) \quad ; \tag{47}$$

2 [Observation] apply the Bayes theorem, i.e. compute the relative weights of the particles:

$$w_{t+1}^i = \bullet\,(\mathbf{b}_{t+1}|\mathbf{j}_{t+1}^i) \quad , \tag{48}$$

and then normalize the weights so that $\sum_{i=1}^{\mathcal{N}_{particles}} w_{t+1}^i = 1$; an approximation to the posterior probability density function is given by

$$\bullet\,(\mathbf{j}_{t+1}|\mathbf{b}_{1:t+1}) \simeq \sum_{i=1}^{\mathcal{N}_{particles}} w_{t+1}^i \bullet (\mathbf{j}_{t+1} - \mathbf{j}_{t+1}^i) \quad ; \tag{49}$$

3 [Resampling] resample the sample set representing the posterior density: extract a new set of particles $\{\tilde{\mathbf{j}}^i_{t+1}\}_{i=1}^{\mathcal{N}_{particles}}$ from the old set $\{\mathbf{j}^i_{t+1}\}_{i=1}^{\mathcal{N}_{particles}}$, in such a way that the probability of drawing the i-th particle is w^i_{t+1} (see Arulampalam et al. (2002) for the details); we get

$$\bullet\,(\mathbf{j}_{t+1}|\mathbf{b}_{1:t+1}) \simeq \sum_{i=1}^{\mathcal{N}_{particles}} \frac{1}{\mathcal{N}_{particles}} \bullet(\mathbf{j}_{t+1} - \tilde{\mathbf{j}}^i_{t+1}) \quad ; \tag{50}$$

go to Step 1.

Remarkably, the combination of Step 1 and 2 can be viewed as an importance sampling.

6.2 Filtering of multiple dipoles with Random Finite Sets

In order to deal with a time-varying and unknown number of sources, in Sorrentino et al. (2009) we have proposed the use of Random Finite Sets as a mathematical tool to model the neural current.

Random Finite Sets (Molchanov, 2005) are generalizations of Random Vectors to a non-fixed dimension case. As the name suggests, realizations of a Random Finite Set are sets containing a random number of random objects. The use of Random Finite Sets for multiple target tracking has been proposed in (Mahler, 2003) for the first time.

In the RFS approach to the MEG problem, the neural current at time t is assumed to be a RFS of current dipoles, denoted by $\mathcal{J}_t = \{\mathbf{D}_{,..,}\mathbf{D}_t^{N_t}\}$, where each $\mathbf{D}^i_t$ is a Random Vector containing the parameters of a single current dipole and the Random Variable N_t represents the number of sources at time t. A realization of $\mathcal{J}_t$ will be denoted as J_t. The model now amounts to:

$$\mathcal{J}_{t+1} = \mathcal{E}(\mathcal{J}_t) \cup \mathcal{B}_{t+1} \tag{51}$$

$$\mathbf{B}_t = \mathbf{B}(\mathcal{J}_t) + W_t \quad . \tag{52}$$

In (51), the dipole set at time $t+1$ is given by the union of the set $\mathcal{E}(\mathcal{J}_t)$, containing the subset of dipoles active at time t which have survived and evolved, and the set of new born dipoles $\mathcal{B}_{t+1}$. In (52), the Random Finite Set of dipoles $\mathcal{J}_t$ produces the data; since the dimension of the data vector is fixed to the number of sensors in the MEG device, the data is represented as a standard Random Vector.

Despite the formulation in terms of Random Finite Sets, single dipole probabilities can be used to describe most of the models as long as individual dipoles are assumed to behave independently on each other . In the following we describe the main features of the model in terms of single dipole probability density functions.

6.2.1 Initializing density

HADES adopts an uninformative initializing density for the multi-dipole states. Let $\bullet_{max}$ be the maximum number of dipoles in a RFS (which we need to fix for computational reasons); then the prior probability of different models is uniform, P$(n_0) = 1/\,(\bullet_{max}+1)$ for $n_0 = 0,...,\bullet_{max}$. Dipoles are assumed to be independent and identically distributed with the same density used for the single-dipole case; the probability density function of each dipole $\mathbf{D}_0 \in \mathcal{J}_0$ is

$$\bullet\,(\mathbf{d}_0|\mathbf{b}_0) \propto \frac{1}{V} \times \exp\left(-\mathbf{q}_0^T \Xi \mathbf{q}_0\right) \tag{53}$$

where we have defined separately the uniform density for the dipole location in the volume V and the zero-mean Gaussian density with covariance matrix Ξ for the dipole moment.

6.2.2 Likelihood function

Due to the linearity of the Biot-Savart equation, the magnetic field produced by a set of sources is given by the linear combination of the magnetic fields produced by the individual dipoles contained in the set. If we denote by $\mathbf{b}(J_t)$ the magnetic measurement produced by the dipole set J_t, under the standard assumption of additive white Gaussian noise, with covariance matrix $\mathbf{\Sigma}$, the likelihood function is

$$\bullet\,(\mathbf{b}_t|J_t) \propto \exp\left(-[\mathbf{b}_t - \mathbf{b}(J_t)]^T\mathbf{\Sigma}^{-1}[\mathbf{b}_t - \mathbf{b}(J_t)]\right) \ . \tag{54}$$

6.2.3 Transition kernel

Lack of knowledge on the true dynamics of the neural sources is coded in a transition kernel based on the random walk. The transition probabilities between sets with different number of dipoles are uniform. The evolution of a dipole set containing n dipoles at time t is governed by the following rules:

- the probability that the dipole set contains n dipoles at time $t+1$ is 1/ 3; the probability that it contains $n+1$ dipoles is 1/ 3; the probability that it contains $n-1$ dipoles is 1/ 3;
- if the dipole set at time $t+1$ contains $n-1$ dipoles, the dipole to be removed is selected randomly from the set;
- if the dipole set at time $t+1$ contains $n+1$ dipoles, the new dipole is drawn from the same distribution of the initializing prior, eq. (53);
- all the surviving dipoles of a dipole set evolve independently according to the single-dipole transition kernel:

$$\bullet\,(\mathbf{d}_{t+1}|\mathbf{d}_t) \propto \mathcal{I}_{B(\mathbf{r}_t)}(\mathbf{r}_{t+1}) \times \exp - \left([\mathbf{q}_{t+1} - \mathbf{q}_t]^T \Xi_{\bullet}^{-1}[\mathbf{q}_{t+1} - \mathbf{q}_t]\right) \ . \tag{55}$$

  where $\mathcal{I}_{B(\mathbf{r})}(\cdot)$ is the indicator function of a ball with center in $\mathbf{r}$ and $\Xi_{\bullet}$ is the covariance matrix for the Gaussian random walk.

6.2.4 Source estimates

Point estimates of the dipole parameters are provided in a three-step automatic procedure. First, the number of sources is estimated from the marginal distribution

$$\mathrm{P}(|J_t| = k) = \int_{S(k)} \bullet\,(J_t|\mathbf{b}_{1:t})\bullet J_t \ , \tag{56}$$

where $S(k)$ is the set of all subsets with k elements; the maximum of the marginal distribution can be used as an estimator:

$$\hat{n}_t = \arg\max_k \mathrm{P}(|J_t| = k) \ . \tag{57}$$

Second, source locations are estimated as the maxima of the marginal quantity often referred to as Probability Hypothesis Density (PHD) in the RFS framework. The PHD is defined as

$$PHD(\mathbf{d}_t) = \int \bullet\,(\{\mathbf{d}_t\} \cup Y)\bullet Y \ , \tag{58}$$

where the integral is a set integral, $\{\mathbf{d}_t\}$ is a single-dipole set and $\bullet\,(\cdot)$ is the probability density function of the Random Finite Set $\mathcal{J}_t$. In a particle filter implementation, the PHD can be approximated by

$$PHD(\mathbf{d}_t) = \sum_{i=1}^{\mathcal{N}_{particles}} w_t^i \left(\sum_{\mathbf{d} \in J_t^i} \bullet (\mathbf{d} - \mathbf{d}_t) \right) \quad . \tag{59}$$

The PHD can also be viewed as the intensity measure of a point process.
Third and last step, once the dipole locations have been estimated the dipole moments are estimated with a linear least squares.

6.3 Rao-Blackwellization

The SIR particle filter described in the previous subsection is very general as it allows approximation of non-Gaussian densities which arise due to the non-linear dependence between the data and the parameters. However, in the MEG case such non-linearity is limited to the parameters describing the location of the sources; on the other hand, the data depend linearly on the dipole moment; this linearity can be in fact exploited using a technique known as Rao-Blackwellization. The main idea is that the posterior density can be split (Campi et al. (2008))

$$\bullet\ (\mathbf{r}_t, \mathbf{q}_t | \mathbf{b}_{1:t}) = \bullet\ (\mathbf{q}_t | \mathbf{r}_t, \mathbf{b}_{1:t}) \bullet\ (\mathbf{r}_t | \mathbf{b}_{1:t}) \tag{60}$$

At the right hand side, the density for $\mathbf{q}_t$ $\bullet$ $(\mathbf{q}_t | \mathbf{r}_t, \mathbf{b}_{1:t})$ conditional on $\mathbf{r}_t$ is a Gaussian density, whose parameters can be tracked with a Kalman filter; on the other hand, the locations parameters must be sampled, which leads to an algorithm that realizes a set of Kalman filters for the dipole moment, one for each sampled location.

6.3.1 Clustering

Due to its dynamic nature, the particle filter described above tends to provide slightly moving estimates of static dipoles. In order to produce a compact description of the estimated dipoles, it can be useful to apply a clustering algorithm to the whole set of estimated dipoles $\{\hat{\mathbf{d}}_1^1, ..., \hat{\mathbf{d}}_1^{\hat{n}_1}, ..., \hat{\mathbf{d}}_t^1, ..., \hat{\mathbf{d}}_t^{\hat{n}_t}\}$. In Sorrentino et al. (2009) we have applied an iterative algorithm based on the k-means (Spath, 1980) to obtain a small set of neural sources. The iterations are needed because the number of clusters is unknown, while the k-means works with a fixed number of clusters: hence, we first cluster the dipoles in a large number of clusters $\mathcal{N}_{clusters}$; then apply the Wilcoxon test (Weerahandi, 1995) and check whether all clusters are significantly diverse; if not, we set $\mathcal{N}_{clusters} = \mathcal{N}_{clusters} - 1$ and try again the clustering procedure; if they are all diverse, the algorithm stops. A similar idea, implemented in a more sophisticated strategy, has been proposed in Clark & Bell (2007).

6.4 HADES

The particle filter described above has been implemented in Matlab, and is currently distributed with a Graphical User Interface, named HADES (Highly Automated Dipole EStimation) (Campi et al. (2011)). The software can be downloaded from http://hades.dima.unige.it. The software is open source and is released under the standard GPL license. Through the MNE toolbox (http://www.nmr.mgh.harvard.edu/martinos/userInfo/data/MNE register/index.php) it supports input/output in Neuromag *.fif*, FreeSurfer *.w* and MNE *.stc* formats, further than the standard Matlab *.mat* format.

7. Conclusion

Localization of brain activity from MEG recordings is a challenging problem which has been solved in a variety of frameworks and using many different algorithms. In this Chapter we have attempted a short review of some of these methods, the ones which seem to be most used in the MEG community, with the aim of describing them in the unifying framework offered by statistics. Interestingly, when described in such framework some clear connections between many of these methods appear naturally. Indeed, it emerges clearly from this review that the only difference between most of these methods, except for the type of source model, relies in the choice of the prior density. It also emerges that the main difference between more recent and previously developed methods is that the recent methods tend to exploit the dynamic nature of the inverse problem by performing regularization in the whole spatio-temporal domain; in statistical terms, this corresponds to providing a priori information on the temporal behaviour of the sources in addition to the a priori information on the spatial distribution. Among these new dynamic methods, we have given particular emphasis to the description of HADES, the multi-dipole particle filter we have been developing in collaboration with our colleagues. We look forward to see how far this new generation of spatio-temporal solvers can reach, and what the next generation will be.

8. Acknowledgements

AS has been supported by the European Union Seventh Framework Programme (FP7/ 2007-2013) under the grant agreement PIEF-GA-2009-252440.

9. References

Antelis, J. & Minguez, J. (2010). DYNAMO: dynamic multi-model source localization method for EEG and/ or MEG, *IEEE Engineering in Medicine and Biology Society Conference Proceedings*, pp. 5141–5144.

Arulampalam, M., Maskell, S., Gordon, N. & Clapp, T. (2002). A tutorial on particle filters for online nonlinear/ non-gaussian bayesian tracking, *IEEE Transactions on Signal Processing* 50(2): 174–188.

Bertero, M. & Boccacci, P. (1998). *Introduction to inverse problems in imaging*, IoP, Institute of Physics Publishing.

Campi, C., Pascarella, A., Sorrentino, A. & Piana, M. (2008). A rao-blackwellized particle filter for magnetoencephalography, *Inverse Problems* 24: 025023.

Campi, C., Pascarella, A., Sorrentino, A. & Piana, M. (2011). Highly automated dipole estimation, *Computational Intelligence and Neuroscience* 2011: 982185.

Cantarella, J., Turck, D. D. & Gluck, H. (2001). The biot - savart operator for application to knot theory, fluid dynamics, and plasma physics, *Journal of Mathematical Physics* 42: 876–905.

Clark, D. & Bell, J. (2007). Multi-target state estimation and track continuity for the particle PHD filter, *IEEE Transactions on Aerospace and Electronic Systems* 43: 1441–1453.

Dale, A., Liu, A., Fischl, B., Buckner, R., Belliveau, J., Lewine, J. & Halgren, E. (2000). Dynamic statistical parametric mapping: Combining fmri and meg for high-resolution imaging of cortical activity, *Neuron* 26: 55–67.

Galka, A., Yamashita, O., Ozaki, T., Biscay, R. & Valdes-Sosa, P. (2004). A solution to the dynamical inverse problem of eeg generation using spatiotemporal kalman filtering, *NeuroImage* 23: 435–453.

Golub, G. & Loan, C. V. (1984). *Matrix Computation*, The Johns Hopkins University Press.
Gramfort, A., Papadopoulo, T., Olivi, E. & Clerc, M. (2011). Forward field computation with openmeeg, *Computational Intelligence and Neuroscience* 2011: 923703.
Hämäläinen, M., Hari, R., Knuutila, J. & Lounasmaa, O. (1993). Magnetoencephalography: theory, instrumentation and applications to non-invasive studies of the working human brain, *Reviews of Modern Physics* 65: 413–498.
Hämäläinen, M. & Ilmoniemi, R. (1984). Interpreting measured magnetic fields of the brain: estimates of current distributions.
Jun, S., George, J., Paré-Blagoev, J., Plis, S., Ranken, D., Schmidt, D. & Wood, C. (2005). Spatiotemporal bayesian inference dipole analysis for MEG neuroimaging data, *NeuroImage* 28: 84–98.
Jun, S., George, J., Plis, S., Ranken, D., Schmidt, D. & Wood, C. (2006). Improving source detection and separation in a spatiotemporal bayesian inference dipole analysis, *Physics in Medicine and Biology* 51: 2395–2414.
Kress, R., Kuhn, L. & Potthast, R. (2002). Reconstruction of a current distribution from its magnetic field, *Inverse Problems* 18: 1127–1146.
Lin, F., Witzel, T., Ahlfors, S., Stufflebeam, S., Belliveau, J. & Hamalainen, M. (2006). Assessing and improving the spatial accuracy in MEG source localization by depth-weighted minimum-norm estimates, *NeuroImage* 31: 160–171.
Long, C., Purdon, P., Temeranca, S., Desai, N., Hämäläinen, M. & Brown, E. (2006). Large scale kalman filtering solutions to the electrophysiological source localization problem - a meg case study, *Proceedings of the 28thIEEE EMBS Annual International Conference*, Vol. 5, pp. 4532–4535.
Mahler, R. (2003). Multitarget bayes filtering via first-order multitarget moments, *IEEE Transactions on Aerospace and Electronic Systems* 39: 1152–1178.
Mohseni, H., Wilding, E. & Sanei, S. (2008). Sequential monte carlo techniques for EEG dipole placing and tracking, *2008 IEEE Sensor array and multichannel signal processing workshop*, pp. 95–98.
Molchanov, I. (2005). *Theory of Random Sets*, Springer-Verlag.
Mosher, J., Baillet, S. & Leahy, R. (2003). Equivalence of linear approaches in bioelectromagnetic inverse solutions, *2003 IEEE Workshop on Statistical Signal Processing* pp. 294–297.
Mosher, J. & Leahy, R. (1999). Source localization using Recursively Applied and Projected (RAP) MUSIC, *IEEE Transactions on Signal Processing* 47: 332–340.
Mosher, J., Lewis, P. & Leahy, R. (1992). Multiple dipole modeling and localization from spatio-temporal MEG data, *IEEE Transactions on Biomedical Engineering* 39: 541–557.
Ou, W., Hämäläinen, M. & Golland, P. (2009). A distributed spatio-temporal EEG/MEG inverse solver, *NeuroImage* 44: 932–946.
Pascarella, A., Sorrentino, A., Campi, C. & Piana, M. (2010). Particle filtering, beamforming and rap-music in the analysis of magnetoencephalography time series: a comparison of algorithms, *Inverse Problems and Imaging* 4: 169–190.
Pascual-Marqui, R. (1999). Review of methods for solving the eeg inverse problem, *Int. J. Bioelectromagnetism* 1: 75–86.
Pascual-Marqui, R. (2002). Standardize low resolution electromagnetic tomography (sLORETA: technical details, *Methods and Findings in Experimental and Clinical Pharmacology* 24: 5–12.

Pascual-Marqui, R., C.Michel & D.Lehman (1994). Low resolution electromagnetic tomography: A new method for localizing electrical activity in the brain, *Int. J. Psycophysiol.* 18: 49–65.

Pursiainen, S., Sorrentino, A., Campi, C. & Piana, M. (2011). Forward simulation and inverse dipole localization with lowest order Raviart-Thomas elements for electroencephalography, *Inverse Problems* p. in press.

Sarvas, J. (1987). Basic mathematical and electromagnetic concepts of the biomagnetic inverse problem, *Phys. Med. Biol.* 32: 11–22.

Sekihara, K., Nagarajan, S., Poeppel, D. & Marantz, A. (2002). Performance of an meg adaptive beamformer technique in the presence of correlated neural activities: effects on signal intensity and time course estimates, *IEEE Transactions on Biomedical Engineering* 49: 1534–1546.

Somersalo, E., Voutilainen, A. & Kaipio, J. (2003). Non-stationary magnetoencephalography by bayesian filtering of dipole models, *Inverse Problems* 19: 1047–1063.

Sorrentino, A. (2010). Particle Filters for Magnetoencephalography, *Archives of Computational Methods in Engineering* 17: 213–251.

Sorrentino, A., Parkkonen, L., Pascarella, A., Campi, C. & Piana, M. (2009). Dynamical MEG source modeling with multi-target bayesian filtering, *Human Brain Mapping* 30: 1911–1921.

Spath, H. (1980). *Cluster Analysis Algorithms for Data Reduction and Classification of Objects*, Halsted Press.

Stoica, P. & Nehorai, A. (1989). MUSIC, Maximum Likelihood and Cramer-Rao bound, *IEEE Transactions on acoustics, speech and signal processing* 37: 720–741.

Uutela, K., Hämäläinen, M. & Somersalo, E. (1999). Visualization of magnetoencephalographic data using minimum current estimates, *NeuroImage* 10: 173–180.

Van Veen, B., van Drongelen, W., Yuchtman, M. & Suzuki, A. (1997). Localization of brain electrical activity via linearly constrained minimum variance spatial filtering, *IEEE Transactions on Biomedical Engineering* 44: 867–880.

Weerahandi, S. (1995). *Exact Statistical Methods for Data Analysis*, Springer-Verlag, New York.

6

An Explicit Method for Inverse Reconstruction of Equivalent Current Dipoles and Quadrupoles

Takaaki Nara
The University of Electro-Communications
Japan

1. Introduction

The purpose of the neuromagnetic inverse problem is to reconstruct primary neural current from measured MEG data. It is known that this inverse problem is ill-posed: uniqueness of the solution to the inverse problem is not guaranteed without *a priori* assumptions on the current source (Fokas et al. (2004)), and, even when using the source model that can be uniquely reconstructed, the obtained solution changes very sensitively depending on the noise contained in MEG data. Thus, employment of a stable algorithm is highly required in order that MEG becomes a non-invasive brain monitoring tool with not only high temporal resolution but also high spatial resolution.

Basically, conventional methods are categorized into two groups: parametric approaches and imaging approaches. See the detailed list of references in Baillet et al. (2001). The former methods assume that the current source can be represented by a relatively small number of equivalent current dipoles (ECDs). This source model is shown to be uniquely reconstructed from radial MEG data, except the radial component of the dipole moment, when the head is assumed to consist of concentric spheres. The usual algorithm for this source model is the non-linear least-squares method that minimizes the squared error of data and the forward solution. An advantage of this algorithm is that the parametric description allows us the accurate estimation of the center position of the activated region. However, the problems of this algorithm are: 1) it requires an initial solution, 2) it requires an iterative computing of forward solution, 3) it is often trapped by the local minimum of the cost function, which gives a solution far from the true one, 4) estimation of the number of ECDs is difficult, and 5) spatial extent of the source is not considered.

The second methods, imaging approaches, assume that there exist current dipoles at the nodes of artificial meshes on the cerebral surface, and solve a system of linear equations for the dipole moments at the fixed positions. An advantage of this method is that it can describe the spatial distribution of the neural current. However, the problems of this algorithm are: 1) the solution is not unique, 2) adding a regularization term often gives a unique but over-smoothed solution, 3) choice of the regularization parameters strongly affects the solution.

Recently, a method with the multipolar representation of the source has been developed that incorporates some of the advantages of the above two methods, and has attracted considerable attention (Irimia et al. (2009); Jerbi et al. (2002; 2004); Nara (2008a); Nolte et al. (1997; 2000)). In this model, instead of expressing the current source by an equivalent current dipole, an equivalent dipole and quadrupole (Jerbi et al. (2002; 2004)) or an equivalent dipole and octopole (Nolte et al. (1997; 2000)) are used where the quadrupole or octopole is determined depending on the spatial extent of the support of the current source. Jerbi et al. (2004) showed that the centroid of the spatially distributed source, which they called a patch source, can be estimated more accurately using the dipole and quadrupole model than using the dipole model by means of the nonlinear least squares method. We considered a two-dimensional (2D) problem using a complex analysis framework and proposed an explicit method to reconstruct the dipole and quadrupole parameters directly from the boundary measurements of the meromorphic function (Nara (2008a)). In Nara (2008b), we proposed an explicit method for 3D case when the dipoles were distributed in a plane parallel to the xy-plane.

The aim of this chapter is to describe explicit methods for the equivalent current dipole model and the equivalent current dipole-quadrupole model in Nara et al. (2007), Nara (2008a), and Nara (2008b) and compare them using numerical simulations. Here, the term 'explicit' means that we have an analytic and explicit form of the solution to the inverse problem. As a consequence, the explicit method for the ECD model can resolve the problems 1)-4) in the parametric approach with the conventional, non-linear least-squares method listed above. That is, without an initial solution and iterative computation of forward solution, the algorithm can reconstruct the ECD parameters. The number of the ECDs can be also estimated. With the explicit reconstruction formula, the sensitivity analysis can be conducted in which the estimation error is evaluated with the noise level. From a practical viewpoint, the solution obtained by the explicit method can be used as a good initial solution close to the true one for the iterative non-linear squares methods. Moreover, in order to resolve the problem 5) in the parametric approach, we show an explicit method for the dipole-quadrupole source model.

The rest of this chapter is organized as follows. In section 2, we introduce the equivalent current dipole and quadrupole source model, and show how it expresses the spatial extent of the current source. In section 3, an explicit method is shown: subsection 3.1 describes an algorithm for the equivalent current dipole model, whereas subsection 3.2 explains a method for the equivalent current dipole-quadrupole source model. In section 4, both the algorithms are compared with numerical simulations.

2. Problem setting

In this chapter, we explain our explicit algorithm using the spherical head model. Let $\Omega_1, \Omega_2, \Omega_3$ and Ω_4 be concentric balls centered at the origin in 3D space, where $\Omega_i \subset \Omega_{i+1}$ for $i = 1, 2, 3$. Here, Ω_1, Ω_2/Ω_1, and Ω_3/Ω_2, represent the brain, skull, and scalp, respectively. Ω_3 represents the head. We assume that the radial component of the magnetic field is measured on the sphere $\Gamma = \bullet\Omega_4$ with the radius of R. Although we use this simple head model as well as the spherical sensor surface, the method can be extended to a more realistic case when the head is modeled by a piecewise homogeneous layered domain and the sensors are set on an arbitrarily shaped surface (Nara et al. (2007)).

Let us assume that the neural current J_p is supported on several domains $D_k(\subset \Omega_1)$ for $k = 1, 2, \cdots, N$. The 'center' position of D_k is denoted by $\boldsymbol{r}_k = (x_k, y_k, z_k)^T$; this is the main parameter to be reconstructed. We express this source equivalently by the current dipoles and quadrupoles:

$$J_p = \sum_{k=1}^{N} p_k \bullet (r - r_k) + \sum_{k=1}^{N} Q_k \nabla \bullet (r - r_k), \tag{1}$$

where

$$p_k \equiv \int_{D_k} J_p(r')dv'$$

is the equivalent current dipole for the source in D_k, and

$$Q_k \equiv \int_{D_k} J_p(r')(r' - r_k)dv' = \begin{pmatrix} q_{xx,k} & q_{xy,k} & q_{xz,k} \\ q_{yx,k} & q_{yy,k} & q_{yz,k} \\ q_{zx,k} & q_{zy,k} & q_{zz,k} \end{pmatrix}$$

is the equivalent current quadrupole for the source in D_k. Note here that p_k does not depend on the size of D_k, while Q_k depends on the spatial extent of J_p around r_k in D_k. Q_k is a 3×3 tensor of order 2 and is called the quadrupole moment tensor.

In this chapter, we assume that Q_k are of the form

$$\begin{pmatrix} q_{xx,k} & q_{xy,k} & 0 \\ q_{yx,k} & q_{yy,k} & 0 \\ 0 & 0 & 0 \end{pmatrix}.$$

In other words, the quadrupoles are parallel to the xy-plane. Extention to general case where all the components of Q_k are not zero is an important aspect of further studies.

The validity of the source model (1) is confirmed as follows. Substituting Eq. (1) into the expression of radial MEG given by the Biot–Savart law

$$r \cdot B(r) = \frac{\bullet_0}{4\bullet} \int_{\Omega_1} \left(\nabla' \frac{1}{|r - r'|} \times r \right) \cdot J_p(r')dv', \tag{2}$$

where $\bullet_0$ is the magnetic permeability assumed to be constant in the whole space, we have

$$r \cdot B(r) = \frac{\bullet_0}{4\bullet} \sum_{k=1}^{N} \left(\frac{(r_k \times p_k) \cdot (r - r_k)}{|r - r_k|^3} + Q_k : \frac{3(r \times r_k)(r - r_k) + |r - r_k|^2 X_r}{|r - r_k|^5} \right). \tag{3}$$

Here, ':' represents the tensor contraction defined by $A : B = \sum_{i=1}^{3} \sum_{j=1}^{3} A_{ij} B_{ij}$ for second order tensors A and B whose (i, j) components are given by A_{ij} and B_{ij}, respectively, and X_r is the cross product tensor defined by

$$X_r a = r \times a,$$

and hence is written as

$$X_r = \begin{pmatrix} 0 & -z & y \\ z & 0 & -x \\ -y & x & 0 \end{pmatrix} \quad \text{for} \quad r = (x, y, z)^T.$$

See Appendix for derivation of Eq. (3). Eq. (3) was given in Eq. (46) in Jerbi et al. (2002) (when $N = 1$), which was obtained by truncating the Taylor series expansion of radial MEG, up to the secondly dominant terms, generated by $\boldsymbol{J}_p$ with spatial extent. The first term in Eq. (3) is the magnetic field created by the equivalent current dipole $\boldsymbol{p}_k$, and the second term is the magnetic field created by the equivalent current quadrupole Q_k. Hence we call Eq. (1) the equivalent current dipole-quadrupole source model.
Using this source model (1), our inverse problem is formulated as follows: reconstruct $\boldsymbol{r}_k, \boldsymbol{p}_k, Q_k$ and N from radial MEG data on Γ. Since estimation of $\boldsymbol{p}_k$ and Q_k is a linear problem if $\boldsymbol{r}_k$ and N are determined, we restrict our interest in this chapter to estimation of $\boldsymbol{r}_k$ and N.

3. Explicit method

In this section, we show an explicit method for the source model (1). In subsection 3.1, a method for the dipole source model (when $Q_k = 0$) is shown. An algorithm for the dipole-quadrupole source model is described in subsection 3.2.
Both the algorithms are based on the multipole expansion of radial MEG: Eq. (2) can be expressed by the multipole expansion

$$\boldsymbol{r} \cdot \boldsymbol{B}(\boldsymbol{r}) = \bullet_0 \sum_{l=0}^{\infty} \sum_{m=-l}^{l} \frac{l+1}{2l+1} M_{lm} \frac{\hat{Y}^*_{lm}(\bullet, \bullet)}{r^{l+1}},$$

where

$$\hat{Y}_{lm}(\bullet, \bullet) = \sqrt{\frac{2l+1}{4\bullet} \frac{(l-m)!}{(l+m)!}} Y_{lm}(\bullet, \bullet) \quad : \text{normalized spherical harmonics},$$

$$Y_{lm}(\bullet, \bullet) = P_l^m(\cos \bullet) e^{im\bullet} \quad : \text{spherical harmonics},$$

and $P_l^m(\cos \bullet)$ are the associated Legendre polynomials. As shown in Eq. (84) in Jerbi et al. (2002), the multipole moment has the following relationship with $\boldsymbol{J}_p$:

$$M_{lm} = \frac{1}{l+1} \int_{\Omega_1} [\nabla' r'^l \hat{Y}_{lm}(\bullet', \bullet')] \cdot \left(\boldsymbol{r}' \times \boldsymbol{J}_p(\boldsymbol{r}')\right) d^3 r'. \tag{4}$$

Substituting Eq. (1) into Eq. (4) and using Eq. (17) gives

$$M_{lm} = \frac{1}{l+1} \sum_{k=1}^{N} \Bigg(\nabla' r'^l \hat{Y}_{lm}(\bullet', \bullet')|_{\boldsymbol{r}'=\boldsymbol{r}_k} \cdot (\boldsymbol{r}_k \times \boldsymbol{p}_k)$$
$$+ Q_k : \left(\nabla'(\nabla' r'^l \hat{Y}_{lm}(\bullet', \bullet') \times \boldsymbol{r}')\right)^T |_{\boldsymbol{r}'=\boldsymbol{r}_k} \Bigg). \tag{5}$$

On the other hand, using the orthogonality of the spherical harmonics, the multipole moment is shown to have another relationship with the radial magnetic field on a spherical surface Γ (Alvarez (1991)):

$$M_{lm} = \frac{2l+1}{\bullet_0 (l+1)} \int_\Gamma \boldsymbol{n}' \cdot \boldsymbol{B}(\boldsymbol{r}') R^l \hat{Y}_{lm}(\bullet', \bullet') dS', \tag{6}$$

where n' is the outward unit normal vector at r' on Γ. Equating Eqs. (5) and (6) for $l \geq m \geq 0$ gives algebraic equations

$$\sum_{k=1}^{N}\left(\nabla' r'^{l}\hat{Y}_{lm}(\bullet',\bullet')\big|_{r'=r_k}\cdot(r_k \times p_k) + Q_k : (\nabla'(\nabla' r'^{l}\hat{Y}_{lm}(\bullet',\bullet') \times r'))^{T}\big|_{r'=r_k}\right)$$
$$= \frac{2l+1}{\bullet_0}\int_{\Gamma} n' \cdot B(r') R^{l}\hat{Y}_{lm}(\bullet',\bullet')dS' \quad (7)$$

relating the unknown parameters of the sources to the radial MEG data.

3.1 Explicit method for the equivalent current dipoles

First, we describe an explicit algorithm for the equivalent current dipole source model ($Q_k = 0$). Let us consider Eqs. (7) for $l = m$, which are called 'sectorial harmonics' components. Since in this case it holds that (Hobson (1931))

$$r^{m}Y_{mm}(\bullet,\bullet) = (2m-1)!!(x+iy)^{m},$$

we have

$$\sum_{k=1}^{N}(r_k \times p_k)\cdot[\nabla(x+iy)^{m}]_{r=r_k} = \frac{2m+1}{\bullet_0}\int_{\Gamma} n \cdot B(r)(x+iy)^{m}d\Gamma, \quad (8)$$

where $[\nabla(x+iy)^{m}]_{r=r_k}$ represents $\nabla(x+iy)^{m}$ evaluated at $r = r_k$. The prime characters in the integrands have been omitted for brevity. Define now the following quantities:

$S_k \equiv x_k + iy_k$: k-th dipole position projected on the xy-plane,

$\bullet_k \equiv r_k \times p_k$: magnetic moment of k-th dipole,

$\bullet_k \equiv [\bullet_k]_{x+iy}$: projection of $\bullet_k$ on the xy-plane,

where $[*]_{x+iy}$ represents (the x-component of the vector $*$)$+i\times$(the y-component of the vector $*$). Then, from the identity

$$\nabla(x+iy)^{m} = m(x+iy)^{m-1}\begin{pmatrix}1\\ i\\ 0\end{pmatrix}, \quad (9)$$

Eq. (8) can be rewritten as

$$\sum_{k=1}^{N}\bullet_k S_k^{m} = c_m, \qquad (m = 0,1,2,\cdots) \quad (10)$$

where

$$c_m \equiv \frac{2m+3}{(m+1)\bullet_0}\int_{\Gamma} n \cdot B(r)(x+iy)^{m+1}d\Gamma.$$

The problem of determining $S_k, \bullet_k$ and N in Eqs. (10) from c_m $(m = 0,1,\cdots)$ appears in many inverse problems such as computed tomography (Golub et al. (1997)), EEG inversion

(El-Badia et al. (2000); Nara et al. (2003)), MEG inversion (Nara et al. (2007)), and locating the zeros of analytic functions (Kravanja et al. (1994)). To this problem, an algebraic algorithm called Prony's method and its modified/extended algorithms have been proposed that enable us to reconstruct the source parameter $S_k, \bullet_k$ and N from c_m.
The essence of Prony's method is as follows (See e.g. Elad et al. (2004)). First, let us assume that N is fixed and known *a priori*. Estimation of N is explained afterwards. For N positions $S_1, \cdots, S_N$, let us define $\bullet_1, \cdots, \bullet_N$ by the coefficients of the polynomial

$$\prod_{n=1}^{N}(\bullet - S_n) \equiv \bullet^N + \bullet_1 \bullet^{N-1} + \cdots + \bullet_N.$$

Then, the following difference equations holds

$$\bullet_1 c_{m+N-1} + \bullet_2 c_{m+N-2} + \cdots + \bullet_N c_m = -c_{m+N}, \quad (m = 0, 1, 2, \cdots). \tag{11}$$

Thus, from the $2N$ linear equations (11) for $m = 0, 1, \cdots, 2N-1$, we have

$$\begin{pmatrix} c_0 & c_1 & \cdots & c_{N-1} \\ c_1 & c_2 & \cdots & c_N \\ \vdots & \vdots & \vdots & \vdots \\ c_{N-1} & c_N & \cdots & c_{2N-2} \end{pmatrix} \begin{pmatrix} \bullet_N \\ \bullet_{N-1} \\ \vdots \\ \bullet_1 \end{pmatrix} = - \begin{pmatrix} c_N \\ c_{N+1} \\ \vdots \\ c_{2N-1} \end{pmatrix}. \tag{12}$$

Here, since the coefficient matrix in Eq. (12) is diagonalized as

$$\begin{pmatrix} c_0 & c_1 & \cdots & c_{N-1} \\ c_1 & c_2 & \cdots & c_N \\ \vdots & \vdots & \vdots & \vdots \\ c_{N-1} & c_N & \cdots & c_{2N-2} \end{pmatrix}$$
$$= \begin{pmatrix} 1 & 1 & \cdots & 1 \\ S_1 & S_2 & \cdots & S_N \\ \vdots & \vdots & \vdots & \vdots \\ S_1^{N-1} & S_2^{N-1} & \cdots & S_N^{N-1} \end{pmatrix} \mathrm{diag}\,(\bullet_1, \bullet_2, \cdots, \bullet_N) \begin{pmatrix} 1 & 1 & \cdots & 1 \\ S_1 & S_2 & \cdots & S_N \\ \vdots & \vdots & \vdots & \vdots \\ S_1^{N-1} & S_2^{N-1} & \cdots & S_N^{N-1} \end{pmatrix}^T,$$

we have

$$\det \begin{pmatrix} c_0 & c_1 & \cdots & c_{N-1} \\ c_1 & c_2 & \cdots & c_N \\ \vdots & \vdots & \vdots & \vdots \\ c_{N-1} & c_N & \cdots & c_{2N-2} \end{pmatrix} = \prod_{k=1}^{N} \bullet_k \prod_{i>j} (S_i - S_j)^2.$$

Hence, when $\bullet_k \neq 0$ and $S_i \neq S_j$, Eqs. (12) can be uniquely solved for $\bullet_1, \cdots, \bullet_N$. Then, S_n are obtained as solutions to the Nth degree equation $\bullet^N + \bullet_1 \bullet^{N-1} + \cdots + \bullet_N = 0$.

Although it is known that Prony's method is numerically unstable, modified versions of Prony's method have been proposed by using the truncated singular value decomposition (Kumaresan et al. (1982)), by the projection method (Cadzow (1988)), or by repeating Prony's method while changing the model order N (Barone et al. (1998)). Methods to transform Eqs. (10) to an eigenvalue problem have also been proposed (Hua et al. (1990), Luk et al. (1997), Golub et al. (1997), El-Badia et al. (2000)). See Elad et al. (2004) for a review.
Onece S_k are determined, $\bullet_k$ can be obtained by solving the linear equations (10).
To determine z_k we use Eqs.(7) for $l = m+1$. Since it holds that (Hobson (1931))

$$r^{m+1}Y_{m+1,m}(\bullet,\bullet) = (2m+1)!!(x+iy)^m z,$$

we have

$$\sum_{k=1}^{N}(m\bullet_k z_k S_k^{m-1} + [\bullet_k]_z S_k^m) = d_m, \qquad (m = 0,1,2,\cdots) \tag{13}$$

where

$$d_m \equiv \frac{2m+3}{\bullet_0}\int_\Gamma \boldsymbol{n}\cdot\boldsymbol{B}(\boldsymbol{r})\,(x+iy)^m z d\Gamma.$$

Hence, after S_k and $\bullet_k$ are obtained, z_k and the z-component of $\bullet_k$ denoted by $[\bullet_k]_z$ can be determined by solving Eqs. (13).
In order to estimate N, we assume that there exist $N'(> N)$ dipoles and estimate $\bullet_1,\cdots,\bullet_{N'}$ using the algorithm mentioned above. Then it would be expected, when the data includes noise, that $\bullet_k$ of the 'spurious' sources $k = N+1,\cdots,N'$ are much smaller than those of the true sources, from which N can be estimated.

3.2 Explicit method for the equivalent current dipoles and quadrupoles

Now we describe an explicit algorithm for the equivalent current dipole and quadrupole source model ($Q_k \neq 0$). Considering again Eqs. (7) for $l = m$, we have

$$\sum_{k=1}^{N}\left(\nabla(x+iy)^m|_{\boldsymbol{r}=\boldsymbol{r}_k}\cdot(\boldsymbol{r}_k\times\boldsymbol{p}_k) + Q_k : \left(\nabla(\nabla(x+iy)^m\times\boldsymbol{r})\right)^T|_{\boldsymbol{r}=\boldsymbol{r}_k}\right)$$
$$= \frac{2m+1}{\bullet_0}\int_\Gamma \boldsymbol{n}\cdot\boldsymbol{B}(\boldsymbol{r})(x+iy)^m dS. \tag{14}$$

It is shown in Nara (2008b) that Eq. (14) is rewritten as

$$\sum_{k=1}^{N}\bullet_k S_k^m + m\sum_{k=1}^{N}\bullet_k S_k^{m-1} = c_m, \quad (m = 0,1,2,\cdots), \tag{15}$$

where

$$\bullet_k = (i(q_{xx,k} - q_{yy,k}) - (q_{xy,k} + q_{yx,k}))z_k.$$

Eq. (15) has the same form as that of Eq. (6) in Nara (2008a), and can be transformed into the simultaneous second degree equations

$$\bullet^T H_{N,m} \bullet = 0, \quad (m = 0, 1, \cdots, 2N-1), \tag{16}$$

where

$$H_{N,m} = \begin{pmatrix} c_m & c_{m+1} & \cdots & c_{m+N} \\ c_{m+1} & c_{m+2} & \cdots & c_{m+N+1} \\ \vdots & \vdots & \vdots & \vdots \\ c_{m+N} & c_{m+N+1} & \cdots & c_{m+2N} \end{pmatrix},$$

and

$$\bullet = (\bullet_N, \bullet_{N-1}, \cdots, \bullet_1, 1)^T.$$

Furthermore, the second degree equations (16) for $m = 0, 1, \cdots, 2N-1$ can be turned into linear equations for $\bullet_1, \cdots, \bullet_N$. (See Nara (2008a)).
An example of the algorithm when $N = 2$ is illustrated in Fig. 1: in Step 1), starting with $\bullet^T H_{N,m} \bullet = 0$ for $m = 0, 1, 2, 3$, we compute their linear combinations to have three equations with the Hankel matrices whose (1,1)-components are zero. In Step 2), the linear combinations of those three equations are computed so that we have two equations with the Hankel matrices whose first and second anti-diagonal components are zero. In Step 3), by computing the linear combinations of those two equations, we arrive at a single equation, which is a linear equation for $\bullet_1$. In Step 4), by substituting the obtained $\bullet_1$ into the equations obtained in Step 2), we have linear equations for $\bullet_2$. This is an example how the algorithm proceeds when $N = 2$. See Nara (2008a) for the detailed algorithm for general N.
Once $\bullet_1, \cdots, \bullet_N$ are obtained, $S_1, \cdots, S_N$ are obtained by solving $\bullet^N + \bullet_1 \bullet^{N-1} + \cdots + \bullet_N = 0$. $\bullet_k$ and $\bullet_k$ for $k = 1, 2, \cdots, N$ are linearly solved using Eqs. (15) for $m = 0, 1, \cdots, 2N-1$. Then, we use Eqs. (7) for $l = m+1$ which leads to the second degree equations for z_k.
To estimate N, following the method for the dipole source model, we assume that there are $N'(> N)$ dipole-quadrupole sources and then estimate S_k as well as $\bullet_k$ and $\bullet_k$ for $k = 1, 2, \cdots, N'$. Then we compute $|\bullet_{k+1}/\bullet_k|$ and $|\bullet_{k+1}/\bullet_k|$ for $k = 1, 2, \cdots, N'-1$, which are expected to be sufficiently small when $k = N$. Practically, we estimate N such that these ratios become smaller than some thresholds set *a priori*. The thresholds should be determined by the ratios of the noise level contained in the data to the dipole and quadrupole strength which can be regarded as a physiologically meaningful source. As for the dipole source model in the 2D problem, the threshold is theoretically evaluated in the context of the Padé approximation (Barone et al. (1998)). A similar theory for the dipole-quadrupole source model, although greatly required, is left for further research; in this paper we show only numerical examples in section 4.

Remark: solving the second degree equations under noisy condition

The algorithm repeating elimination might be sensitive to noise contained in data due to the cancellation. To avoid or reduce it, we can alternatively solve the simultaneous second degree equations (16) by means of the Gröbner bases. For example, when $N = 1$, we solve Eq. (16) for $m = 0$ so that we have a set of two projected positions, say $A = \{S^{(1)}, S^{(2)}\}$, and then solve Eq. (16) for $m = 1$ giving the other set, $B = \{S^{(3)}, S^{(4)}\}$. Theoretically, the true position

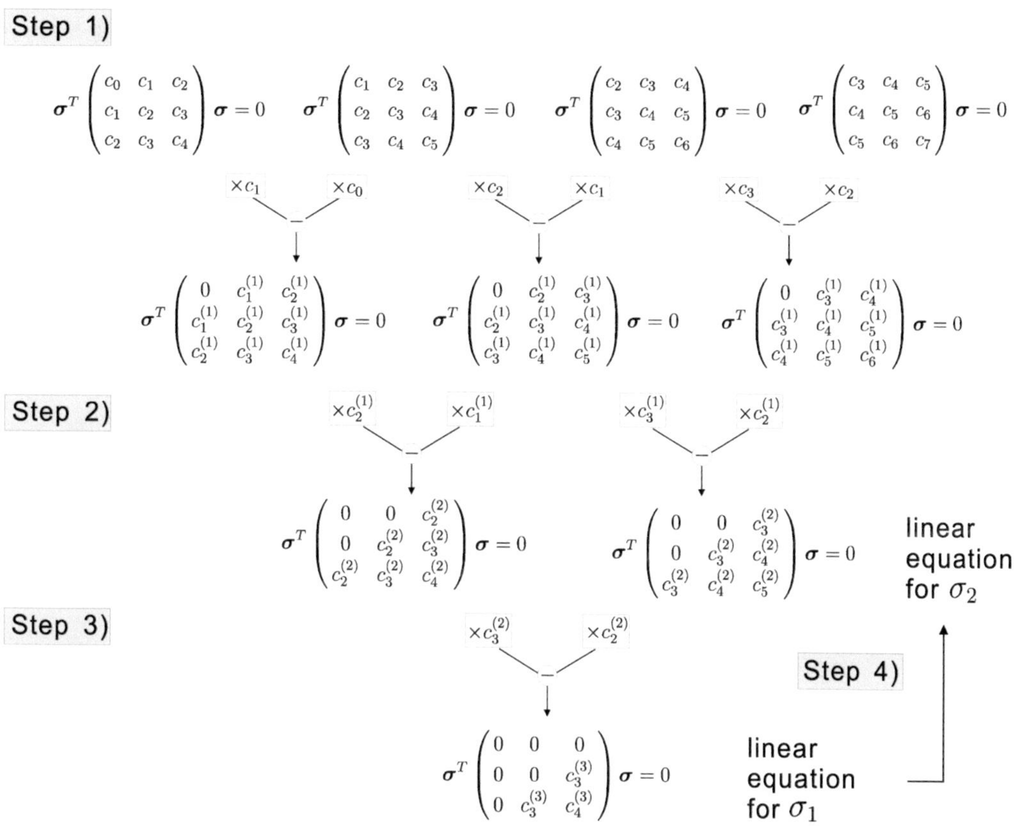

Fig. 1. Example of transformation of the second degree equations to the linear equations for $\bullet = (\bullet_2, \bullet_1, 1)^T$ when $N = 2$.

is included in both A and B. When the data includes noise, we choose an element in A and B, say $S^{(1)}$ and $S^{(3)}$, such that the distance between them, $|S^{(1)} - S^{(3)}|$, is smaller than the distance between the other pair, $|S^{(2)} - S^{(4)}|$, and estimate the projected position S by $\frac{S^{(1)}+S^{(3)}}{2}$. In the simulations in section 4, we use this algorithm.

4. Numerical simulations

In this section, we compare the explicit method assuming the dipole-quadrupole model (DQM) with the explicit method assuming the dipole model (DM). To model dipoles on cerebral convolutions, we assume that dipoles are placed on a mesh on a half cylinder with a radius of $r = 5$mm and a height of $h = 5$ mm, as shown in Fig. 2. There are six dipoles in the circumferential direction by five in the longitudinal direction, and hence a total of 30 dipoles on the half cylinder. All the dipoles are aligned perpendicular to the surface of the cylinder to model the fact that the dipoles are perpendicular to the cerebral convolutions (Hämäläinen et al. (1993)). We examined the following three cases:

- case (i) A single half-cylinder source at $\boldsymbol{r}_1 = 70(\sin\bullet_1\cos\bullet_1, \sin\bullet_1\sin\bullet_1, \cos\bullet_1)$ mm, where $\bullet_1 = \frac{10}{180}\bullet$ and $\bullet_1 = \bullet$. The vectors which determine the posture of the cylinder, $\boldsymbol{e}_{12}$ and $\boldsymbol{e}_{11}$, are set to be $(0,0,1)$ and $(1,0,0)$, respectively. See Fig. 3 left. In this case, the total dipole moment $\boldsymbol{p}_1$ is nearly parallel to $\boldsymbol{r}_1$; the angle between them is 9.8 degrees. Since a radial dipole is a silent source for radial MEG (Hämäläinen et al. (1993)), this cylindrical source is regarded as being almost quadrupolar.

- case (ii) A half-cylinder at $\boldsymbol{r}_1 = 70(\sin \bullet_1 \cos \bullet_1, \sin \bullet_1 \sin \bullet_1, \cos \bullet_1)$ where $\bullet_1 = \frac{70}{180}\bullet$ and $\bullet_1 = 0$. $\boldsymbol{e}_{12} = (0,0,1)$ and $\boldsymbol{e}_{11} = (1,0,0)$. See Fig. 3 center. In this case, the angle between $\boldsymbol{r}_1$ and $\boldsymbol{p}_1$ is 78 degrees, so that the source has a detectable equivalent dipole moment as well as the equivalent quadrupole moment.
- case (iii) Two half-cylinder sources of cases (i) and (ii). See Fig. 3 right. The source at $\boldsymbol{r}_1$ is almost quadrupolar and that at $\boldsymbol{r}_2$ is a dipole-quadrupole source.

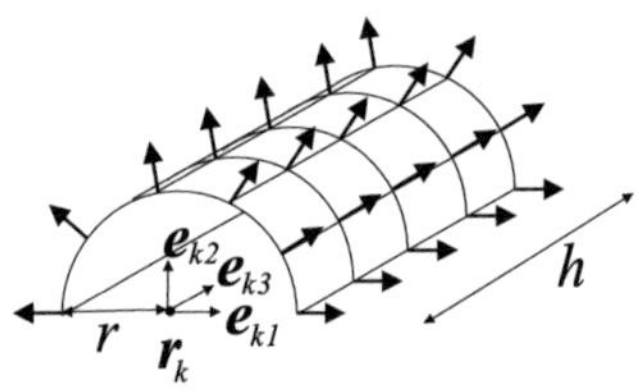

Fig. 2. 'Cylindrical source': distributed dipoles on a half cylinder modeling the cerebral convolutions.

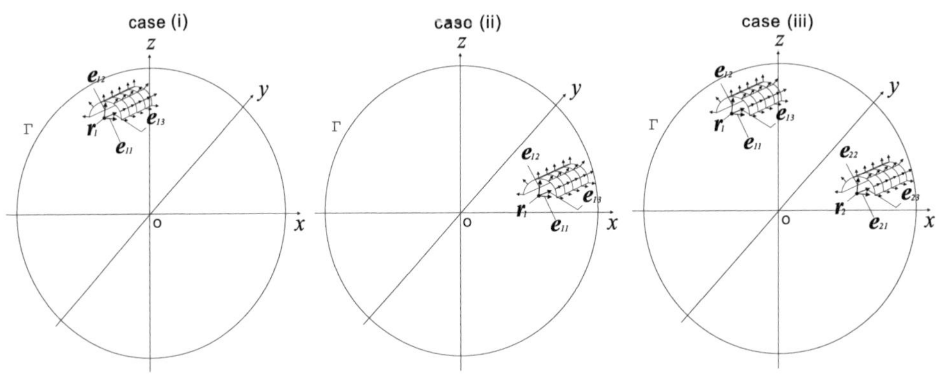

Fig. 3. Case (i) a single cylindrical source where $\boldsymbol{r}_1$ is nearly parallel to the equivalent current dipole $\boldsymbol{p}_1$ (the angle between them is 9.8 degrees); this cylindrical source is almost quadrupolar. Case (ii) a single cylindrical source where $\boldsymbol{r}_1$ is nearly perpendicular to $\boldsymbol{p}_1$ (the angle between them is 78 degrees); this cylindrical source has a detectable equivalent dipole moment as well as the equivalent quadrupole moment. Case (iii) two cylindrical sources (combination of cases (i) and (ii)).

We computed the forward solution generated by the 30 (case (i) and (ii)) or 60 (case (iii)) elemental dipoles using Eq. (2). Note that Eq. (3) was not used to compute the theoretical data. The radius of a head was set to be 100 mm. We assumed that the radial component of the magnetic field was measured at $M = 361$ points distributed uniformly on a sphere with $R = 120$ mm using the spherical t-design (Saff97 et al. (1997)); it is a set of M points on Γ such that the integral of any polynomial of degree t or less over Γ is equal to the average value of the polynomial over the set of M points. We used $M = (t+1)^2 = 361$ points ($t = 18$) given by Chen et al. (2009). Based on this property, for numerical integration, the integrand values on the N points were summed with equal weights $\frac{4\bullet}{M}$.

To validate our algorithm for the dipole-quadrupole model, we assumed that the data was available on the whole sphere which enclosed the source. Simulations using sensors on a part of the sphere is left for future studies. To this end, the so-called Signal Space Separation method proposed by Taulu et al. (2005) or the method for stable data continuation from data on the upper hemisphere to those on the lower hemisphere proposed by Popov (2002) could be very useful.

Gaussian noise was added to the theoretical forward solution, where the noise level defined by the ratio of the standard deviation of the noise to the root mean squares of the data was 5%. 10 data sets with the different noise added were used for reconstruction.

First we show the reconstruction result when N is know *a priori*. Table 1 shows the error between the true position and the mean estimated position using 10 data sets. The true and estimated positions projected on the xy-plane are depicted in Fig. 4. We observe that in case (i) the method using DM cannot estimate the source accurately, while the method using DQM can estimate it within an error of 2 mm. This is because the source is almost quadrupolar.

In case (ii), the result using DM is better than that using DQM.

In case (iii), the maximum error about the xy-projected positions using DQM is 7.6 mm, whereas that using DM is 110 mm (for the almost quadrupolar source). However, the z-coordinates is not accurately obtained even when using DQM. This is because the z-coordinates are estimated using the obtained x- and y-coordinates.

	2D-DM (mm)	2D-DQM (mm)	3D-DM (mm)	3D-DQM (mm)
case (i)	3.0e1	3.1e-1	3.0e1	1.4e0
case (ii)	8.9e-1	6.5e0	1.7e0	6.6e0
case (iii)	1.1e2, 8.3e0	7.6e0, 6.3e0	1.1e2, 8.9e0	5.7e1, 6.3e0

Table 1. 2D and 3D localization error when using DM and DQM. '2D' means the error projected on the xy-plane.

Next, we show the case when N is not known *a priori*. Fig. 5 shows the reconstruction result when assuming $N' = 2$ in cases (i) and (ii) and $N' = 3$ in case (iii). In case (i), when using DQM where $N' = 2$, the two positions are estimated: one is close to the true one, and another is far from the true one (In Fig. 5 top left, the estimated position far from the true position is not seen, since it is out of the figure.) Numbering them 1 and 2, we have $|\bullet_2/\bullet_1| = 5.3e-4$ and $|\bullet_2/\bullet_1| = 9.9e-4$. From this, we can reasonably judge that the second source is spurious due to the noise, and there is a single dipole-quadrupole source. In contrast, when using DM where $N' = 2$, $|\bullet_2/\bullet_1| = 4.3e-1$; $\bullet_1$ and $\bullet_2$ are almost the same order, and hence we judge that there are two dipoles. The estimated dipoles are close to the side walls of the half cylinder. However, the distance between them is larger than the diameter of the cylinder as in Fig. 5 top left.

In case (ii), when using DQM where $N' = 2$, $|\bullet_2/\bullet_1| = 9.7e-4$ and $|\bullet_2/\bullet_1| = 6.5e-3$. Also, when using DM where $N' = 2$, $|\bullet_2/\bullet_1| = 4.1e-3$. Hence, both DQM and DM can estimate the number of the sources.

In case (iii), when using DQM where $N' = 3$, $|\bullet_3/\bullet_2| = 9.5e-4$ and $|\bullet_3/\bullet_2| = 9.0e-4$, from which we can judge that $N = 2$. In contrast, when using DM where $N' = 3$, $|\bullet_3/\bullet_2| = 1.1e-1$; the third source is not much smaller than the second one. Also we observe that, for almost the quadrupole source, the estimated two dipoles are too separated.

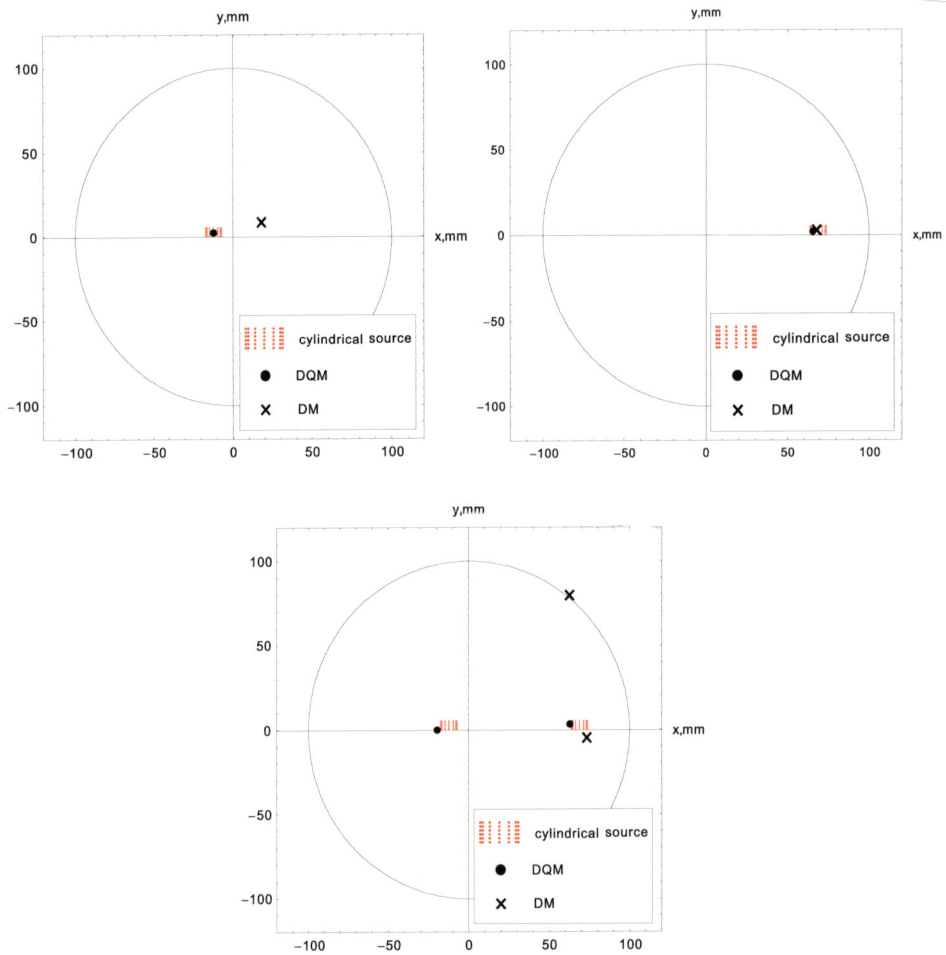

Fig. 4. The reconstruction result projected on the xy-plane. In this figure, N is assumed to be known *a priori*. (top left) In case (i), the equivalent dipole is almost directed to the radial direction, and the source is almost quadrupolar. As a result, when using DM with $N = 1$, the cylindrical source is not at all localized, while DQM with $N = 1$ well estimates the center of the source. (top right) In case (ii), the equivalent dipole is almost perpendicular to the radial direction. In this case, both DM and DQM can well localize the source. (bottom) In case (iii), both the sources are well estimated when using DQM, while almost the quadrupole source is not at all estimated when using DM.

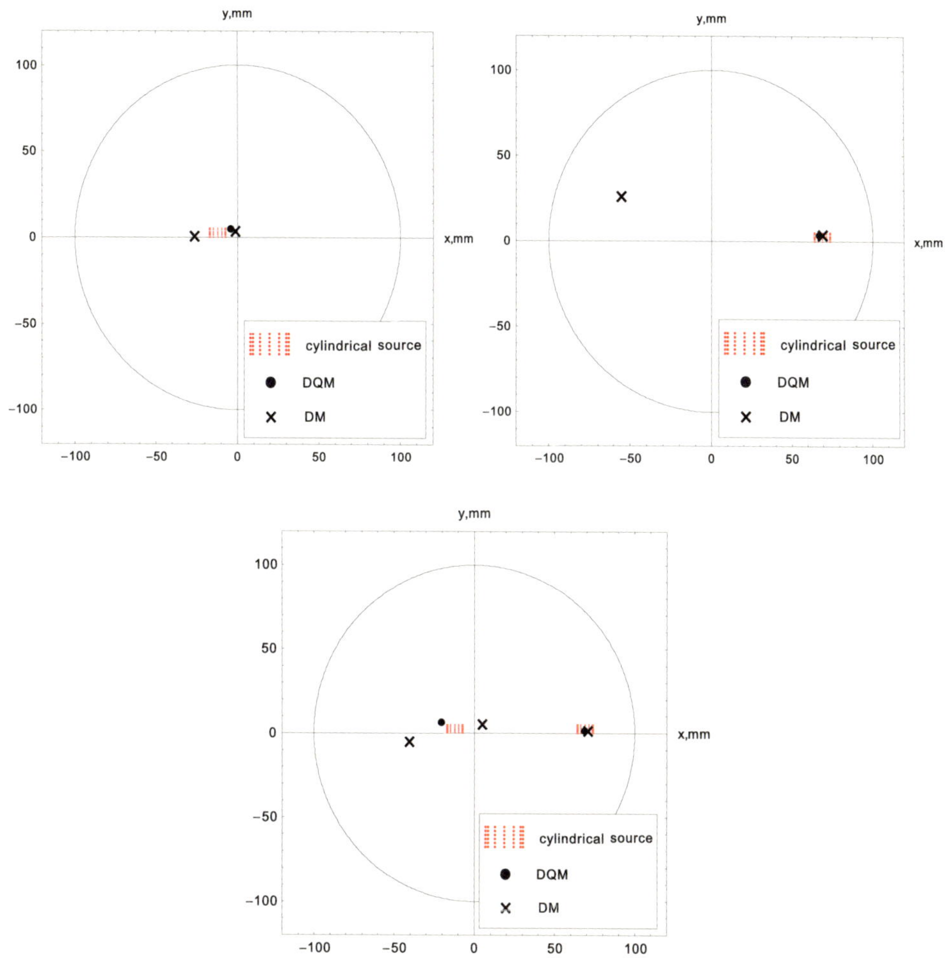

Fig. 5. The result when N is not known *a priori*. (top left) Reconstruction result in case (i) when assuming $N' = 2$. When using DQM, the estimated source far from the true position (which is out of the figure and is not depicted) has much smaller dipole and quadrupole moments than the estimated source close to the true position. In fact, $|\bullet_2/\bullet_1| = 5.3e-4$ and $|\bullet_2/\bullet_1| = 9.9e-4$, from which we can judge $N = 1$. In contrast, when using DM, $|\bullet_2/\bullet_1| = 4.3e-1$ from which we judge that there are two dipoles. Although two dipoles are estimated close to the side walls of the cylindrical surface, the distance between them is larger than the diameter of the cylinder. (top right) In case (ii), $|\bullet_2/\bullet_1| = 9.7e-4$ and $|\bullet_2/\bullet_1| = 6.5e-3$ when using DQM where $N' = 2$. Also, $|\bullet_2/\bullet_1| = 4.1e-3$ when using DM. Hence, both DQM and DM can estimate the number of the sources. (bottom) In case (iii), $|\bullet_3/\bullet_2| = 9.5e-4$ and $|\bullet_3/\bullet_2| = 9.0e-4$ when using DQM where $N' = 3$, from which we can judge that $N = 2$. In contrast, when using DM where $N' = 3$, $|\bullet_3/\bullet_2| = 1.1e-1$; the third source is not much smaller than the second one. Also we observe that, for almost the quadrupole source, the estimated two dipoles are too separated.

5. Conclusion

In this chapter, we introduced the equivalent current dipole-quadrupole source model which has a potential to parametrically represent the spatial extent of the neural current in MEG inverse problem. Then, explicit methods for the equivalent dipole-quadrupole source model as well as the equivalent dipole source model were shown, that enables us to reconstruct the dipole-quadrupole parameters explicitly with MEG data. In numerical simulations, it was suggested that the dipole-quadrupole source model would be useful especially when the elemental dipoles are distributed on the surface of a half cylinder modeling the cerebral convolution such that the equivalent dipole is parallel to the radial direction.

6. Appendix

It is easy to obtain the dipole terms. For the quadrupole terms, we use the identity

$$\int_{\Omega_1} \boldsymbol{a}(\boldsymbol{r}') \cdot Q_k \nabla' \bullet (\boldsymbol{r}' - \boldsymbol{r}_k) dv' = Q_k : (\nabla' \boldsymbol{a}(\boldsymbol{r}'))^T|_{\boldsymbol{r}'=\boldsymbol{r}_k} \tag{17}$$

for an arbitrary vector field $\boldsymbol{a}(\boldsymbol{r}') = (a_x(\boldsymbol{r}'), a_y(\boldsymbol{r}'), a_z(\boldsymbol{r}'))^T$, where T represents the transpose. When inserting the quadrupole terms in Eq. (1) into Eq. (2), we have from Eq. (17)

$$\int_{\Omega_1} (\nabla' \frac{1}{|\boldsymbol{r} - \boldsymbol{r}'|} \times \boldsymbol{r}') \cdot Q_k \nabla' \bullet (\boldsymbol{r}' - \boldsymbol{r}_k) dv' = Q_k : (\nabla' (\nabla' \frac{1}{|\boldsymbol{r} - \boldsymbol{r}'|} \times \boldsymbol{r}'))^T|_{\boldsymbol{r}'=\boldsymbol{r}_k}.$$

Here, it holds that

$$\nabla'(\nabla' \frac{1}{|\boldsymbol{r} - \boldsymbol{r}'|} \times \boldsymbol{r}') = \nabla' \frac{\boldsymbol{r} \times \boldsymbol{r}'}{|\boldsymbol{r} - \boldsymbol{r}'|^3} = (\nabla' \frac{1}{|\boldsymbol{r} - \boldsymbol{r}'|^3})(\boldsymbol{r} \times \boldsymbol{r}') + \frac{\nabla'(\boldsymbol{r} \times \boldsymbol{r}')}{|\boldsymbol{r} - \boldsymbol{r}'|^3}$$

$$= \frac{3(\boldsymbol{r} - \boldsymbol{r}')(\boldsymbol{r} \times \boldsymbol{r}')}{|\boldsymbol{r} - \boldsymbol{r}'|^5} + \frac{1}{|\boldsymbol{r} - \boldsymbol{r}'|^3} \begin{pmatrix} 0 & z & -y \\ -z & 0 & x \\ y & -x & 0 \end{pmatrix},$$

and hence

$$(\nabla'(\nabla' \frac{1}{|\boldsymbol{r} - \boldsymbol{r}'|} \times \boldsymbol{r}'))^T|_{\boldsymbol{r}'=\boldsymbol{r}_k} = \frac{3(\boldsymbol{r} \times \boldsymbol{r}_k)(\boldsymbol{r} - \boldsymbol{r}_k)}{|\boldsymbol{r} - \boldsymbol{r}_k|^5} + \frac{X_r}{|\boldsymbol{r} - \boldsymbol{r}_k|^3}.$$

Thus we have Eq. (3).

7. References

Hobson, E. W. (1931). *The theory of spherical and ellipsoidal harmonics*, Cambridge University Press.

Alvarez, R. E. (1991). Filter functions for computing multipole moments from the magnetic field normal to plane, *IEEE Transactions on Medical Imaging*, Vol. 10, No. 3, pp. 375-381, 1991.

Baillet, S.; Mosher, J. C.; Leahy, R. M. (2001). Electromagnetic brain mapping, *IEEE Signal Processing Magazine*, Vol.18, pp.14-30, 2001.

Barone, P.; March, R. (1998). Some properties of the asymptotic location of poles of Pade approximants to noisy rational functions, relevant for modal analysis, *IEEE Trans. Signal Process.*, Vol.46, pp. 2448–2457, 1998.

Cadzow, J. A. (1988) Signal enhancement - a composite property mapping algorithm, *IEEE Trans. Acoust., Speach, Signal Process.*, Vol.36, pp. 49–62, 1988.

Chen, X.; Womerlsy, R. (2009). Spherical t-design with $d = (t+1)^2$ points, http://www.polyu.edu.hk/ama/staff/xjchen/sphdesigns.html.

Elad, M.; Milanfar, P.; Golub, G.H. (2004). Shape from moments — an estimation theory perspective, *IEEE Trans. Signal Process.*, 52, pp. 1814–1829, 2004.

El-Badia, A.; Ha-Duong, T. (2000). An inverse source problem in potential analysis, *Inverse Problems*, Vol. 16, No. 3, pp. 651-663, 2000.

Fokas, A. S.; Kurylev, Y.; Marinakis, V. (2004). The unique determination of neuronal currents in the brain via magnetoencephalography, *Inverse Problems*, Vol. 20, pp. 1067-1082, 2004.

Golub, G. H.; Milanfar, P.; Varah, J. (1997). A stable numerical methods for inverting shape from moments *SIAM Journal of scientific computing*, Vol. 21, No. 4, pp. 1222-1243, 1999.

Hämäläinen, M; Hari, R.; Ilmoniemi, R.J.; Knuutila, J.; Lounasmaa, O. V. (1993). Magnetoencephalography - theory, instrumentation, and applications to noninvasive studies of the working human brain *Review of Modern Physics*, Vol.65, pp. 413-497, 1993.

Hua, Y.; Sarkar, T. K. (1990). Matrix pencil method for estimating parameters of exponentially damped/undamped sinusoids in noise, *IEEE Trans. Acous., Speech, and Signal Process.*, 38, pp. 814–824, 1990.

Irimia, A.; Swinney, K. R.; Wikswo, J. P. (2009). Partial independence of bioelectric and biomagnetic fields and its implications for encephalography and cardiography, *Physical Review E*, Vol. 79, 051908, 2009.

Jerbi, K.; Mosher, J. C.; Bailet, S.; Leahy, R. M. (2002). On MEG forward modelling using multipolar expansions, *Physics in Medicine and Biology*, Vol. 47, pp. 523-555, 2002.

Jerbi, K.; Baillet, S.; Mosher, J. C.; Nolte, G.; Garnero, L.; Leahy, R. M. (2004). Localization of realistic cortical activity in MEG using current multipoles, *NeuroImage*, Vol. 22, pp. 779-793, 2004.

Kumaresan, R.; Tufts, D. W. (1982). Estimating the parameters of exponentially damped sinusoids and pole-zero modeling in noise, *IEEE Trans. Acoust. Speech and Signal Process.*, Vol.30, pp. 833–840, 1982.

Kravanja, P.; Sakurai, T.; Barel, M. V. (1994). On locating clusters of zeros of analytic functions *BIT* Vol. 39, pp. 646-682, 1994.

Luk, F.T.; Vandevoorde, D. (1997). Decomposing a signal into a sum of exponentials, Iterative methods in scientific computing, Springer-verlag, pp. 329–357, 1997.

Nara, T.; Ando, S. (2003). A projective method for an inverse source problem of the Poisson Equation *Inverse Problems* Vol. 19, No. 2, pp. 355-369, 2003.

Nara, T.; Oohama, J.; Hashimoto, M.; Takeda, T.; Ando, S. (2007). Direct reconstruction algorithm of current dipoles for vector magnetoencephalography and electroencephalography, *Physics in Medicine and Biology*, Vol. 52, pp. 3859-3879, 2007.

Nara, T. (2008). An algebraic method for identification of dipoles and quadrupoles, *Inverse Problems*, Vol. 24, 025010 (19pp), 2008.

Nara, T. (2008). Reconstruction of the number and positions of dipoles and quadrupoles using an algebraic method, *Journal of Physics : Conference Series*, International Conference on Inverse Problems in Engineering, 012076, 2008.

Nolte, G.; Curio. G. (1997). On the calculation of magnetic fields based on multipole modeling of focal biological current source, *Biophysical Journal*, Vol. 73, pp. 1253-1262, 1997.

Nolte, G.; Curio. G. (2000). Current multipole expansion to estimate lateral extent of neuronal activity: a theoretical analysis, *IEEE Trans. Biomedical Engineering*, Vol. 47, No. 10, pp. 1347-1355, 2000.

Popov, M. (2002). Data continuation for the explicit solution of an inverse biomagnetic problem, *IEEE Trans. Magnetics*, Vol. 38, pp. 3620-3632, 2002.

Saff, E. B.; Kuijlaars, A. B. J.; Distributing many points on a sphere, *Mathematical Intelligencer*, Vol. 19. pp. 5-11, 1997.

Taulu, S.; Kajola, S. (2005). Presentation of electromagnetic multichannel data: The signal space separation method, *Journal of Applied Physics*, Vol. 97, 124905, 2005.

Part 3

Current State of the Art: Phase-Related Phenonmenon

7

Detection of Artifacts and Brain Responses Using Instantaneous Phase Statistics in Independent Components

Jürgen Dammers and Michael Schiek
Institute of Neuroscience and Medicine, Research Centre Jülich, Jülich,
Central Institute for Electronics, Research Centre Jülich, Jülich,
Germany

1. Introduction

Multichannel recordings of magnetoencephalography (MEG) are usually comprised of repetitive events (e.g. external stimuli) in order to evoke the relatively weak magnetic fields of brain responses to a specific task. The analysis of the underlying electrophysiological brain activity of such unaveraged signals is notoriously challenging. During MEG experiments environmental and other external noise sources derogate the signal of interest. Furthermore, brain activity which is not involved in the task processing and therefore not of prime interest (often termed as "brain noise") also interfere with the weak brain responses.

In order to increase the signal-to-noise ratio (SNR) of the recorded data a widely common strategy is to perform signal averages. Assuming white[1] noise that is temporally uncorrelated across trials, the SNR improvement gained by the averaging process over N trials scales theoretically with $\sqrt{N}$. In practice the noise reduction is a little less than $1/\sqrt{N}$ since, the evoked activity usually varies in its signal strength over time. An important aspect to bear in mind when performing averages is, that it will reveal the most prominent neuromagnetic correlates of brain responses, only. In this way information about weaker brain activity is largely suppressed, especially when multiple strong and weaker sources acting in a coordinated manner. Additionally, the temporal dynamics of each individual response will not be preserved. In contrast, single-trial analysis retains the temporal dynamics of the neuromagnetic responses, but suffers from poor signal-to-noise ratio (SNR), and is therefore rarely applied.

Multichannel MEG recordings are usually comprised of a mixture of the underlying brain activity and field components originated from noise and artifact sources. In MEG, as well as in electroencephalography (EEG), the most prominent biological artifacts originate from eye blinks/movements (ocular artifacts, OA), heart beats (cardiac artifacts, CA) and muscle activity (MA). The signal strength of such biological artifacts may be several orders of magnitude higher than the signal of interest. Therefore, the analysis of MEG/EEG signals

---

[1]In analogy to white light (visible light), where all types of visible wavelengths are represented, the term „white" is used for types of signal (or noise), where the power spectral density of the signal is uniform. This means the power spectral density of the signal is the same at all frequencies.

requires the identification and elimination of the artificial signals prior to analysis. Independent component analysis (ICA), for example, is widely used to separate brain signals from noise and artifact components. Effective removal of noise and biological artifacts was reported in various publications (Dammers et al., 2010; Escudero et al., 2011; Mantini et al., 2008; Nikulin et al., 2011; Ting et al., 2006).

Most of the proposed ICA based source separation methods are performed to identify and exclude artifacts from the recorded signal, while only a few studies have been performed to elicit brain responses from the decomposed signals (Dammers et al., 2010; Hild & Nagarajan, 2009; Nikulin et al., 2011). Reliable classification of noise, artifacts and brain activity in decomposed MEG signals is not an easy task to do. However, separating brain responses due to an external stimulus from unwanted signal contributions (i.e., the remaining signal components which are not related to the signal of interest, such as brain noise) in unaveraged multichannel MEG recordings, is even more challenging due to the weak signal strength. Artifact signals, such as eye blinks, eye movements, muscle artifacts or the field contribution from the heart are types of signals that are usually much stronger in amplitude than brain signals are. This is one of the reasons why most of the applied artifact identification routines are based on amplitude statistics of the decomposed MEG signal. In previous reports, it has been shown that in the case of cardiac artifacts the ICA decomposition may reveal multiple independent components (ICs), where peak amplitudes of the cardiac artifact components vary quite substantially across the components, and is therefore, difficult to identify by amplitude based methods (Dammers et al., 2008; Sander et al., 2002).

When trying to identify brain responses from independent components different strategies are indispensable. In the last decade, the number of channels in whole head MEG systems has increased quite substantially. Meanwhile modern MEG systems are comprised with about 250 or more channels to cover most of the human head. For source reconstruction a dense inter-channel spacing has a favorable effect on the spatial resolution of the localized activity. On the other hand, higher channel densities require smaller pick-up loops (i.e., the size of the field measuring coil is smaller), which in turn has the effect of measuring a smaller amount of underlying brain activity. If we assume the same amount of environmental noise at each channel, the measured signal will have a smaller SNR when the size of the pick-up loop decreases.

In particular, when [2]magnetometers are used to detect the neuromagnetic activity, such brain responses must be really strong to be identified by visual inspection. Therefore, the high dimensionality of the data and the poor signal-to-noise ratio (SNR) are the two most inviting challenges in MEG single-trial analysis. In order to overcome these problems different strategies have been proposed. Guimaraes and colleagues, for example, used well-known classification methods to identify brain responses in MEG raw signals or signal decompositions (Guimaraes et al., 2007). In this study single-trial classification of MEG recordings have been applied utilizing two different classifier, the linear discriminant classification (LDC) and support vector machine (SVM). Both strategies were applied to classify single-trial brain responses to auditory and visual presentations of words. Another and novel approach utilizing the frequency domain for the identification of neural oscillations from MEG measurements based on spatio-spectral decompositions was recently introduced by Nikulin and colleagues (Nikulin et al., 2011). The method optimizes the

[2]Magnetometers pick-up coils are in principle much more sensitive to magnetic field changes than gradiometers are, and therefore, they are also more sensitive to noise.

spectral SNR by maximizing the signal power at certain peak frequencies, while simultaneously minimizing the power at the neighboring frequency bins. In this way, the method allows to identify components with a "peaky" spectral profile, which is typical for oscillatory processes (Nikulin et al., 2011).

A different way of detecting strong and weak oscillatory neuromagnetic activity is to incorporating the phase dynamics of the data into the analysis (Gross et al., 2006; Matani et al., 2010; Schyns et al., 2011; Tass et al., 1998; Vairavan et al., 2010; Yoshino et al., 2002). Numerical studies have shown that the analysis of phase dynamics reveals synchronization patterns even in cases of weak or absent amplitude correlation (Rosenblum et al., 1996). In 2008, Dammers and colleagues introduced a fully automated approach using cross trial phase statistics (CTPS) for the identification of cardiac artifacts in phase space from decomposed MEG signals (Dammers et al., 2008). In this study, the authors demonstrated that CTPS is a highly sensitive method, which is capable of identifying not only strong but also weak cardiac artifacts that hardly can be identified by visual inspection. Recently, the same method has been applied to extract brain responses that are highly correlated to an external stimulus from a set of decomposed MEG signals in a user-independent fashion (Dammers et al., 2010). Using a single statistical measure the method automatically extracts the components of interest, with respect to repetitive events. When focusing on brain responses, CTPS leads to an enhanced signal-to-noise ratio and therefore enables single-trial data analysis including source localization with improved spatial resolution.

2. Artifact or signal of interest?

According to the experimental design and the neuroscientific question behind the MEG investigation the number and types of stimuli may vary for each experiment. Quite often, within one MEG experiment several conditions (i.e., different stimuli are presented to invoke different brain areas) are employed, where the subject has to cope with different tasks during the experiment. Depending on the duration of the experiment and the number of different conditions used within one experiment, the number of stimuli for each condition may be in the range of a few tens only. In such cases, averaging is less effective to reduce the noise. In addition to noise, the measured activity in all MEG experiments represents a signal mixture comprised of field contributions originating from different brain areas and artifact sources, such as, ocular, muscle and cardiac activity. In addition, the signal strength of such biological artifacts may be several orders of magnitude higher than the signal of interest. Although the signal strength of ocular artifacts (e.g., eye blinks and eye movements) is less compared to the signal of cardiac activity, ocular artifacts are one of the strongest biological artifact signals in MEG due to the close eye-to-sensor distance. Contrary to ocular and muscle artifacts (e.g. swallow and mimic), the cardiac signal is more frequent and cannot be avoided or prevented. In unfavorable cases, the artifact signal (e.g. ocular or cardiac activity) may occur just around the time of the stimulus. It is therefore advisable, and whenever possible, to avoid stimuli intervals, which do have the same frequency rate as the heart beat. However, even when the experimental design includes variable stimuli intervals (often called as stimulus onset asynchrony, SOA) in many MEG experiments it is observed that subjects do perform eye blinks straight after a visual or auditory stimulation. In terms of source localization, this is a severe problem. The artifact signal will be highly correlated with the signal of interest so that even averaging of hundreds of trials may not prevent the source location being shifted towards to source of the artifact. In Fig. 1 the upper row shows strong magnetic field contributions, which are highly correlated with the onsets of auditory stimuli as indicated by the blue vertical lines. Superposition of the EOG signal reveals that the recorded signal is related to ocular artifacts (eye blinks). The bottom row of the figure shows an example of strong but stimulus uncorrelated field contributions from cardiac activity. In either case, the analysis of MEG signals requires the identification and elimination of the artificial signals prior to analysis.

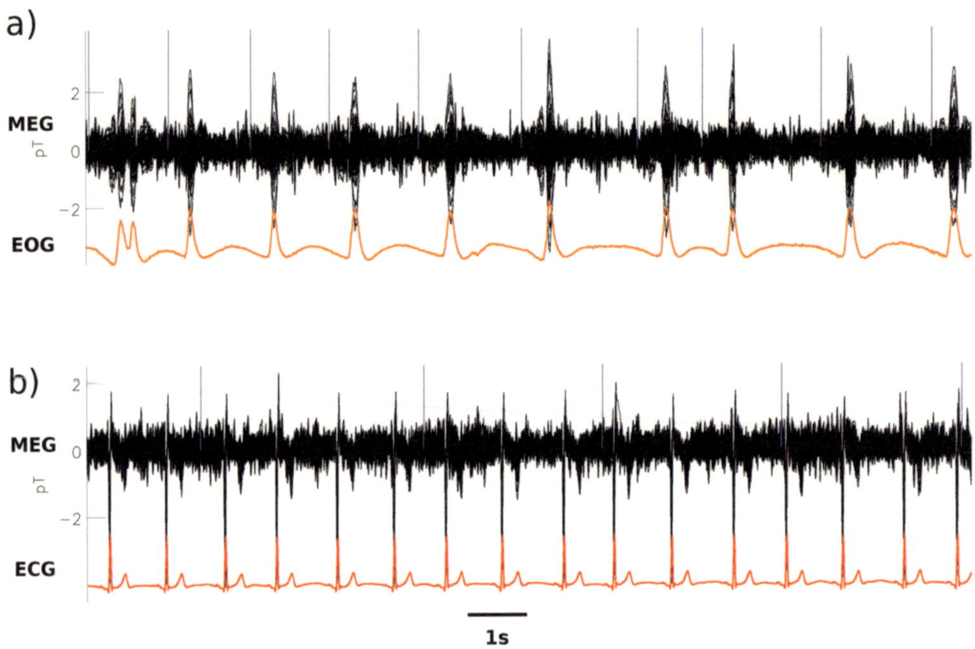

Fig. 1. Signal of interest or artifact?
In a) strong magnetic field contributions appear to be highly correlated with the onsets of the auditory stimuli (blue vertical lines). A superposition of the EOG signal (in orange) reveals that the recorded signal is related to ocular artifacts. In b) an example of strong but stimulus uncorrelated field contributions from cardiac activity (in red) is shown.

3. Methodological concepts of signal separation and classification

In the following sections we will give a brief introduction to the basic principles of signal decomposition utilizing independent component analysis (ICA), followed by an introduction to the basic concepts of cross trial phase statistics (CTPS).

3.1 A short introduction to independent component analysis (ICA)

As described in the previous section the recorded signal at each detector consists of field components originating from the acting brain, noise and artifact sources. A variety of methods for the identification and separation of noise and artifacts from the signal of interest have been proposed over the last ten years to overcome this problem. The rejection of corrupted epochs or trials by visual inspection is however still widely applied. The major disadvantage of this method is that it results in loss of data. Apart from the fact that visual inspection cannot be objective, if the number of trials for averaging is low or the analysis must be performed on single-trials, a rejection of corrupted epochs is not an option.

Independent component analysis (ICA) is widely used to separate brain signals from artifact components using utilizing both semi- and fully automated procedures (Dammers et al., 2008; Escudero, et al., 2010, 2011; Hironaga & Ioannides, 2007; Li, et al., 2006; Mantini et al., 2008; Ossadtchi et al., 2004; Ting et al., 2006). Independent component analysis was developed for solving the blind source separation (BSS) problem with the basic assumption, that the recorded data in a sensor array are linear sums of temporally independent components originating from spatially fixed sources (Bell & Sejnowski, 1995; Comon, 1994; Herault & Jutten, 1986; Hyvärinen, 1999). The general idea of ICA based source analysis methods is to separate the signal of interest from unwanted noise and artifact signals, before source localization is applied to a few number of selected components. The challenge here is to recover N independent source signals $\mathbf{s}(t) = [s_1(t), s_2(t), ..., s_N(t)]^T$ from N linearly mixed observed signals $\mathbf{x}(t) = [x_1(t), x_2(t), ..., x_N(t)]^T$ recorded by N detectors. Let $\mathbf{A}$ denote the mixing matrix the system to be solved can be formulated as

$$\mathbf{x} = \mathbf{A}\mathbf{s} \tag{1}$$

If M is the number of data points in $\mathbf{x}$ (t) at time t using N detectors the mixing matrix $\mathbf{A}$ will be of dimension NxN. The key problem in ICA is to find an unmixing matrix $\mathbf{W}$ (similar to a pseudo-inverse $\mathbf{A}^{-1}$, with $\mathbf{W} \approx \mathbf{A}^{-1}$) while imposing that the sources in $\mathbf{s}$ are statistically independent

$$\mathbf{c} = \mathbf{W}\mathbf{x} \tag{2}$$

ICA transforms an N-sensor data array into an N-dimensional component space, where each of the components in $\mathbf{c}$ carries a minimum amount of mutual information with respect to the temporal dynamic and thus is maximally independent. The independent components are stored in rows of $\mathbf{c}$. Assuming the model is valid each row in $\mathbf{c}$ reflects the time courses of the true source, except that scale, sign and order will not be preserved. For solving equation (2), the method makes no assumption about the mixing process except that it is linear including the restriction that the number of sources is less or equal N. The estimated full rank square matrix $\mathbf{W}$ in (2) can be treated as a spatial filter matrix which linearly inverts the mixing process. It is important to note that independence is not equivalent to uncorrelatedness, as it would be for Gaussian distributions. In fact estimating independent components is based on maximization of the non-gaussianity of $\mathbf{Wx}$ (Hyvärinen & Oja, 2000). However, if $\mathbf{A}$ is sufficiently determined (i.e., by solving $\mathbf{W}^{-1}$) one can remove the mixing effect by applying $\mathbf{W}$ to $\mathbf{x}$.

After signal decomposition the problem now is to objectively identify components of interest in such high dimensional data sets, as it is the case for modern MEG systems. Different strategies have been proposed to exactly tackle the problem of unsupervised component extraction to find either artifacts (Dammers et al., 2008; Escudero et al., 2011; Li et al., 2006; Mantini et al., 2008) or signal of interest (Dammers et al., 2010; Hild & Nagarajan, 2009; Nikulin et al., 2011; Vairavan et al., 2010).

Apart from time series analysis applied to the independent components for the identification of the source of interest, it might be helpful to look at the so-called place map of each temporally independent component. Such maps can be constructed from the columns of $\mathbf{W}^{-1}$. Since each column of matrix $\mathbf{W}^{-1}$ has N entries a projection of the signal onto

the sensor arrangement gives rise to the location of the detectors showing strong signal contributions for the associated component.
Once all components of interest are identified, the separation from unwanted components is done by zeroing all columns of $\mathbf{W}^{-1}$ except those which correspond to the signal of interest. The zeroing results in a new matrix $\hat{\mathbf{W}}^{-1}$ which filters out the unwanted source contributions, while leaving the signal of interest. The ICA filtering (i.e., artifact removal or extraction of components of interest) of the measured data is then performed by back transformation of $\mathbf{c}$ using the filter matrix $\hat{\mathbf{W}}^{-1}$

$$\mathbf{x}' = \hat{\mathbf{W}}^{-1}\mathbf{c} \tag{3}$$

3.2 A short introduction to cross trial phase statistics

Phase space methods are well established in non linear time series analysis; a good overview can be found in (Kantz & Schreiber, 2003). These methods are based on the famous Takens' Theorem stating that the dynamics of a system can be reconstructed from a single signal measured with a constant sampling rate (Takens, 1981). The concept based on these methods to concentrate on phase dynamics while neglecting amplitude dynamics has proven to be very powerful in analyzing noisy data of nonlinear or even chaotic systems (M. Rosenblum et al., 1996). As physiological systems very often show these features, phase based methods have been widely applied in this field. Especially the research on physiological oscillators and their mutual synchronization has a long tradition (Holst, 1937) and phase based methods for synchronization analysis have contributed a lot to this field of research (Glass, 2001; Mosekilde et al., 2002; Schiek et al., 1998; P. Tass, 1999), while the improvement of these methods still continues (Ocon et al., 2011; Wacker & Witte, 2011; Wagner et al., 2010).
To define instantaneous phases of a signal of interest one starts to transform the signal s using a rotational process by introducing an additional but related signal $\hat{s}$ as a second coordinate in the so called embedding plane. The most common method to obtain these related signals is the Hilbert transform (Bracewell, 1999). Alternative, if one knows the characteristic period length τ of the process of interest the following definition is also an appropriate choice (Schiek et al., 1998)

$$\hat{s}(t) = s(t - \tau/4) \tag{4}$$

A precondition for both methods is to band pass filter the original signal, where the filter limits being defined by the frequency of interest. In the following we will use the discrete approximation of the Hilbert transform:

$$\hat{s}(t) = 1/\pi \sum_{k=1}^{\infty} \frac{s(t-k)-s(t+k)}{k} \tag{5}$$

with t denoting the time step.
This leads to the following phase definition as the rotational angle around the origin within the two-dimensional embedding space:

$$\varphi(t) = \arctan\frac{\hat{s}(t)}{s(t)} \tag{6}$$

The idea of the cross trial phase statistics (CTPS) is to test for changes within the phase dynamics induced by the recurring events. Therefore the time series of the instantaneous phase is split into windows, where the center is defined by the event itself. In CTPS the statistics of these cross trial phases are analyzed. Stereotypic responses of a signal to stimuli for example, will reveal itself as a single cluster of phases short after the occurrence of the stimulus. Non stereotypic responses may also be detected by the method, as long as there are only a limited number of possible responses, and furthermore, this number is small compared to the number of stimuli. Two different responses for example would lead to two clusters within the cross trial phase plot. In systems without any stimuli related responses no phase clustering will be observed. In such a case, the phase values will form a more or less uniform distribution (Fig. 2D). Three examples for phase clustering (Fig. 2A-C) and one for a uniform phase distribution are shown in Fig. 2. The differences between the large or weak coupled signals can be detected by visual inspection very easily. With no difficulty one is able to differentiate between rather strict responses (Fig. 2A) or more weak responses (Fig. 2B-C), where the phase clustering is more broad. Such a moderate phase clustering may be caused by measurement noise and/or by weak or irregular coupling.

In order to quantify these findings (i.e. to quantify the strength of the response to the stimuli) the so called Kuiper test is used. This statistical test is a refinement of the more common Kolmogorow-Smirnow test (KS test). The KS test is widely accepted to quantify the probability that two data sets are samples of the same distribution. As a preparatory step, the two data sets have to be transformed to their normalized cumulative distribution. A good introduction to both tests can be found in (Press et al., 2001). The application of these tests in phase resetting analysis is described in (Tass, 2004). To check for stimuli related phase responses we compare the cross trial phase distribution $g(\Phi)$ with the uniform distribution $u(\Phi)$.

Let $s(t)$ be the original signal, $\Phi(t)$ be the instantaneous phase, normalized by 2π (i.e., the phase values range from 0 to 1), $g(\Phi)$ being the normalized cumulative cross trial phase distribution ($g(\Phi)$ ~ relative number of cross trial phases smaller than Φ, and g ranging from 0 to 1), and $u(\Phi) = \Phi$ being the uniform density distribution. Using the absolute maximal difference between the two cumulative distribution

$$D = \max_{0 \leq \Phi \leq 1} | g(\Phi) - u(\Phi) | \tag{7}$$

the KS-test calculates the probability of error for rejecting the null hypothesis that g and u are samples of the same distribution with

$$P_{KS}(\lambda) = 2 \sum_{k=1}^{\infty} (-1)^{k-1} e^{-2k^2\lambda^2} \tag{8}$$

with $\lambda = V(\sqrt{N} + 0.155 + 0.24/\sqrt{N})$ and N being the number of data points.

The disadvantage of the KS-test is that the accuracy decreases in case where the largest difference D is located close to the tails, i.e. $\Phi=0$ or $\Phi=1$. This however is considered in the Kuiper test by defining D in the following way

$$D = \max_{0 \leq \Phi \leq 1} [g(\Phi) - u(\Phi)] + \max_{0 \leq \Phi \leq 1} [u(\Phi) - g(\Phi)] \tag{9}$$

and by using a modified probability statistic that reads

$$P_K(\lambda) = 2 \sum_{k=1}^{\infty} (4k^2\lambda^2 - 1) e^{-2k^2\lambda^2} \tag{10}$$

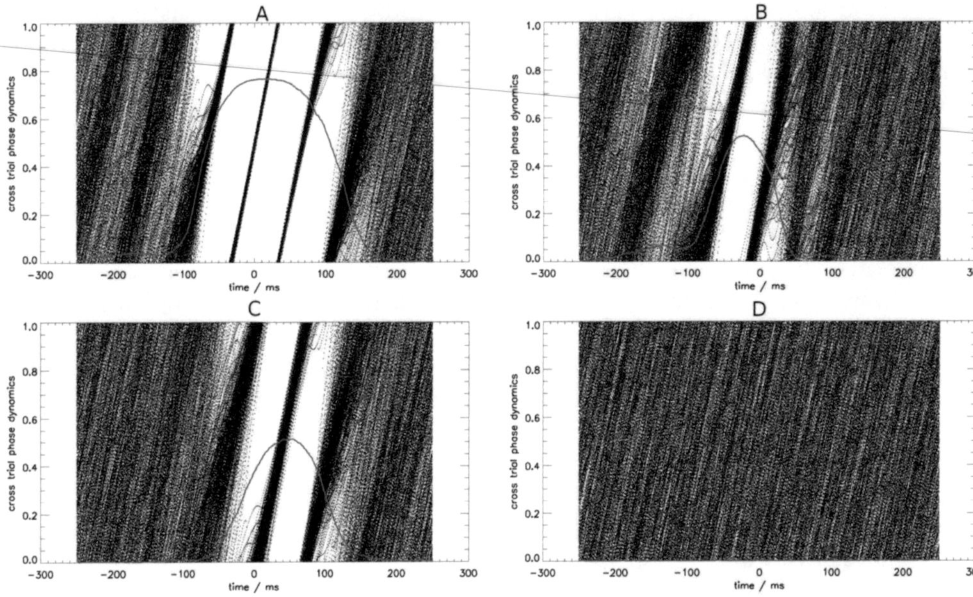

Fig. 2. Cross trial phase statistics of strong (A), moderate (B-C) and non-coupled (D) signal responses.

In the case of a disproof of the null hypothesis (i.e. g(Φ) has a non-uniform distribution), P_K becomes 0 in the limit of D→1. Since P_K becomes very small for D→1, we introduced the negative logarithmic value

$$p_K = -\log_{10}(P_K)/N_T \tag{11}$$

with N_T being the number of trials used. This is done to quantify the strength of the response to the stimuli independently from the number of trials used. It is a consequence of the applied statistical method that the test statistic $-\log_{10}(P_K)$ increases the more events (i.e. stimuli) are taken into account for the analysis. In order to have comparable results the test statistic is normalized to the number of trials used, so that the p_K value is ranging between 0 and 1.

4. CTPS based cardiac and ocular artifact rejection

For automatic identification of cardiac and ocular artifact using CTPS data segments (trials) from the decomposed MEG signals needs to be defined around the event of interest (e.g., the R-peak of the QRS-complex or the peak of an eye blink). The window length should be large enough to cover the artifact signal and may be set to about 0.5s and 1s for the cardiac and eye blink artifact, respectively. Each window (trial) should be centered around the (main) peak of the artifact of interest The peak latencies for the two types of artifacts can easily be extracted from auxiliary ECG and EOG channels, while for R-peak detection an ECG channel may not be necessary, as shown by Escudero and colleagues (Escudero, et al., 2011). For a reasonable definition of the instantaneous phases a bandpass filter should be applied to the ECG and EOG signals, which covers the main energy of the QRS power spectrum. The normal duration of the QRS-complex is typically in the range of about 0.06 – 0.10 s,

while for normal subjects the QRS duration should be ≤ 0.12s (Kashani & Barold, 2005). The total eye blink duration (closing and opening of the eye lid) is even more variable and depends on the subject's condition and the task demands. Under normal condition the full blink duration d_{blink} is often reported to be in the range of $0.1s < d_{blink} < 1s$ (Benedetto et al., 2011). Therefore, reasonable frequency ranges for the CTPS analysis to reveal field contributions from the QRS-complex and eye blinks in independent components are 10-20 Hz and 1-5 Hz, respectively. Slight (!) variations in the selection of the frequency range will not result in a complete failure of the method, but may reduce the significance level of the test statistic.
In Fig. 3 typical cardiac and eye blink artifacts are shown for one subject after signal decomposition using the Infomax algorithm (Bell & Sejnowski, 1995). In the first three rows components related to the cardiac artifact are shown, while the last component highly correlates (by means of Pearson's linear correlation coefficient c, with c=0.98) with the subject's eye blink activity. All components in red shown in Fig. 3 were automatically identified using different second and higher order statistics as described in (Dammers et al., 2008). Note, the third cardiac component (in grey) has much weaker amplitudes compared to the first two components and was identified by CTPS analysis only. Previous reports showed that the cardiac activity often splits into multiple components after ICA decomposition, where the signal strength of each IC can vary quite substantially (Dammers et al., 2008; Sander et al., 2002) However, it has been shown that CTPS is capable of identifying weak artifact components, where second and higher order statistics (including correlation analysis) failed (Dammers et al., 2008).

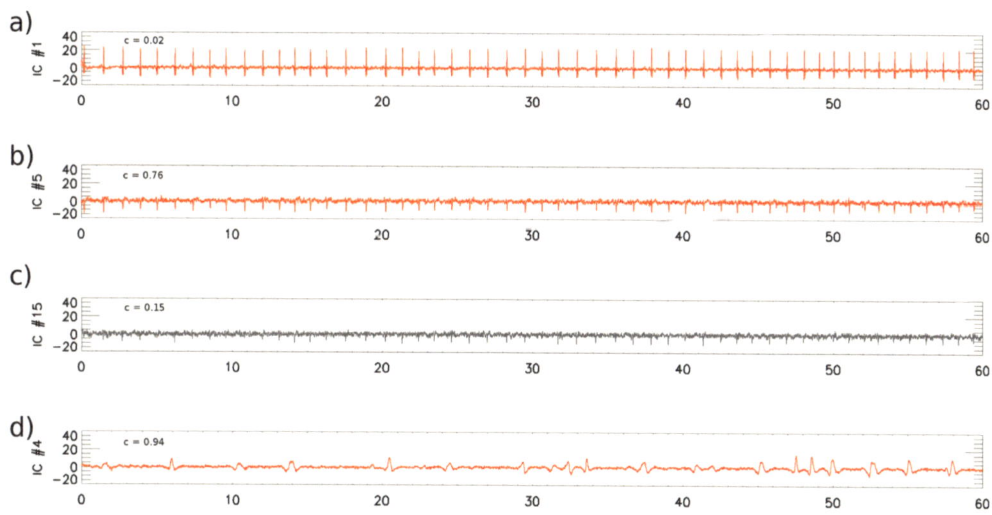

Fig. 3. Identification of ocular and cardiac artifacts.
Typical examples of independent components (ICs) showing cardiac (a-c) and ocular (d) artifacts in one subject, during the first minute of an MEG experiment. ICs shown in red were identified using second or higher order statistics, or correlation analysis. In contrast to the amplitude based methods, CTPS analysis was able to identify all four components (a-d). Note, the poor correlation of IC#1 (a) and IC#15 (c) to the ECG signal, where correlation coefficient was 0.02 and 0.15, respectively. In contrast, both ICs were perfectly identified using CTPS analysis (significance level ≥ 0.5).

The number of components related to cardiac activity depends on the subject's individual electrical heart axis and the position of the MEG sensor array (e.g., seated or supine position). Therefore, during analysis one may observe that the latencies across the cardiac components are shifted with respect to the R-peak latencies of the ECG. In such cases, it is much more difficult to identify cardiac components by correlation analysis, even if the amplitude of the signal is large.
Such an example is shown in Fig. 3, where the first cardiac component (IC#1, Fig. 3a) has an absolute correlation coefficient of c=0.02 only, even though this component has the largest amplitude. Further analysis showed that the peak latencies of component IC#1 (Fig. 3a) and IC#15 (Fig. 3c) are correlated to the Q- and S-peak of the ECG signal, respectively (Fig. 4). Therefore, for both components the [3]correlation analysis failed, while the two ICs were identified with no problem as cardiac artifacts using CTPS. The reason here is that CTPS analysis is applied to a predefined time window (e.g., around the R-peak) to search for non-uniform phase distributions. As long as at one latency within the time window, the cross trial phase distribution differs significantly from a uniform distribution, CTPS will be able to identify such a component that is synchronized with the event of interest.

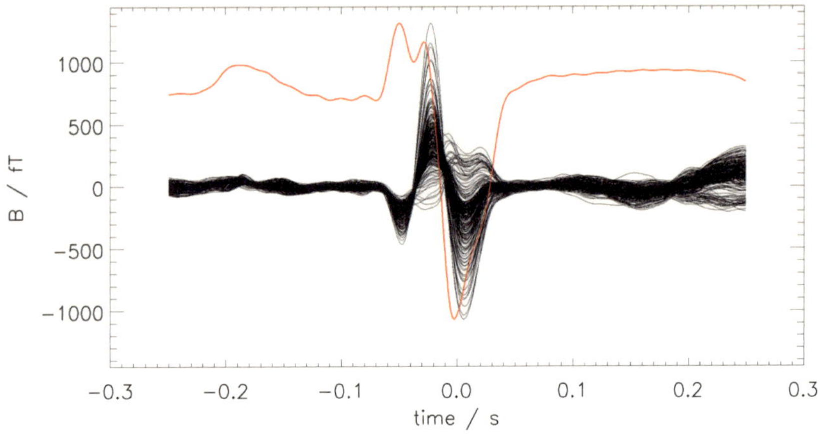

Fig. 4. Additional cardiac component identified by CTPS.
Magnetic fields constructed (black) from IC#15 (cf. Fig. 3) are averaged to the onset of the R-peak. For comparison the ECG signal average is superimposed in red. Note the time shift between the R-peak onset (at time t=0s) and the peak latency of the magnetic signal reconstructed from component #15. The maximum field strength of this IC is even more than 180 ft at the MEG sensor level, while the maximum signal strength of IC#15 (7.8 a.u.) is about one order less compared to IC#1 (78.6 a.u.). This artifact component was solely identified by CTPS, while the applied amplitude based methods failed.

An estimation of how well the CTPS based (or any other) artifact rejection method performs, the artifact signal removal can easily be visualized (Fig. 5). For the example described above, the MEG signals are aligned to the onset of the R-peak and the peak latency of the eye blink.

[3]The correlation of both signals can be increased by allowing a time dependent lag, but with the expense of being much more sensitive to non-cardiac or noise components.

Cross trial averages of the MEG signal will enhance the content of the artifact before and after artifact rejection (Fig. 5). For quantification of the artifact removal one can use the rejection performance measure as introduced in (Dammers et al., 2008).

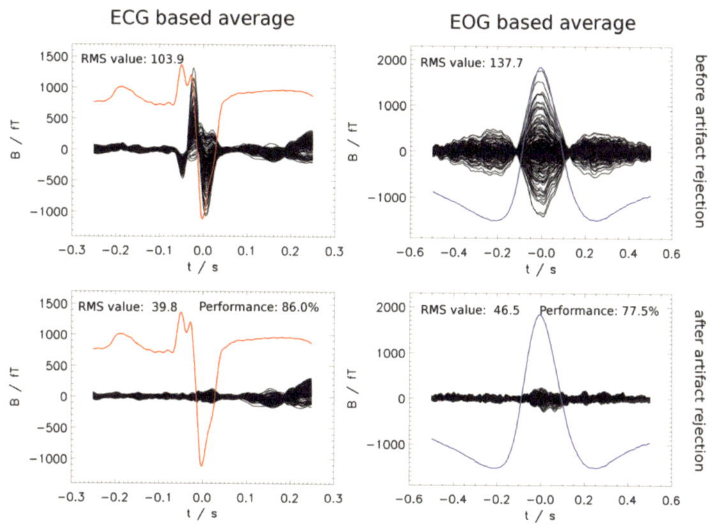

Fig. 5. Artifact rejection performance.
MEG signals averaged with respect to the R-peak of the ECG (left) and the eye blink signal (right) before (top row) and after (bottom row) CTPS based artifact removal. The respective reference signal is superimposed in red and blue (in arbitrary scaling) for the cardiac and ocular artifact, respectively. The RMS based rejection performance (bottom row) indicates the quality of the artifact cleaning process, using the performance measure described in (Dammers et al., 2008). The MEG data were recorded using the MAGNES WH3600 from 4D-neuroimaging.

5. CTPS based identification of strong and weak brain responses

In most cases unaveraged neuromagnetic brain responses are too weak (or too noisy) to be reliably identified by its amplitude statistic only. Averaging on the other hand will enhance the most prominent brain activity by suppressing uncorrelated noise, with the expense of not preserving the temporal dynamics of each individual brain response.

In the previous sections we showed that the analysis of the cross trial phase dynamics in decomposed MEG signals discloses artifact components that are highly correlated to the phase dynamics from trials of a reference signal. Such a reference signal may be the QRS-complex or the eye blink signals recorded by the ECG and EOG channel, respectively. In principal, CTPS analysis can be applied to any other event of interest in order to investigate the phase dynamics of signals and its dependency to predefined points in time. For example, burst onsets in the electromyogram (EMG) or stimulus onsets in the trigger channel may be used to define trials of interest for CTPS analysis. In this way, even weak but stimulus dependent brain responses can be disclosed by its phase clustering around the event of interest, while at the same time, the temporal dynamics of the underlying sources will be remained. The CTPS based identification of stereotypic brain responses in MEG data is best performed if the effect of signal mixtures is removed. Therefore, the decomposition of the MEG data using for example independent component analysis (ICA) is a mandatory requisite.

5.1 CTPS analysis applied to auditory cued MEG signals

For evaluation the method is applied to decomposed MEG data (MAGNES 2500WH, 4D-Neuroimaging) from a simple auditory experiment. About 300 click tones (1 kHz, 50 ms duration, SOA of 1.5 s ± 0.5 s) were presented to both ears of a male volunteer. ICA (Infomax) was applied separate noise and artifacts from brain activity. The trigger onset latencies were used to define 300 trials using a time window ranging from stimulus onset to 150 ms post stimulus. From the MEG raw data (frequency range 1-200 Hz) only, one can be rather vague about stimulus dependent activity (Fig. 6a). After source separation (i.e., by means of ICA) a stimulus related component is identified by CTPS analysis (Fig. 6a). Since analysis of phase dynamics requires a frequency band of interest, either prior knowledge of the frequency components or multiple frequency ranges should be used for CTPS analysis. Therefore, within the frequency ranges of 2–4, 4–8, 8–12, 12–16, and 16–20 Hz we scanned for the largest p_K value in all ICs. The component with the highest significance level of the

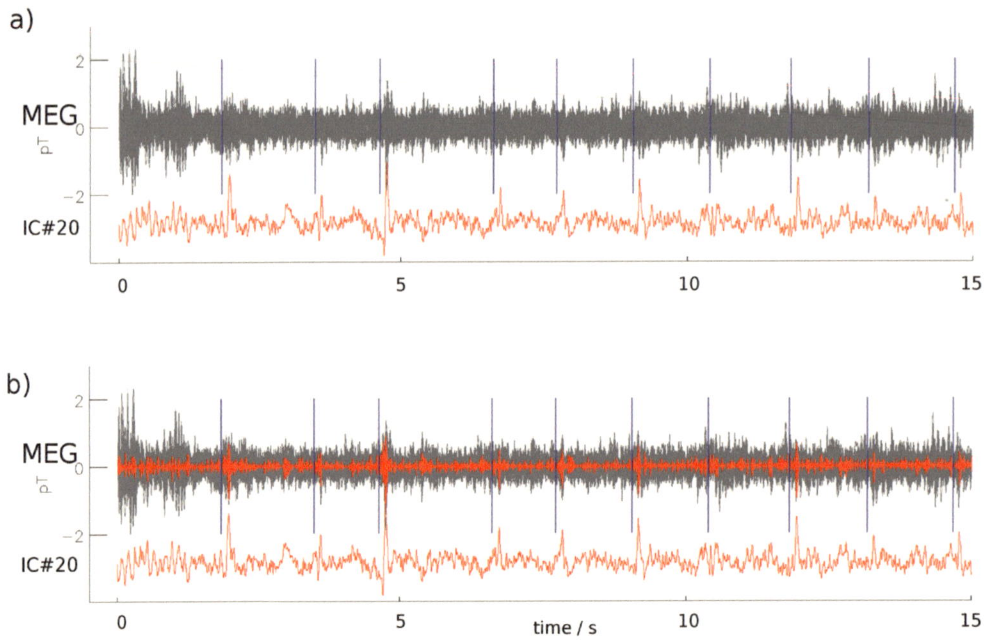

Fig. 6. CTPS based source identification.
In a) unaveraged MEG raw signals (gray) are shown for the first 15 s of an auditory experiment. All 148 MEG signals are superimposed, while the blue lines indicate the stimulus onset times. The independent component (IC#20 in red) with the maximum significance level after CTPS analysis is plotted below the MEG signal. The peaked activity of this component reflects brain activity that is highly synchronized with the stimulus. In b) the MEG raw signals (gray) are shown together with MEG signals after back-transformation of the identified component (red). The amplitude varies, but stimulus dependent brain activity is now obvious.

test statistic (Eq. 11) was found in IC#20 at a frequency range of 4–8 Hz ($p_{K,max}$=0.45), while for the frequency ranges 8–12 and 12–16 Hz the maximum p_K value was still about 0.44. Typically, p_K values of ICs related to brain responses are smaller compared to ICs which are related to cardiac activity (where p_K values typically are above 0.5). The reason is that we do not precisely know the latencies of the trial-by-trial brain activity. For example, for auditory cued brain responses we expect strong evoked activity around 100 ms after stimulus onset. The latencies of the true brain responses however jitter a few milliseconds from trial to trial, with the effect, that the phase clustering around the average response latency is not as narrow as it is e.g. for cardiac activity. Nevertheless, the maximum p_k value of IC#20 was found to be $p_{K,max}$=0.452, while the mean value across all ICs was $p_{K,mean}$=0.016 ±0.038.

Back-transformation of the identified signal component to the MEG sensor space revealed stimulus dependent evoked activity with a much better signal-to-noise ratio (Fig. 6b). Subsequent source analysis of the identified component revealed that the corresponding signal was localized in the primary auditory cortices. In Fig. 7 five trials (trial #6-10) are shown before and after CTPS based source extraction. Compared to trials of the MEG raw signal the signal-to-noise ratio after back-transformation of the identified source component (IC#20) is much better. With such an improvement in SNR CTPS analysis enables source localization on the single-trial level.

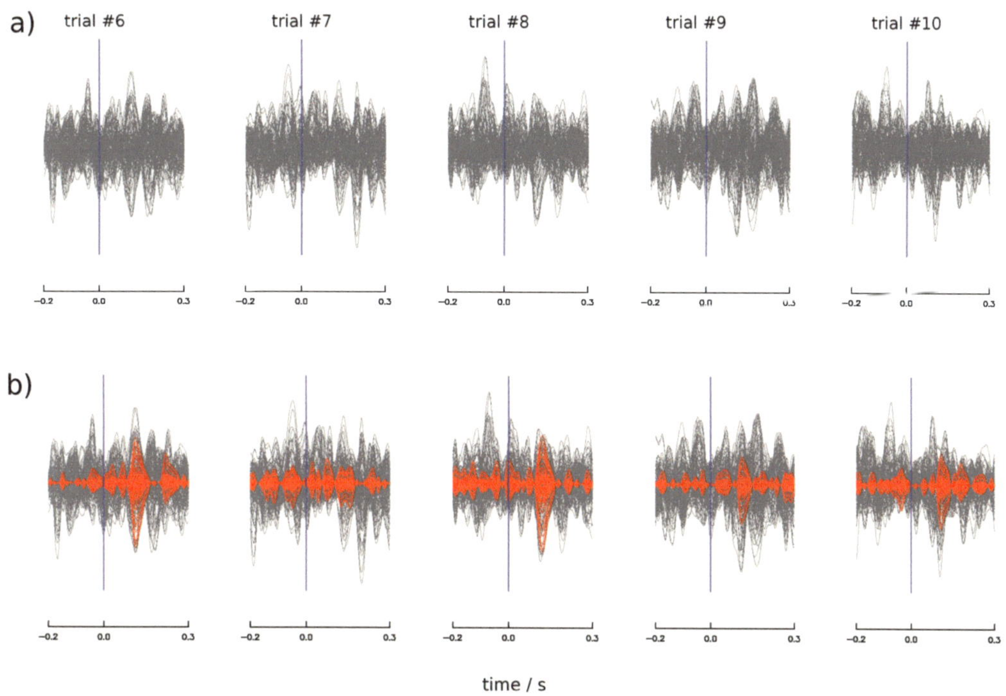

Fig. 7. Signal enhancement in MEG single-trials.
Selected single-trials from an auditory MEG experiment. In a) trials of unprocessed MEG raw signals (gray) are shown. In b) single-trials of MEG signals after back-transformation (in red) of one source component (IC#20 in Fig. 6) as identified by CTPS analysis. The blue lines indicate the stimulus onset times of the auditory click tones.

5.2 CTPS analysis on MEG signals evoked by voluntary finger movements

In the following experiment CTPS analysis is applied to search for stereotypic brain responses with respect to voluntary finger movements. The MEG data of one subject were recorded using a 248 magnetometer whole head MEG system from 4D-Neuroimaging (MAGNES 3600WH). The right handed subject voluntarily lifted up and down the right index finger 117 times. Between two subsequent finger lifts the subject was asked to perform a short rest of about 1–2 s.

After ICA decomposition cross trial phase distributions were calculated for each IC within a time window of 600 ms centered around the movement onset detected by a photoelectric barrier. We have analyzed the phase dynamics of all ICs within different frequency bands (cf. section 5.1). Results from CTPS analysis revealed that the phase dynamics for different frequency bands qualitatively resemble, therefore the results presented here are limited to the frequency band corresponding to the largest p_K value (Fig. 8).

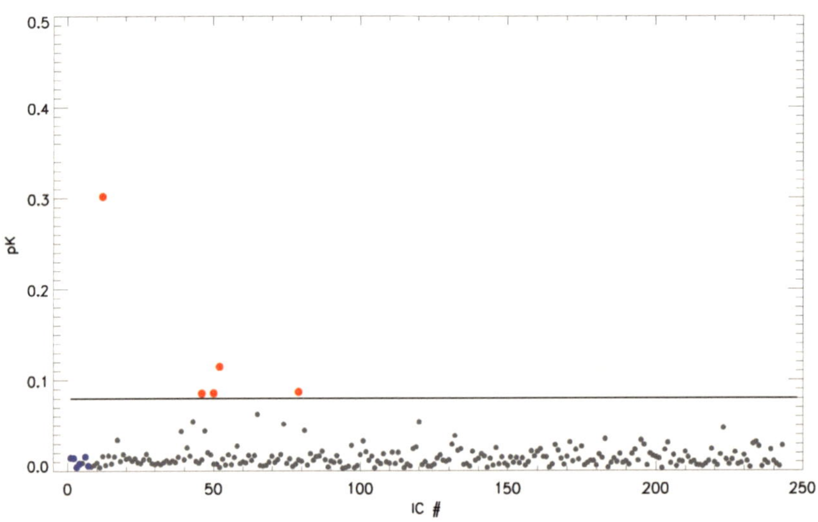

Fig. 8. Significance level of components related to voluntary finger movement.
CTPS analysis applied to a voluntary finger movement experiment. ICs with p_k values greater or equal the 98th percentile of all p_k values (indicated by the black horizontal line) are marked in red. ICs that have been identified as artifacts are shown in blue.

For subsequent single-trial data analysis, only ICs related to significant brain responses (as defined by large p_k values in Fig. 8) were back-transformed into the MEG signal space. The separation of these components from other contributions results in a much better SNR in the single-trial data as illustrated in Fig. 9. On average the strongest peak in the MEG signal is found at the time t=0 ms, when the finger is just lifted (Fig. 9a), while the peak latencies of the individual brain responses may vary as indicated by the red arrow in Fig. 9.

For the same experiment, current source localization was then performed to single-trial MEG data, as well as to signal averages aligned to the onsets of voluntary finger movements. The difficulty here is that two nearby sources, i.e. the primary motor (MI) and the somatosensory cortex (SI), are activated at the same time, where a separation of the two focal sources is challenging for any source analysis. Here we used magnetic field tomography (MFT, Ioannides et al., 1990) to reveal source localizations of the underlying neuromagnetic activity from both averaged and single-trial data (Fig. 10). Source reconstruction based on standard averaging revealed distributed activity over both motor and somatosensory areas (Fig. 10a) for the time indicated by the red arrow as depicted in Fig. 9.

In Fig. 10b-c localization results of a single epoch (trial #5, cf. Fig. 9b) are illustrated, while in Fig. 10c the reconstruction was applied to MEG signals derived from the IC with the maximum p_K value (IC#12, cf. Fig. 8). Due to the poor signal-to-noise ratio for this single-trial the reconstructed activity shown in Fig. 10b is widely distributed over the brain, while its maximum was found to be close to the cerebellum (not shown). In contrast, the CTPS based source localization of the components with the strongest p_K value (IC#12) reveals a more focal source pattern for this single-trial, while its maximum activity (in red) is located in MI (Fig. 10c). For comparison, localization results based on signal averages are shown in (Fig. 10a). Although uncorrelated noise is fairly suppressed after signal averaging, the maximum activity here is distributed over both areas, the motor and somatosensory cortex, since both areas are activated at the same time.

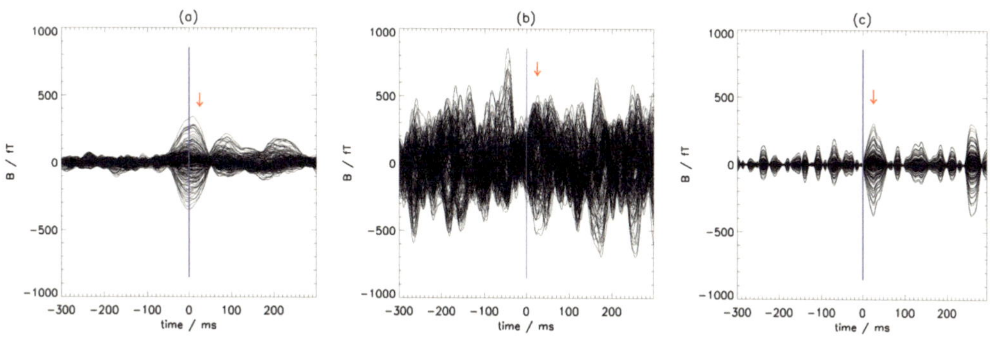

Fig. 9. MEG signal averages vs. single-trial analysis.
In a) MEG signal averages aligned to the onset of voluntarily finger movements (indicated by the blue line). In b). unaveraged MEG signals are shown for one selected trial (trial #5). The signal-to-noise ratio does not allow to make any statements about the stimulus related activity. For the same trial the MEG signal derived from the IC with the maximum p_K value is shown in c) (cf. Fig. 8). Note, the shift in peak latency (indicated by the red arrow) of the individual response in trial#5 (b-c) compared to the averaged peak latency in a). The improvement in the SNR after CTPS analysis as shown in c) is evident compared to b).

Localization of the 2nd to 5th strongest components (with respect to their p_K value, cf. Fig. 8) revealed "independent" somatosensory activity (by means of statistical independence as defined by ICA), where the origin of the maximum activity was found to be within the somatosensory cortex, as indicated by the location of the central sulcus (Fig. 11). By adding the current densities of each localized component, the resulting activation pattern closely resemble the activation one gets, when localizing the fields constructed from all four components. However, the major advantages in CTPS based source analysis is i) the method is capable of identifying components that are highly synchronized to an event of interest and ii) nearby sources which are activated at the same time can be separated, where standard averaging based methods may fail.

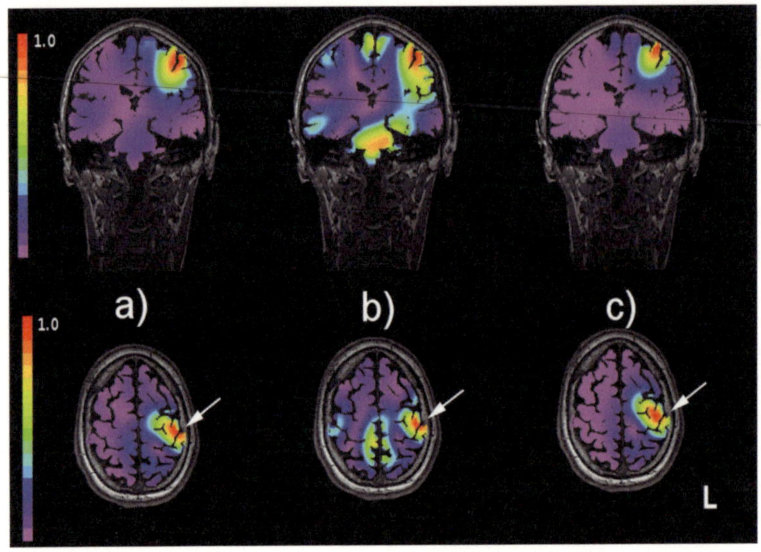

Fig. 10. Source reconstruction of signal averages vs. single-trial data.
All localization results are shown for the latency indicated by the red arrow in Fig. 9. Standard averaging source analysis (a) shows that the activity is distributed in both motor and somatosensory areas. The white arrow indicates the central sulcus. The reconstructed current density distribution of the unaveraged data in b) is fairly widespread over the entire brain, while the strongest activity was found to be in the cerebellum (not shown). In c) the CTPS based source localization of the signal shown in Fig. 9c is much more focal and its maximum activity (in red) is located in the primary motor cortex.

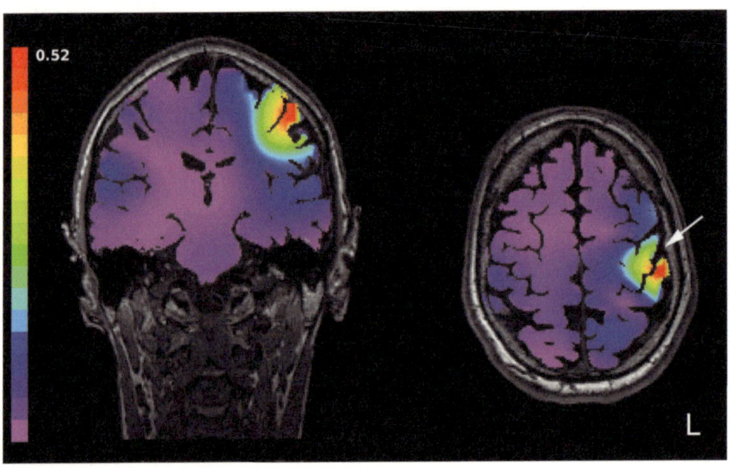

Fig. 11. CTPS based source reconstruction.
Source localization of magnetic fields constructed from ICs with p_K values ranging from $0.12 \leq p_K < p_{Kmax}$ as identified by CTPS analysis (cf. Fig. 8). The localization of the corresponding single-trial MEG signal shows that the activity can be attributed to a weak stimulus related somatosensory response, which could not be isolated using averaging based localization (cf. Fig. 10). The white arrow indicates the central sulcus.

6. Conclusion

Cross trial phase statistics (CTPS) applied to decomposed MEG signals allows for both, user independent identification of artifacts, as well as the extraction of strong and weak event related brain responses. With respect to cardiac artifact (CA) rejection, the ICA decomposition of the recorded MEG signal often shows multiple independent components (ICs) that can be attributed to CA. Since, the amplitudes of CA components can vary quite substantially; it is therefore difficult for any automatic procedure that exclusively relies on amplitude information alone. In contrast, CTPS based identification of CA related components is very sensitive. Even in cases of weak signal strength, the method identifies multiple components that can be attributed to cardiac activity, where amplitude based methods fail (Figs. 3-4). For ocular artifacts, CTPS as well as second and higher order statistics are able to identify eye blink components due to its larger amplitudes (Fig. 3). In any case, the performance of the artifact rejection can be visualized (Fig. 5) and estimated using the rejection performance metric described in (Dammers et al., 2008).
Within CTPS analysis the information about the occurrence of an event is of importance. Phase clustering of an event related signal is enhanced if trials of the phase dynamics are perfectly aligned to the time of the event. In the case of cardiac artifact rejection the CTPS based identification is very accurate, since all trials can precisely be aligned by extracting the R-peak latencies of the QRS-complex signal from the ECG signal.
Since CTPS is a highly sensitive approach for extracting weak event-related fields, the same strategy can also be used for the identification of stereotypic brain responses. For this, time information about the occurrence of each brain response must be available. Therefore, the latencies of the brain responses which do correlate to an external event are estimated by make use an external reference signal, such as the trigger or response channel. These channels provide time information about a stimulus presentation or a subject's response to a stimulus (e.g. a button press). However, the delay between for example a stimulus and the event related brain activity is not strictly fix. This results in a drop of p_K values (p_K describes the significance of a component being synchronized to an event of interest) when compared to values of CTPS based cardiac artifact rejection. Nevertheless, as long as the brain responses jitter a few milliseconds only, CTPS is able to identify event related brain activity in unaveraged decomposed MEG data (Figs. 6,10,11).
In this way the method enables single-trial data analysis by providing reconstructed MEG signals with sufficient SNR (cf. Fig. 7) for single-trial source reconstruction. The CTPS based single-trial source localization provides equal or even improved spatial accuracy compared to standard averaging techniques (Fig. 10). Reconstruction of identified single (or a group of) components have the advantage of being able to separate nearby sources although they are activated at the same time (Figs. 10c, 11). Therefore, if single-trial brain dynamics or the source separation of nearby sources is of interest, CTPS based source reconstruction seems to be a promising tool for the identification of event related brain activity in unaveraged decomposed MEG data.

7. References

Bell, A. J., & Sejnowski, T. J. (1995). An information-maximization approach to blind separation and blind deconvolution. *Neural computation*, 7(6), 1129-59. MIT Press.

Benedetto, S., Pedrotti, M., Minin, L., Baccino, T., Re, A., & Montanari, R. (2011). Driver workload and eye blink duration. *Transportation Research Part F: Traffic Psychology and Behaviour, 14*(3), 199-208. doi:10.1016/j.trf.2010.12.001

Bracewell, R. N. (1999). *The Hilbert transform. The Fourier Transform and Its Applications.* (Brace, Ed.) (3rd ed., pp. 267-272). McGraw-Hill.

Comon, P. (1994). Independent Component Analysis - a new concept? *Signal Processing, 36,* 287-314.

Dammers, J., Schiek, M., Boers, F., Silex, C., Zvyagintsev, M., Pietrzyk, U., & Mathiak, K. (2008). Integration of amplitude and phase statistics for complete artifact removal in independent components of neuromagnetic recordings. *IEEE transactions on bio-medical engineering, 55*(10), 2353-62. doi:10.1109/TBME.2008.926677

Dammers, J., Schiek, M., Boers, F., Weidner, R., Chen, Y.-H., Mathiak, K., & Shah, N. J. (2010). Localization of stereotypic brain responses detected by instantaneous phase statistics from independent components. *Frontiers in Neuroscience. Conference Abstract. 17th International Conference on Biomagnetism. 2010.*

Escudero, J., Hornero, R., & Abásolo, D. (2010). Consistency of the blind source separation computed with five common algorithms for magnetoencephalogram background activity. *Medical engineering & physics, 32*(10), 1137-44. doi:10.1016/j.medengphy.2010.08.005

Escudero, J., Hornero, R., Abásolo, D., & Fernández, A. (2011). Quantitative Evaluation of Artifact Removal in Real Magnetoencephalogram Signals with Blind Source Separation. *Annals of biomedical engineering,* 1-13-13. Springer Netherlands. doi:10.1007/s10439-011-0312-7

Glass, L. (2001). Synchronization and rhythmic processes in physiology. *Nature, 410*(6825), 277-84. doi:10.1038/35065745

Gross, J., Schmitz, F., Schnitzler, I., Kessler, K., Shapiro, K., Hommel, B., & Schnitzler, Alfons. (2006). Anticipatory control of long-range phase synchronization. *The European journal of neuroscience, 24*(7), 2057-60. doi:10.1111/j.1460-9568.2006.05082.x

Guimaraes, M. P., Wong, D. K., Uy, E. T., Grosenick, L., & Suppes, P. (2007). Single-trial classification of MEG recordings. *IEEE transactions on bio-medical engineering, 54*(3), 436-43. doi:10.1109/TBME.2006.888824

Herault, J., & Jutten, C. (1986). Space or time adaptive signal processing by neural network models. *AIP Conference Proceedings, 151*(1), 206-211. doi:10.1063/1.36258

Hild, K. E., & Nagarajan, S. S. (2009). Source localization of EEG/MEG data by correlating columns of ICA and lead field matrices. *IEEE transactions on bio-medical engineering, 56*(11), 2619-26. doi:10.1109/TBME.2009.2028615

Hironaga, N., & Ioannides, A. A. (2007). Localization of individual area neuronal activity. *NeuroImage, 34*(4), 1519-34. doi:10.1016/j.neuroimage.2006.10.030

Holst, E. (1937). Vom Wesen der Ordnung im Zentralnervensystem. *Die Naturwissenschaften, 25*(40), 641-647. Springer Berlin / Heidelberg. doi:10.1007/BF01496358

Hyvärinen, A. (1999). Fast and robust fixed-point algorithms for independent component analysis. *IEEE transactions on neural networks / a publication of the IEEE Neural Networks Council, 10*(3), 626-34. doi:10.1109/72.761722

Hyvärinen, A., & Oja, E. (2000). Independent component analysis: algorithms and applications. *Neural networks : the official journal of the International Neural Network Society, 13*(4-5), 411-30.

Ioannides, A. A., Bolton, J. P. R., & Clarke, C. (1990). Continuous probabilistic solutions to the biomagnetic inverse problem. *Inverse Problems, 6*, 523-542. doi:10.1088/0266-5611/6/4/005

Kantz, H., & Schreiber, T. (2003). *Nonlinear Time Series Analysis*. Cambridge, UK: Cambridge Univerity Press.

Kashani, A., & Barold, S. S. (2005). Significance of QRS complex duration in patients with heart failure. *Journal of the American College of Cardiology, 46*(12), 2183-92. doi:10.1016/j.jacc.2005.01.071

Li, Yandong, Ma, Z., Lu, W., & Li, Yanda. (2006, April). Automatic removal of the eye blink artifact from EEG using an ICA-based template matching approach. *Physiological measurement*. doi:10.1088/0967-3334/27/4/008

Mantini, D., Franciotti, R., Romani, G. L., & Pizzella, V. (2008). Improving MEG source localizations: an automated method for complete artifact removal based on independent component analysis. *NeuroImage, 40*(1), 160-73. doi:10.1016/j.neuroimage.2007.11.022

Matani, A., Naruse, Y., Terazono, Y., Iwasaki, T., Fujimaki, N., & Murata, T. (2010). Phase-compensated averaging for analyzing electroencephalography and magnetoencephalography epochs. *IEEE transactions on bio-medical engineering, 57*(5), 1117-23. doi:10.1109/TBME.2009.2038363

Mosekilde, E., Maistrenkio, Y., & Postnov, D. (2002). *Chaotic synchronization: applications to living systems*. River Edge, NJ :: World Scientific Singapore.

Nikulin, V. V., Nolte, G., & Curio, G. (2011). A novel method for reliable and fast extraction of neuronal EEG/MEG oscillations on the basis of spatio-spectral decomposition. *NeuroImage, 55*(4), 1528-35. doi:10.1016/j.neuroimage.2011.01.057

Ocon, A. J., Medow, M. S., Taneja, I., & Stewart, J. M. (2011). Respiration drives phase synchronization between blood pressure and RR interval following loss of cardiovagal baroreflex during vasovagal syncope. *American journal of physiology. Heart and circulatory physiology, 300*(2), H527-40. doi:10.1152/ajpheart.00257.2010

Ossadtchi, A., Baillet, S., Mosher, J. C., Thyerlei, D., Sutherling, W., & Leahy, R. M. (2004). Automated interictal spike detection and source localization in magnetoencephalography using independent components analysis and spatio-temporal clustering. *Clinical neurophysiology : official journal of the International Federation of Clinical Neurophysiology, 115*(3), 508-22. doi:10.1016/j.clinph.2003.10.036

Press, W. H., Vetterling, W. T., Teukolsky, S. A., & Flannery, B. P. (2001). *Numerical Recipes in C++: the art of scientific computing* (2nd ed., pp. 626-627). Cambridge Univerity Press.

Rosenblum, M., Pikovsky, Arkady, & Kurths, Jürgen. (1996). Phase Synchronization of Chaotic Oscillators. *Physical Review Letters, 76*(11), 1804-1807. doi:10.1103/PhysRevLett.76.1804

Sander, T. H., Wübbeler, G., Lueschow, A., Curio, G., & Trahms, L. (2002). Cardiac artifact subspace identification and elimination in cognitive MEG data using time-delayed decorrelation. *IEEE transactions on bio-medical engineering, 49*(4), 345-54. doi:10.1109/10.991162

Schiek, M., Drepper, F., Engbert, R., Abel, H. H., & Suder, K. (1998). Cardiorespiratory synchronization. In H. Kantz, J Kurths, & G. Mayer-Kress (Eds.), *Nonlinear Analysis of Physiological Data*. (pp. 191-209). Berlin: Springer.

Schyns, P. G., Thut, G., & Gross, J. (2011). Cracking the Code of Oscillatory Activity. (M. Fahle, Ed.)*PLoS Biology, 9*(5), e1001064. doi:10.1371/journal.pbio.1001064

Takens, F. (1981). Detecting strange attractors in turbulence. In D. A. Rand & L. S. Young (Eds.), *Dynamical Systems and Turbulence* (Vol. 898, pp. 366-381). Springer.

Tass, P. (1999). *Phase resetting in medicine and biology.* Berlin: Springer.

Tass, P. (2004). Transmission of stimulus-locked responses in two coupled phase oscillators. *Physical Review E, 69*(5). doi:10.1103/PhysRevE.69.051909

Tass, P. A., Rosenblum, M. G., Weule, J., Kurths, J., Pikovsky, A., Volkmann, J., Schnitzler, A., et al. (1998). Detection of n:m Phase Locking from Noisy Data: Application to Magnetoencephalography. *Physical Review Letters, 81*(15), 3291-3294. doi:10.1103/PhysRevLett.81.3291

Ting, K. H., Fung, P. C. W., Chang, C. Q., & Chan, F. H. Y. (2006). Automatic correction of artifact from single-trial event-related potentials by blind source separation using second order statistics only. *Medical engineering & physics, 28*(8), 780-94. doi:10.1016/j.medengphy.2005.11.006

Vairavan, S., Eswaran, H., Preissl, H., Wilson, J. D., Haddad, N., Lowery, C. L., & Govindan, R. B. (2010). Localization of spontaneous magnetoencephalographic activity of neonates and fetuses using independent component and Hilbert phase analysis. *Conference proceedings : ... Annual International Conference of the IEEE Engineering in Medicine and Biology Society. IEEE Engineering in Medicine and Biology Society. Conference, 2010*, 1344-7. doi:10.1109/IEMBS.2010.5626753

Wacker, M., & Witte, H. (2011). On the stability of the n:m phase synchronization index. *IEEE transactions on bio-medical engineering, 58*(2), 332-8. doi:10.1109/TBME.2010.2063028

Wagner, T., Fell, J., & Lehnertz, K. (2010). The detection of transient directional couplings based on phase synchronization. *New Journal of Physics, 12*(5), 053031. doi:10.1088/1367-2630/12/5/053031

Yoshino, K., Takagi, K., Nomura, T., Sato, S., & Tonoike, M. (2002). MEG responses during rhythmic finger tapping in humans to phasic stimulation and their interpretation based on neural mechanisms. *Biological cybernetics, 86*(6), 483-96. Springer Berlin / Heidelberg. doi:10.1007/s00422-002-0314-5

8

Epoch Filters: Analyses of Phase–Related Phenomena of MEG

Ayumu Matani[1,2], Aya Ihara[2], Yasushi Terazono[1], Norio Fujimaki[2] and Hiroaki Umehara[2]
[1]*The University of Tokyo,*
[2]*National Institute of Information and Communication Technology*
Japan

1. Introduction

When MEG researchers measure an MEG time series in a well magnetically shielded environment and view their measurements on a real-time monitor, they see an amplitude- and frequency-modulated rhythmic wave and make no judgement about whether the rhythmic wave is a signal or noise. MEG-detectable magnetic fields by themselves reflect macroscopic electrophysiological collective phenomena in the brain, which are generated by a large number (ten thousand or more) of spatially (including directionally) and temporally localized neurons. That is, even rhythmic MEGs are already results of not a random spatiotemporal synchronization. Phase is more important than amplitude when it comes to the synchronization of rhythmic MEGs.

1.1 Phase-related phenomena

1.1.1 Event-related desynchronization (ERD) and event-related synchronization (ERS)

Rhythmic MEGs are distinguished by frequency bands: e.g., the delta band (1-4 Hz), theta band (4-8 Hz), alpha band (8-13 Hz), beta band (13-26 Hz), and gamma band (26- Hz). There are occasionally slight differences in the above frequency ranges (e.g., separation of beta and gamma bands) and naming (e.g., mu and tau bands). In the arousal state, the alpha-band MEG is largest in amplitude. As is well-known, it increases when subjects are relaxed and has their eyes closed, and hence, it might relate to an inactive state. Alpha-band suppression is observed in event-related experiments; i.e., the alpha-band MEG decreases when subjects receive stimuli and/or executes motor tasks. During this suppression, gamma- and/or beta-band MEGs sometimes increase in amplitude. Decreases and increases in MEG activity relative to that in the resting state might be caused by populations of synchronizing neurons and are called event-related desynchronizations (ERDs) and synchronizations (ERSs), respectively. ERD is a kind of the suppression of MEG in a specific frequency band, and the ERD of the alpha band is often observed in MEG recordings. On the other hand, ERS is not as distinctly observed because of its short-lived and poor time-locked characteristics. The word ERS seems to be used in context with ERD. In fact, appearances of ERD and ERS would be much more complicated (Lopes da Silva, 2006, Pfurtscheller, 2006, Herrmann et al., 2005, Başar, 1998). ERD and ERS are often mentioned in the literature of EEG-based brain-computer interfaces (BCIs) (Dornhege et al., 2007). In particular, it has been found that well-trained BCI users can use imagery to control ERD/ERS.

The event-related field (ERF) is the MEG version of the event-related potential (ERP), the only difference being the sort of measurement. Of course, there is an intrinsic difference between EEG and MEG; i.e., only MEG can detect intracellular current flows. Many stimuli are typically presented to subjects in ERF experiments. MEG data clip out according to the triggers of stimuli.

In what follows, we denote $x_{mq}[n]$ to be the ERF of the mth channel (m=0, 1, …, M–1), nth time sample (n=N_{pre}, N_{pre}+1, …, N_{post}–1, N_{post}; n=0 means the trigger timing), and qth epoch (q=0, 1, …, Q–1). This is the determination of ERF in this chapter. Do not confuse the ERFs with the following averages; $x_{mq}[n]$ is averaged over epoch to enhance a signal-to-noise (S/N) ratio:

$$\bar{x}_m[n] = \frac{1}{Q}\sum_{q=0}^{Q-1} x_{mq}[n]. \tag{1}$$

Equation (1), or conventional averaging, is related to the supposition that the stimulus-locked additive activity is the most important object of analysis, and this supposition has remained implicit in most of the ERP and ERF literature. Additive activities are similar to impulse responses in the system theory, and they are thought to appear only as a result of stimuli and/or motor executions. In fact, conventional averages are experiment-dependent and (mostly) subject-independent; most of the rhythmic activities are averaged out. It is thus natural to think that conventional averages would have important information and rhythmic activities would not. But is this really the case? For instance, do conventional averages converge to additive activities when the number of epochs becomes large? A much more elementary question arises as to whether additive activities actually exist or not. The conventional averages (1) are just mean values in the mathematical sense. Moreover, 'stimulus-locked' in the sense of conventional averaging means 'phase-locked' to stimuli, and additive activities are often referred as evoked activities.

ERD and ERS researchers are interested in rhythmic activities. Therefore, they often initially calculate the power-spectrograms of MEG epochs, $P_{mq}[n,k]$ (k: discrete frequency), and then average the power-spectrograms over epoch:

$$\begin{aligned} X_{mq}[n,k] &= \mathrm{WT}\{x_{mq}[n]\}, \\ P_{mq}[n,k] &= \left|X_{mq}[n,k]\right|^2, \\ \bar{P}_m[n,k] &= \frac{1}{Q}\sum_{q=0}^{Q-1} P_{mq}[n,k], \end{aligned} \tag{2}$$

where WT{·} means a continuous wavelet transform, the mother wavelet of which is the complex Morlet (modulated Gaussian) (Tallon-Baudry et al., 1999). The wavelet transform can be replaced by other time-frequency methods (e.g., the Wigner distribution or the short-time Fourier transform) and the Hilbert transform (frequency-wise). The power calculation of eq. (2) is a simple but nonlinear operation to eliminate stimulus-unlocked phase differences. Therefore, power-spectrogram averaging (2) can reflect ERD and ERS. Note that power-spectrogram averages are usually frequency-wise normalized by the mean power for a pre-trigger duration to enhance the ERD (ERS) changes. Power-spectrogram averaging indeed has played an important role in making researchers notice that a portion of the rhythmic activities are actually event-related. However, power-spectrogram averages may also contain additive activities, if they actually exist. Moreover, if the phases of ERFs are also event-related, another important piece of information regarding the phases in the brain processing is unfortunately lost. 'Stimulus-locked' in power-spectrogram averaging means only 'time-locked to stimuli' (not care for 'phase-locked'), and time-locked rhythmic activities are often referred to as induced activities.

Averaging methods for analysing event-related phases have been also proposed. The phase-locking factor (PLF) for a single channel phase synchronization analysis is expressed as

$$X_{mq}[n,k_0] = r_{mq}[n,k_0]\exp\left(\mathrm{j}\psi_{mq}[n,k_0]\right),$$
$$\mathrm{PLF}_m[n,k_0] = \frac{1}{Q}\left|\sum_{q=0}^{Q-1}\exp\left(\mathrm{j}\psi_{mq}[n,k_0]\right)\right|, \tag{3}$$

where j is the imaginary unit (Tallon-Baudry et al., 1996). PLF is the absolute value of the average of a specific-frequency k_0 ERF on the complex unit circle, $\exp(\mathrm{j}\psi_{mq}[n,k_0])$, avoiding the amplitude term $r_{mq}[n,k_0]$. PLF is one if the instantaneous phases are perfectly locked to the stimuli whereas it is zero if they are independent of the stimuli. PLF requires a complex-valued $X_{mq}[n,k]$, whereas power-spectrogram averaging does not. Therefore, the calculation procedure to obtain $X_{mq}[n,k]$ would be restricted to the wavelet transform with the complex Morlet and the Hilbert transform. Regarding the use of the wavelet transform, the frequency of interest in PLF spreads around k_0 in the form of the Gaussian that is the Fourier transform of the Gaussian of the complex Morlet corresponding to k_0. Therefore, the frequency band around k_0 is included in the PLF analysis. On the other hand, regarding the use of the Hilbert transform, k_0 is only k_0, and hence it does not have a frequency spread. If one needs a frequency band in PLF when using a Hilbert transform, one should just add some $X_{mq}[n,k]$ to construct a frequency band, of say, $X_{mq}[n,k_0-1]+X_{mq}[n,k_0]+X_{mq}[n,k_0+1]$.

So far, we have explained three averaging methods (1)-(3) for a single channel and their related technical terms. In fact, their applicability to the problem at hand may still be somewhat confusing. In particular, the term 'phase-locked activities' includes in its meaning both additive activities and phase-locked rhythmic activities. Accordingly, the conventional averaging (1) picks up both of these activities, and PLF (3) also picks them up, even if the number of epochs is sufficiently large. Moreover, phase-locked activities are just subsets of time-locked activities, and hence, these two activities cannot be separated either. Power-spectrogram averages (2) include not only the above-mentioned activities but also phase-unlocked rhythmic activities.

1.1.2 Long distance synchronization and phase resetting

Why is the phase of ERF modulated if it is actually modulated? It could be that an oscillator is unilaterally drawn to phase synchronization with another oscillator or two are bilaterally drawn to their halfway phase point or a third oscillator's phase. Long distance synchronization refers to phase synchronization between distant brain areas (Rodriguez et al., 1999). The phase synchronization of two channels would be meaningful when the distance between two phase-synchronized brain areas is large in the sense of the MEG pattern (not only their locations but also their orientations are relevant). The phase-locking value (PLV) was proposed (Lachaux et al., 1999) as a way to analyze cross-channel (between two channels m and l) phase synchronization:

$$\mathrm{PLV}_{lm}[n,k_0]=\frac{1}{Q}\left|\sum_{q=0}^{Q-1}\exp\left(\mathrm{j}\left(\psi_{lq}[n,k_0]-\psi_{mq}[n,k_0]\right)\right)\right|. \tag{4}$$

PLV is sometimes referred as the phase-locking index (PLI). PLV is apparently a cross-channel version of PLF and is also distributed from zero to one. Unlike PLF, the significance of PLV can be statistically tested with a surrogate method as follows. i) Make surrogate sets of phases by random permutation of $\psi_{mq}[n,k_0]$ over q. ii) Calculate the PLV of $\psi_{lq}[n,k_0]$ for each surrogate set. iii) Rank the actual PLV value in the surrogate PLVs. Such significance testing is very important in actual ERF analyses, e.g., comparison among conditions. One may find differences to suit one's preference if one performs many kinds of analyses. Results are difficult to discuss without knowing their significances.

The single-trial phase-locking index (SPLI) For a cross-channel single epoch analysis is (Lachaux et al., 2000)

$$\mathrm{SPLI}_{lm}=\frac{1}{T}\left|\sum_{n=n_0-T/2}^{n_0+T/2-1}\exp\left(\mathrm{j}\left(\psi_l[n,k_0]-\psi_m[n,k_0]\right)\right)\right|, \tag{5}$$

where T is the single period of n corresponding to the frequency k_0. While PLV is an average over epoch, SPLI is an average over time.

Phase resetting is another way of picturing phase modulation. Long-distance synchronization is based on the cross-channel phase relationship. Phase resetting refers to the phenomenon wherein the phase of an oscillator jumps to a specific value in a short period of time. Since the specific value is not determined by another running oscillator, phase resetting is not a cross-channel phenomenon. If stimuli produce phase resetting, nonzero activities will appear in the conventional averages. Probably because of this, phase-resetting has been discussed in the context of whether activities are additive or not. For instance, i) visual ERFs were divided into two bins by post-stimulus alpha amplitude and ERFs were averaged for each bin. ii) the amplitudes of the averages inherited the post-stimulus alpha-band amplitudes (Makeig et al., 2002). This simple fact could provide strong evidence for the existence of phase resetting.

There is a counterexample. The phase preservation index (PPI) is expressed by

$$\mathrm{PPI}_m[n,k_0]=\frac{1}{Q}\left|\sum_{q=0}^{Q-1}\exp\left(\mathrm{j}\left(\psi_{mq}[n,k_0]-\psi_{mq}[n_0,k_0]\right)\right)\right| \tag{6}$$

for evaluating how much the phase of a specific pre-stimulus time n_0 and frequency k_0 are preserved in the post-stimulus duration (Mazaheri & Jensen, 2006). The results of a PPI analysis showed that the alpha-band phase was preserved, or not reset. This would be a very simple but strong evidence for the existence of additive activity. Taken together, these results could reveal the existence of a phase resetting component or an additive component in the conventional average without rejecting the existence of the other component. Therefore, there is a possibility of these components coexisting.

Finally, we would like to point out that i) indices (3)-(6) discard the amplitude terms, ii) they are not MEG activities, which can be further analyzed with subsequent methods, but rather indices, and iii) the cross-channel indices (4) and (5) are undirectional.

1.2 Simulation: Phase modulation

This section describes a simple simulation performed to investigate the influence of only phase-locked rhythmic activities on the three averages (1)-(3).

A 10-Hz stable sinusoid with an initial phase θ is expressed as $\cos(2\pi 10t+\theta)$, where t is continuous time. For channel 0, θ_{0q} (q=0, 1, …, Q–1, Q=200) is a random phase uniformly distributed from 0 to 2π and ERF is $x'_{0q}(t)=\cos(2\pi 10t+\theta_{0q})$. The ERF for channel 1 is $x_{1q}(t)=\cos(2\pi 10t+\theta_{1q})$, where θ_{1q} is a separately generated random phase. Note that the cosine can be replaced by the sine without any essential difference, since both θ_{0q} and θ_{1q} are uniformly distributed. Now, every pair of $2\pi 10t+\theta_{0q}$ ($t\le 0.1$) and $2\pi 10t+\theta_{1q}$ ($t\ge 0.3$) is connected by a straight line for a duration of $0.1<t<0.3$ (top-left, Fig. 1). The cosines of these connected phases produce a new ERF $x_{0q}(t)$ (top-right, Fig. 1). ERF $x_{0q}(t)$ is thus initially $x'_{0q}(t)$ ($t\le 0.1$) and finally $x_{1q}(t)$ ($t\ge 0.3$), and it is unilaterally drawn to phase synchronization with $x_{1q}(t)$ for the middle duration ($0.1<t<0.3$). Note that $x_{0q}(t)$ has no additive activity.

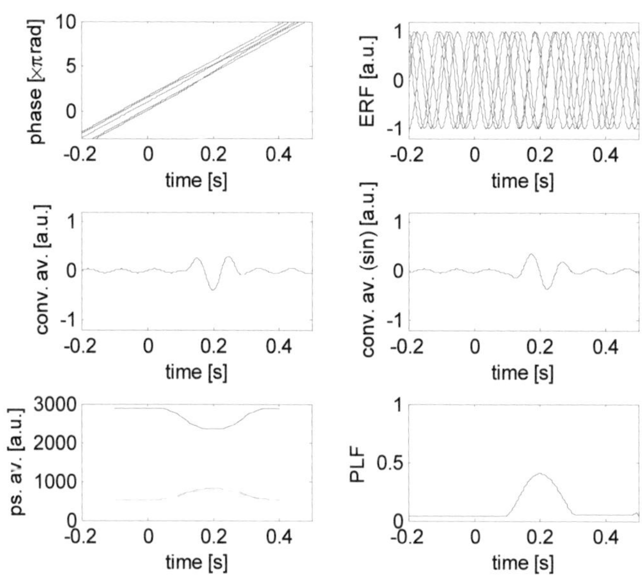

Fig. 1. Simulation of a phase-drawing phenomenon. Top-left) Given phases of five samples (out of 200). The fundamental basic slope is 10 Hz. Top-right) Given ERFs of the five samples, or the cosines of the five given phases. Middle-left) The conventional average of the 200 ERFs. Middle-right) The conventional average of the sines of the phases. Bottom-left) Power-spectrogram averages (dashed: 5 Hz, solid: 10 Hz, and dotted: 15 Hz). The lines for 5 and 15 Hz mostly overlap. Bottom-right) PLF of the 200 ERFs.

One might be interested in the conventional average of $x_{0q}(t)$ (middle-left, Fig. 1). Significant activity occurs in the middle duration, although activities are mostly averaged out in the other durations. Moreover, one repeatedly sees essentially the same activity for any uniformly distributed initial phase combination. This is a demonstration that the conventional average is not necessarily equal to, or rather, does not necessarily converge to, an additive activity (even if it actually exists). The power-spectrogram average shows ERD

for 10 Hz and ERS for 5 and 15 Hz in the middle duration (bottom-left, Fig. 1). PLF shows a phase bias, or an amount of phase-locking, in the middle duration (bottom-right, Fig. 1).
Let us now investigate whether there is any difference between using the cosine and sine in the simulation setup of the initial $x_{0q}(t)$. The fact is that the sine of the connected phases results in a significant activity in the conventional average (middle-right, Fig. 1), which is different from the cosine result. These two are $\pi/2$ rad apart. The shape of the sine is also reproducible for any uniformly distributed initial phase combination. This means there is an essential difference between cosine and sine for the simulation setup of the final $x_{0q}(t)$ despite such a random phase connection. The reason is in the final quantity discarded when calculating PLF. PLF provides a phase just before absolute calculation (3). The phase at the extreme of PLF (t=0.2 in this case) (bottom-right, Fig. 1) is not a random value but highly likely to be a specific value (π in this case). Accordingly, the line segments consisting of the phases of $x_{0q}(t)$ in the middle duration have similarly constricted envelopes for any uniformly distributed initial phase combination.

2. Epoch filter

ERF is a function of time, channel, and epoch (Fig. 2). There are huge variations for time, or temporal, filters (e.g., bandpass filter, wavelet transform, and Hilbert filter) and for channel, or spatial, filters (e.g., beamformer, Laplacian filter, principal component analysis (PCA), and independent component analysis (ICA)). These filters have their own benefits. Now let us turn to the question of epochs. As shown in the figure, we can consider a third filter for the epoch axis.

2.1 Concept

Let us begin with an interpretation of the three averaging methods (1)-(3) as possible epoch filters. PLF (3) is significantly different from conventional averaging (1) and power-spectrogram averaging (2). The most conspicuous difference from an epoch filter viewpoint is that PLF treats epochs as a series; i.e., instantaneous phases give epochs their own order. The instantaneous phases also serve as an order for a series for indices (4)-(6). PLF is a weighted average of ones (in the absolute value sense), to which the ERF amplitudes are normalized at all time sampling points. The weight is derived from the instantaneous phase of ERF. More precisely, it is the filter kernel of PLF (3), $\exp(j\psi_{mq}[n,k_0])/Q$. Accordingly, the filter kernels of the other two averaging methods (1) and (2) (having non-normalized amplitudes) are $1/Q$, which does not require the epochs to have an order. Thus, the other two methods can be interpreted as 'averaging filters'.
The most essential reason for the temporal and spatial filters is that time and channel have own orders based on physical properties. Since time and channel have orders, they are not always assigned the same weights (filter kernels). Epoch filters would be possible if epochs can be given an order, even if this order does not have an unequivocal physical meaning. PLF has built a small bridge to epoch filters.
Filters, in general, have pass- and stop-bands. Although bands might fit in frequency very well (namely, frequency band), bands should be treated here as just subsets. Filters are designed by taking one of the two bands into account. Since the three averaging methods (1)-(3) are not originally designed as epoch filters, they do not handle pass- and stop-bands very well. There is no appropriate band concept corresponding to time-locked and phase-locked activities for epoch filters.

The question thus is can ERFs have bands? Rhythmic activities, which are sometimes referred to as ongoing spontaneous activities, always exist and are amplitude- and/or frequency-modulated. Since phase modulation can be done in place of frequency modulation, it may be fruitful to separate the rhythmic activities into amplitude-modulated (AM) and phase-modulated (PM) components. In addition to these components, additive activities (AD), which are template-like activities corresponding to individual inputs (stimuli) and outputs (motor executions), may exist. Accordingly, let us treat AD, AM, and PM as bands, and let one purpose of epoch filters be to pass one of these bands and to stop the others.

Another purpose of epoch filters is illustrated by the simulation described in section 1.2. In that simulation, the phase of $x_{0q}(t)$ was unilaterally drawn to phase synchronization with $x_{1q}(t)$ for the middle duration, and hence, $x_{0q}(t)$ directionally phase-synchronized with $x_{1q}(t)$. Such a directional phase synchronization should be quantitatively evaluated. In fact, undirectional and free-amplitude phase synchronizations have so far been evaluated with indices (5) and (6).

Let us introduce a quantity that gives epochs an order. For the above-mentioned two purposes, phase is surely important. Therefore, as the first attempt to design an epoch filter, let us use the instantaneous phase to give an order to epochs, and let us discuss independence of the instantaneous phase as an aside. An epoch is defined as the integer number of stimuli/motor executions that make up an ERF recording. Therefore, an epoch is definitely an independent variable. Although instantaneous-phase-sorted epochs are, however, distinguished by the original numbers, they differ by the other independent variables: time and channel.

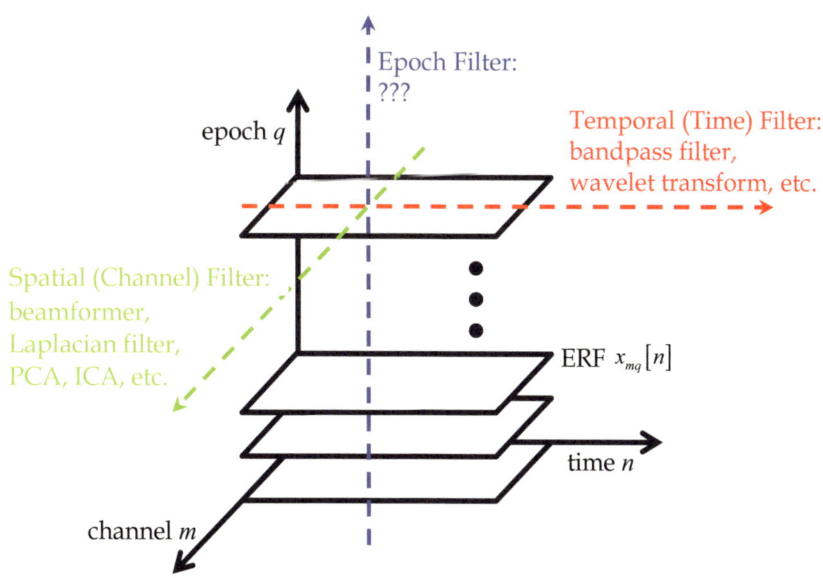

Fig. 2. Concept of epoch filter. Epoch filter could be a third filter for ERF processing.

Finally, we have a perhaps subjective feeling about filters. We wonder if the inputs and outputs of most of the existing filters might belong to the same category. This means the outputs of epoch filters should not be indices and should be spatiotemporal-structure-preserved ERFs. In other words, the outputs of epoch filters can be used as inputs to spatial and temporal filters.

2.2 Preliminary: Temporal filtering

Before explaining the methodologies of epoch filtering, we should mention frequency-selective temporal filtering.
The instantaneous phase will play an important role in ordering epoch filters. To determine the instantaneous phase, we often perform a discrete Hilbert transform (Oppenheim & Schafer, 2007), which retains the real part of the sequence as is and only generates the imaginary part of the sequence under the constraint that the total complex sequence consists of only positive frequency terms; namely, the total complex sequence is analytic. The discrete Hilbert transform consists of i) a discrete Fourier transform, ii) doubling of positive frequency terms (except the DC and Nyquist frequency terms) and zero-padding of negative frequency terms, and iii) an inverse discrete Fourier transform. Therefore, we usually embed temporal filtering in the Hilbert transform by padding zeros to stop-frequency-band terms. Even in the case that only temporal filtering is necessary and an analytic sequence is not, we should perform the pair-wise forward and inverse discrete Fourier transforms and halfway stop-band zero padding for consistency. The need for consistency relates to the fact that the discrete Fourier transform treats a sequence as periodic. In other words, we should not cross-process two sequences, one of which is generated by a convolution (not a periodic procedure) and the other of which is generated by a Hilbert transform (a periodic procedure). Instead of using a Hilbert transform, one can perform a wavelet transform and convolution-based temporal filtering and maintain consistency. However, in so doing, one may encounter difficulty in obtaining a wide-frequency-band-limited analytic sequence. In addition, the wavelet transform with the complex Morlet also generates an analytic sequence unless one takes care about the negative frequency terms for the complex Morlet.

2.3 Phase-interpolated averaging

Phase-interpolated averaging, which is an epoch filter, has been proposed for separately extracting AD, AM, and PM and for reducing noise in the averaging sense (Matani et al., 2011). It is originated from the phase-series analysis for echography (Matani et al., 2006).

2.3.1 Methodology

Time and channel, which are independent variables of ERF, are discrete samples of continuous variables in a computer; needless to say about time, channels are actually input coils and hence are spatial samples. On the other hand, an epoch is ordered according to the instantaneous phase. Phase is continuous, and therefore, an epoch can be virtually treated as a sample. However, phase sampling intrinsically has unavoidable jitter. Another characteristic is that phase has a period of 2π, or more precisely, has an uncertainty of integral multiples of 2π. Phase-interpolated averaging consists of two stages: I) interpolation of ERF by eliminating phase sampling jitter and II) a discrete Fourier transform of the interpolated ERF over the epoch.

Stage I) Interpolation of ERF

Let us recall ERF, and suppose it is first frequency-band I limited, $x_{mq}^{I}[n]$. Frequency band I can be selected to be, say, wide band: 0.1-50 Hz, alpha band: 8-13 Hz, etc. Since phase-interpolation is a nonlinear procedure as a whole, frequency-selective filtering should be done first, if necessary. Now, consider the analytic signal of $x_{mq}^{I}[n]$:

$$\tilde{x}_{mq}^{I}[n] = r_{mq}^{I}[n]\exp\left(\mathrm{j}\psi_{mq}^{I}[n]\right). \tag{7}$$

$x_{mq}^{I}[n]$ can be regarded as ordered-phase samples $x_{mn}^{I}[q']$, where q' has a one-to-one correspondence with q such that $\psi_{mn}^{I}[q']$ is sorted in ascending order from 0 to 2π. Note that the variable in [·] means the one of current interest and, for instance, $x_{mq}^{I}[n]$ and $x_{mn}^{I}[q]$ are identical to each other but are treated as time and epoch series, respectively. Since $\psi_{mn}^{I}[q']$ is not at the start on a phase-grid, $x_{mn}^{I}[q']$ has an unavoidable phase-sampling jitter. Now, let us virtually introduce a continuous phase ϕ to be jitter-sampled as $\psi_{mn}^{I}[q']$. The ERF in terms of ϕ can be approximated by a Fourier series, as

$$x_{mn}^{I}(\phi) \simeq \sum_{k=-K}^{K} c_{mn}[k]\exp(\mathrm{j}k\phi), \tag{8}$$

where

$$c_{mn}[k] = \frac{1}{2\pi}\int_{-\pi}^{\pi} x_{mn}^{I}(\phi)\exp(-\mathrm{j}k\phi)\,\mathrm{d}\phi. \tag{9}$$

The pair of $+k$ and $-k$ correspond to bipolar same-frequency terms and k=0 corresponds to the DC term. Therefore, the number of ks must be an odd number $2K+1$.

Since phase is intrinsically periodic, $c_{mn}[k]$ can be replaced by

$$c_{mn}^{\mathrm{G}}[k] = \frac{1}{2K+1}\sum_{l=0}^{2K} x_{mn}^{I}\left(\frac{2\pi l}{2K+1}\right)\exp\left(-\mathrm{j}\frac{2\pi kl}{2K+1}\right). \tag{10}$$

The superscript 'G' means grid-sampling.

The periodic version of the sampling theory is expressed as

$$\begin{aligned} x_{mn}^{I}(\phi) &\simeq \sum_{k=-K}^{K} c_{mn}^{\mathrm{G}}[k]\exp(\mathrm{j}k\phi) \\ &= \sum_{l=0}^{2K} x_{mn}^{I}\left(\frac{2\pi l}{2K+1}\right)\mathrm{diric}_{2K+1}\left(\phi - \frac{2\pi l}{2K+1}\right), \end{aligned} \tag{11}$$

where

$$\mathrm{diric}_{2K+1}(\phi) = \frac{\sin\frac{2K+1}{2}\phi}{(2K+1)\sin\frac{\phi}{2}} \tag{12}$$

is the Dirichlet kernel of the $2K$+1th order.

Therefore, the jittered and unjittered (grid-on) phase-sample interface can be formulated as

$$\boldsymbol{x}_{mn}^{\mathrm{J}} \simeq \boldsymbol{\Xi}_{mn}\boldsymbol{x}_{mn}^{\mathrm{G}}, \tag{13}$$

where

$$\boldsymbol{x}_{mn}^{\mathrm{J}} = \left[x_{mn}^{I}\left(\psi_{mn}^{\mathrm{J}}[0]\right)\cdots x_{mn}^{I}\left(\psi_{mn}^{\mathrm{J}}[q']\right)\cdots x_{mn}^{I}\left(\psi_{mn}^{\mathrm{J}}[Q-1]\right)\right]^{\mathrm{T}},$$
$$\boldsymbol{x}_{mn}^{\mathrm{G}} = \left[x_{mn}^{I}(0)\cdots x_{mn}^{I}\left(\frac{2\pi l}{2K+1}\right)\cdots x_{mn}^{I}\left(\frac{2\pi 2K}{2K+1}\right)\right]^{\mathrm{T}}, \tag{14}$$
$$\Xi_{mn} = \left[\xi_{mq'l}\right], \xi_{mq'l} = \mathrm{diric}_{2K+1}\left(\psi_{mn}^{\mathrm{J}}[q'] - \frac{2\pi l}{2K+1}\right).$$

The superscript 'J' means jittered-sampling. Note that both $\boldsymbol{x}^{\mathrm{J}}_{mn}$ and $\boldsymbol{x}^{\mathrm{G}}_{mn}$ are real-valued and their independent variable is only phase (channel m and time n are treated as constants here). Now, $2K+1$ is the number of interpolated epochs. By setting K such that $2K+1<Q$, we can interpolate the unjittered phase samples by using the least squares solution:

$$\hat{\boldsymbol{x}}_{mn}^{\mathrm{G}} = \left[\Xi_{mn}^{\mathrm{T}}\Xi_{mn} + \lambda^2\mathbf{I}_{2K+1}\right]^{-1}\Xi_{mn}^{\mathrm{T}}\boldsymbol{x}_{mn}^{\mathrm{J}}. \tag{15}$$

Stage II) Discrete Fourier transform

The interpolated ERF is then discrete Fourier transformed. However, so far, we need only the 0th and 1st terms:

$$\bar{x}_{m0}[n] = \frac{2}{2K+1}\sum_{l=0}^{2K}\hat{x}_{mn}^{\mathrm{G}}\left(\frac{2\pi l}{2K+1}\right),$$
$$\bar{x}_{m1}[n] = \frac{2}{2K+1}\mathrm{Re}\left\{\sum_{l=0}^{2K}\hat{x}_{mn}^{\mathrm{G}}\left(\frac{2\pi l}{2K+1}\right)\exp\left(-\mathrm{j}\frac{2\pi l}{2K+1}\right)\right\}. \tag{16}$$

They are respectively called the 0th and 1st phase-interpolated averages.
As will be shown in the next simulation, the 0th and 1st phase-interpolated averages are to separately extract the AD activity and the AM component, respectively. The condition number of Ξ_{mn}, which quantitatively indicate a difficulty of the interpolation, is to reflect the PM component. One may have doubts about the origin of the two 2s as multipliers in eq. (16). These multipliers were numerically determined by simulation (Matani et al., 2011).
Finally, we would like to stress that phase-interpolated averaging is performed for each time sampling point and each channel (not for cross-channel).

2.3.2 Simulation: Separation ability

In the simulation in section 1.2, only PM occurred in the middle duration ($0.1<t<0.3$). On the other hand, in the simulation described here, AD and AM also simultaneously occurred in the middle duration. AD consisting of two bipolar Gaussians was added to the ERFs (top-left, Fig. 3). The envelope of AM was a Gaussian (middle-left, Fig. 3). The rhythmic activities were thus not only amplitude- but also phase-modulated (bottom-left, Fig. 3). Note that the instantaneous phases, which play a very important role in phase-interpolated averaging, were not given ones for this simulation but were actually calculated from the given ERF with the Hilbert transform.
The condition number monotonically increases with the number of interpolated epochs, $2K+1$(=3, 5, 7, 9), in eqs. (8)-(16) (bottom-right, Fig. 3). This indicates that increasing K increases the difficulty of the interpolation. The condition number increases in the middle

duration, and thereby, PM is successfully evaluated. The 0th (top-right, Fig. 3) and 1st (middle-right, Fig. 3) phase-interpolated averages mostly overlap for K=2 and 3. The overlapping averages successfully extract the AD and AM. This indicates that the stably extracted AD and AM overlap with a certain range of K. In practice, one should perform phase-interpolated averaging for some Ks and then check such an overlap. On the other hand, the conventional average shows a PM-contaminated AD (gray line, top-right, Fig. 3).

The above-mentioned stability depends on not only the instantaneous phase bias but also the amplitude of AD. This simulation was of a difficult case in which the amplitudes of AD and the rhythmic activities (including AM) were comparable. As mentioned in section 3, also as the common experience, AD (if it actually exists) is usually smaller than the rhythmic activities. If this is not the case, no one tries to perform conventional averaging. Thus, we can say that actual phase interpolation is not so difficult.

One may wonder about strange surges at the ends of the 1st phase-interpolated averages and the condition numbers. This is a transient phenomenon caused by the discrete Hilbert transform, which treats the objective series as periodic. To avoid it, we can set the time duration of interest to the center before the analysis and cut off both ends after the analysis. (We would have done so if this article were for journal papers.) Although we think this treatment is sufficient, such transients can in any event be avoided with Hamming-windowing.

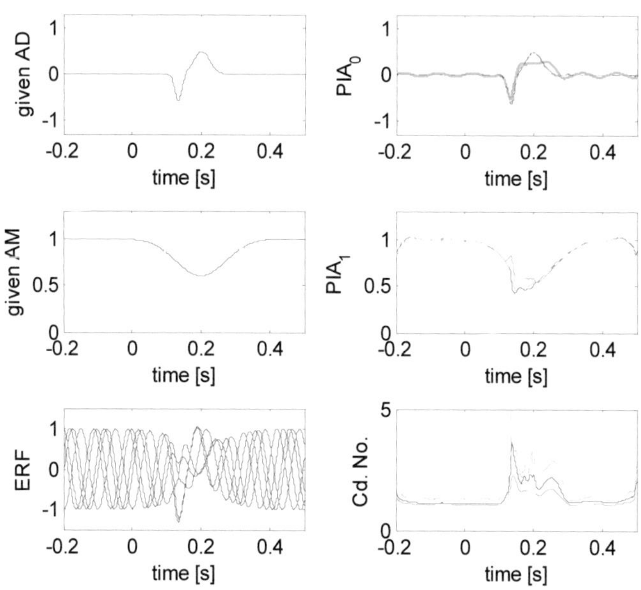

Fig. 3. Simulation of phase-interpolated averaging. Top-left) Given AD (common to all ERFs). Middle-left) Given AM (common to all ERFs). Bottom-left) ERFs of the five samples (out of 200). Top-right) 0th phase-interpolated average superimposed on the conventional average (gray line). Middle-right) 1st phase-interpolated average. Bottom-right) Condition numbers. The line textures for the right column are; dashed: K=1, solid: K=2, dotted: K=3, and dashed-dotted: K=4.

Consequently, phase-interpolated averaging works as an epoch filter to pass only one of AD, AM, and PM bands and to stop the others.

2.4 Phase-compensated averaging

Phase-compensated averaging, which is an epoch filter, has been proposed for visualizing directional phase synchronization between channels and for reducing noise in the averaging sense (Matani et al., 2010).

2.4.1 Methodology

Phase-compensated averaging consists of filter kernel design and actual filtering.
Regarding the filter kernel design, let a narrow-frequency-band N limited analytic ERF of channel m be

$$\tilde{x}_{mq}^{N}[n] = r_{mq}^{N}[n]\exp\left(\mathrm{j}\psi_{mq}^{N}[n]\right). \tag{17}$$

The filter kernel of phase-compensated averaging is $\exp\left(-\mathrm{j}\psi_{mq}^{N}[n_0]\right)$, where n_0 is a reference time that one can specify freely. The other instantaneous phases and the residual terms in eq. (17) are not used.
Regarding the actual filtering, we can use a wide-frequency-band W limited analytic ERF of channel l:

$$\tilde{x}_{lq}^{W}[n] = r_{lq}^{W}[n]\exp\left(\mathrm{j}\psi_{lq}^{W}[n]\right). \tag{18}$$

The phase-compensated averaging is expressed as

$$\begin{aligned}\bar{x}_{l|m}[n] &= \frac{1}{Q}\sum_{q=0}^{Q-1}\tilde{x}_{lq}^{W}[n]\exp\left(-\mathrm{j}\psi_{mq}^{N}[n_0]\right)\\ &= \frac{1}{Q}\sum_{q=0}^{Q-1}r_{lq}^{W}[n]\exp\left(\mathrm{j}\left(\psi_{lq}^{W}[n]-\psi_{mq}^{N}[n_0]\right)\right).\end{aligned} \tag{19}$$

Thus, $x_{lq}^{W}[n]$ is phase-compensated by $\psi_{mq}^{N}[n_0]$ and then averaged. The notation of 'channel A | channel B' that is used below indicates the average of channel A (to be filtered) phase-compensated by channel B (used for the kernel design). Phase-compensated averaging creates two averages. Channel m for the kernel filter design and channel l to be filtered can be different from each other. As names for the correlation function, the case of $m=l$ is called the auto-average and that of $m\neq l$ is the cross-average. Note that the cross-averages are directional; i.e., $\bar{x}_{l|m}[n] \neq \bar{x}_{m|l}[n]$.
Phase-compensated averages are complex valued. They should be represented by their absolute values and phases (if necessary) rather than their real and imaginary parts. This is because they usually appear as modulated complex sinusoids having a single center frequency (they look like a synchronization burst), and therefore, the absolute value representations contain the envelopes of the phase-compensated averages, which are the most useful for characterization.
Regarding the significance test, we shall fundamentally adhere to the statistical test of PLV (Lachaux et al., 1999). A surrogate method is used for evaluating the significance, as follows.

i) Surrogates are generated by random permutation of $\exp\left(j\psi_{mq}^{N}[n_0]\right)$ over q. ii) The phase-compensated average for each surrogate is calculated. iii) The absolute values of the averages are ranked for each time sampling point. iv) The $p<0.05$ levels are determined. For this significance measure, phase-compensated averages are represented by their absolute values. If one statistically tests the difference between two phase-compensated averages, the difference in the absolute values of two sets of surrogates should be both one-sided ranked. Thus, there is a hidden merit associated with phase-compensated averaging and the surrogate method: For a single run of ERF recording, which generates only one conventional average, phase-compensated averaging provides many auto- and cross-averages with significance measures.

Finally, we would like to point out a number of methodological differences between phase-interpolated averaging and phase-compensated averaging: i) The filter kernel of the former is calculated for each time sampling point, whereas that of the latter is calculated for only a reference time sampling point n_0. ii) The former is performed for individual channels, whereas the latter is performed for auto- and cross-channels. iii) The former nominally requires the same frequency bands (indicated by I) for the filter kernel and the sequence to be filtered, whereas the latter does not care (indicated by N and W). The most important difference is, of course, that each averaging has its own purpose.

2.4.2 Simulation: Directional synchronization

We will again refer to the ERFs $x_{0q}(t)$ and $x_{1q}(t)$ of the simulation described in section 1.2. We would like to confirm that they first oscillated independently ($t \leq 0.1$), then $x_{0q}(t)$ was unilaterally drawn to phase synchronization with $x_{1q}(t)$ ($0.1<t<0.3$ is called the middle duration), and they eventually became synchronized with each other ($t \geq 0.3$). That is, $x_{0q}(t)$ changed and $x_{1q}(t)$ remained unchanged.

Phase-compensated averaging of the given ERF is performed for reference times $t_0=0$ (top-row, Fig. 4), 200 (middle-row, Fig. 4), and 400 ms (bottom-row, Fig. 4). Since these averages are intrinsically complex-valued, they are represented as absolute values. Note that the instantaneous phases are not given ones for this simulation but were actually calculated from the given ERF with the Hilbert transform and frequency-band N and W are not specified because the given ERF is already frequency-band-limited.

The significance levels ($p<0.05$) of the phase-compensated averages are generated by 1000 surrogates. Two auto-averages and two cross-averages are represented by their absolute values. Each of average has its own significance level (dotted lines: channel 0, dashed and dotted lines: channel 1, Fig. 4). The following results are valid since each phase-compensated average exceeds the corresponding significance level.

The auto-averages of channel 1 are always a constant value because channel 1 has an independent oscillation (dashed lines in right column, Fig. 4). Note that the phases of channel 1 over q are essentially the same for any of the time sampling points (only circularly shifted). The cross-averages of channel 1 | channel 0 increase as phase drawing to channel 1 increased (solid lines in right column, Fig. 4). On the other hand, the auto-averages of channel 0 are all short-lived. Each one has a peak only around its own reference time (solid lines in left column, Fig. 4). The cross-averages of channel 0 | channel 1 have the same shape, which indicates that channel 0 is unilaterally drawn to phase synchronization with channel 1 (dashed lines in left column, Fig. 4). As an aside, transient phenomena occur at the ends of period (These were not included in the analysis).

These results show that phase-compensated averaging works as an epoch filter to pass a phase-synchronized band and to stop the other bands.

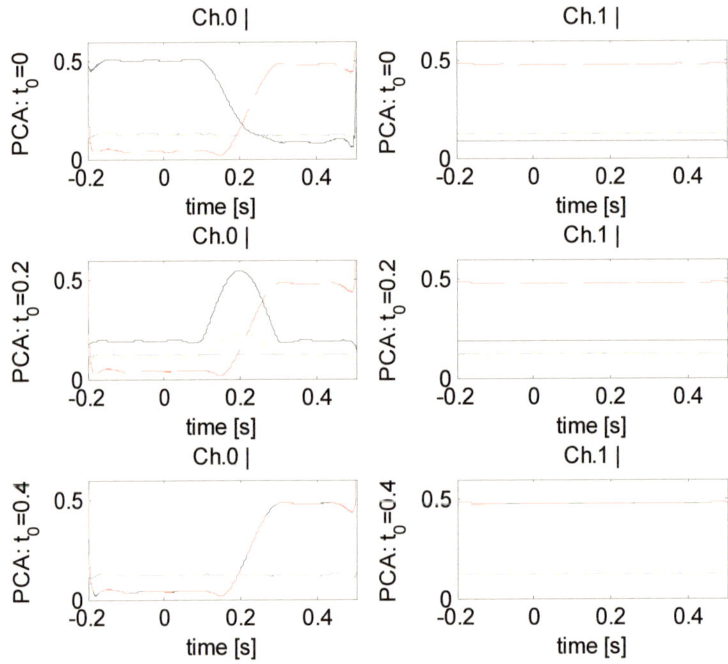

Fig. 4. Simulation of phase-compensated averaging (absolute values). Left-column) Phase-compensated averages of channel 0. Right-column) Phase-compensated averages of channel 1. Top-row) Reference time: 0 ms. Middle-row) Reference time: 200 ms. Bottom-row) Reference time: 400 ms. The line textures are; solid: compensated by channel 0, dashed: compensated by channel 1, dotted: $p<0.05$ significance level for channel 0, dashed and dotted: $p<0.05$ significance level for channel 1.

3. Actual ERF analysis with epoch filters

We shall explain the practical issues affecting the use of epoch filters by illustrating an analysis of the ERF of an actual semantic priming experiment (Ihara et al., 2007). In typical semantic priming experiments, a pair of words (prime and target) is sequentially presented to a subject and a task (e.g., button-pressing) is required to be performed only on the target word. Reaction time differs depending on whether or not there is a semantic relationship between the prime and target words. ERF sometimes is recorded during priming experiments as a physiological index. Now, although the objective of this priming experiment originally addressed a somewhat complicated issue, or selection of a meaning of a target word having semantic ambiguities through a context with the paired prime, it included a typical semantic priming experiment as a control experiment. Hence, for the sake of this discussion, we will illustrate only the epoch filtering of the ERF from the typical portion.

3.1 Semantic priming ERF

The main topic of this chapter is to introduce epoch filters. Here, we will briefly explain the procedures of a sematic priming experiment and the reconstruction of the signal source activities. Such a reconstruction is fraught with problems, due to the ill-posedness of the MEG inverse problem. Although the problems affect the overall performance of epoch filtering, we would believe that this matter should be dealt with as a separate problem from the one at hand.

All the prime and target words are Japanese nouns written with two morphograms (kanji) and three to five syllabograms (kana), respectively (left-panel, Fig. 5). The target words are either semantically related (related condition) or unrelated (unrelated condition) to the prime words. One hundred word pairs for each condition are visually presented in random order with a stimulus onset asynchrony of 1000 ms; the duration of each word is 300 ms. We ask subjects to judge whether the prime and target words are semantically related or not and to press a button after the delayed cue.

MEG in a frequency bandwidth of 0.1-200 Hz is recorded with a sampling frequency of 678 Hz using a 148-channel whole-head system (Magnes 2500WH, BTi). ERFs occasioned upon miss-pressed buttons and eye-blink artifacts are excluded from each condition. From our experience, eye-blinks often cause phase-resets, and therefore, these artifacts must be excluded when analyzing phase-related phenomena.

Dipole activities are tentatively estimated by means of the selective minimum-norm (SMN) method, which obtains minimum L1-norm solutions (Matsuura and Okabe, 1996). The SMN is applied to the conventional averages for a duration of 0-700 ms (target onset: 0 s) for all conditions. All dipoles, the amplitude of which exceeded the noise level of five times the root mean squares of the magnetic fields for a pre-trigger duration of –0.2-0 s, are gathered, neglecting the neighbors within 20 mm (Fujimaki et al., 2002). Thus, approximately 60 dipoles, which span most of the conventional average space, are selected.

The current distribution forms a vector field, and thereby, each discretized site has three orientations. The target time series of the epoch filters should have its related orientation fixed, e.g., parallel to the axons of pyramidal cells in the site. A simple way to fix the orientation with only ERF is to perform a PCA of the three dipole activities for each site. The projection vector corresponding to the first principal component is used for the orientation-fixed dipoles; i.e., three orientations of each site are projected onto the eigenvector corresponding to the largest eigenvalue of the covariance matrix of the three dipole activities in the site.

Up to this point in the experiment, only the dipoles to be fitted have been selected. In the methodological sense, a leadfield matrix, which is based on a real head shape with ASA (ANT Software B.V.), is determined. The epoch-wise (orientation-fixed) dipole activities, which are objects of the epoch filters, are subsequently estimated with least squares fitting.

We shall describe epoch filtering for a typical subject. Fifty-one orientation-fixed dipoles are used for building the leadfield matrix and 12 dipoles (Dipoles 1-12) out of the 51 are selected. Note that these 12 dipole activities showed conditional differences (Ihara et al., 2007). Each of these 12 dipoles belongs to one of six regions of interest (ROIs) (right-side, Fig. 5); the left anterior inferior frontal cortex (LaIFC: Dipoles 1 and 2), the left posterior inferior frontal cortex (LpIFC: Dipole 3), the anterior medial temporal lobe (LaMedT: Dipole 4), the left anterior middle and inferior temporal areas (LaT: Dipoles 5-7), and the left posterior superior temporal and the inferior parietal areas (LpST1: Dipoles 8-11, LpST2: Dipole 12).

The dipole activity version of the ERF is epoch filtered from the next subsection.

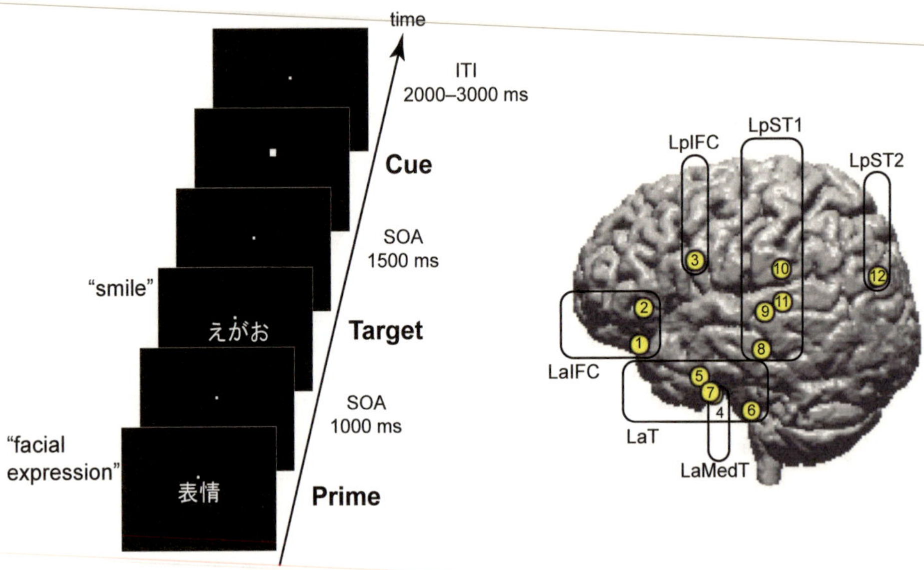

Fig. 5. ERF recording. Left) Schematic diagram of the stimulus sequence. The prime and target words were presented with a stimulus onset asynchrony (SOA) of 1000 ms, and the cue for subjects to respond with related or unrelated by pressing a button was presented 1500 ms after the onset of the target word. The inter-trial interval (ITI) between the onset of the cue and the next prime was randomly set at 2000-3000 ms. Right) Locations of the estimated dipoles and ROIs (LaIFC: Dipoles 1, 2; LpIFC: Dipole 3; LaMedT: Dipole 4; LaT: Dipoles 5-7; LpST1: 8-11; LpST2: Dipole 12).

3.2 Phase-interpolated averages

First, we will show how phase interpolation works. As a typical example, we will choose the source activity of LaT (Dipole 6) for the related condition. The actual dipole activities for the first seven epochs show rhythmic activities, and the conventional average of the all 98 epochs seem to run through the approximate center (top row, Fig. 6). It is of interest to determine whether the wave (spike is not clear for LaT) of the conventional average come from AD or PM. As shown in the simulation in section 1.2, even only PM can generate nonzero activity in the conventional average. While the instantaneous phases at 0 ms are almost uniformly distributed, those at 200 and 400 ms are clearly biased (second row, Fig. 6). Therefore, the dipole activities seem to at least partially come from PM. The phase interpolation is performed for K=3. The seven (=2K+1) interpolated dipole activities are not rhythmic compared with the original activities (third row, Fig. 6). This is because of the phase interpolation that placed instantaneous phases on the seven-phase-grid at any time sampling point (bottom row, Fig. 6). The reason a rhythmic wave is rhythmic is that its instantaneous phase rotates. Conversely, if an instantaneous phase is fixed, its waveform will be a straight line with an occasional small fluctuation. If AD exists, the interpolated dipole activities shift in the same direction. Slight upward shifts are observed for the 200-450 ms duration. Thus, the 0th phase-interpolated average, which is the twice the average of the interpolated activities as shown in eq. (16), shows a slight AD (third row, Fig. 6). Note that while the instantaneous phases for the real dipole activities are calculated, those for the interpolated dipole activities are just phase-grids for *K* and are not recalculated from the interpolated dipole activities.

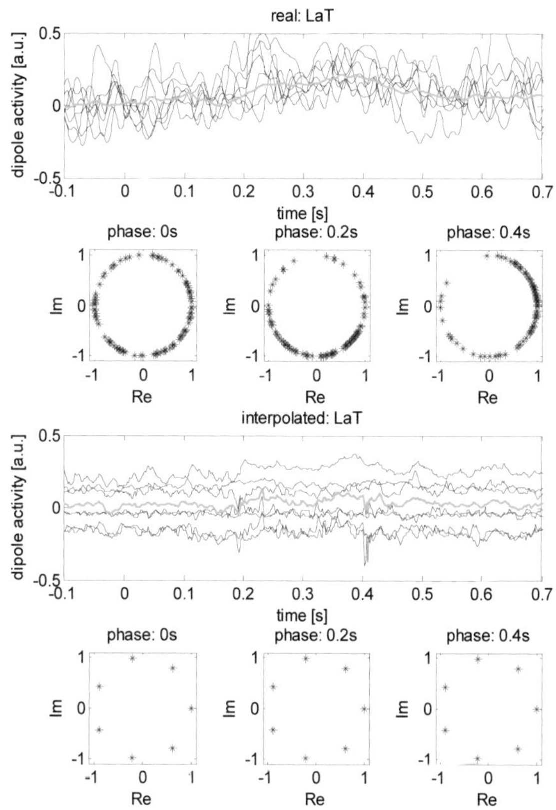

Fig. 6. Phase interpolation of actual ERF. Top row) Seven samples of actual dipole activities at LaT: Dipole 6 (black lines). The conventional average of all valid (98) samples (gray line). Second row) Instantaneous phase distributions of the actual dipole activities at 0, 200, and 400 ms. Third row) Interpolated dipole activities (black lines). The 0th phase-interpolated average for *K*=3 (gray line). Bottom row) Instantaneous phase distributions of the interpolated dipole activities at 0, 200, and 400 ms.

Next, we perform phase-interpolated averaging (*K*=2, 3, 4) on six dipoles for the related condition; one dipole is selected from each of the ROIs. The overlap of the 0th and 1st phase-interpolated averages implies that the analysis is stable, whereas spike-like changes in the condition numbers indicates that these averages at the corresponding time are somewhat unreliable. Each 0th phase-interpolated average looks like a low-amplitude replica of the corresponding conventional average (first and fourth columns, Fig. 7). The residual amplitude of the conventional average comes from PM, which is evaluated with condition numbers (third and sixth columns, Fig. 7). Such an amplitude relationship between two averages is often observed for other ERFs. Therefore, the conventional averages would be due to both AD and PM. Regarding the ratio of AD and PM, sometimes, the 0th phase-interpolated averages are very small. This indicates that PM might be dominant. However, we must point out that imprecise instantaneous phases are apt to yield very small 0th phase-interpolated averages. Phase-interpolated averaging, which is more or less fail-safe, does not generate phantom ADs. Therefore, the fact that the 0th phase-interpolated averages even very slightly inherit the trace of the conventional averages cannot deny the existence of AD. On the other hand, the 1st phase-interpolated averages do not show characteristics common to all ROIs.

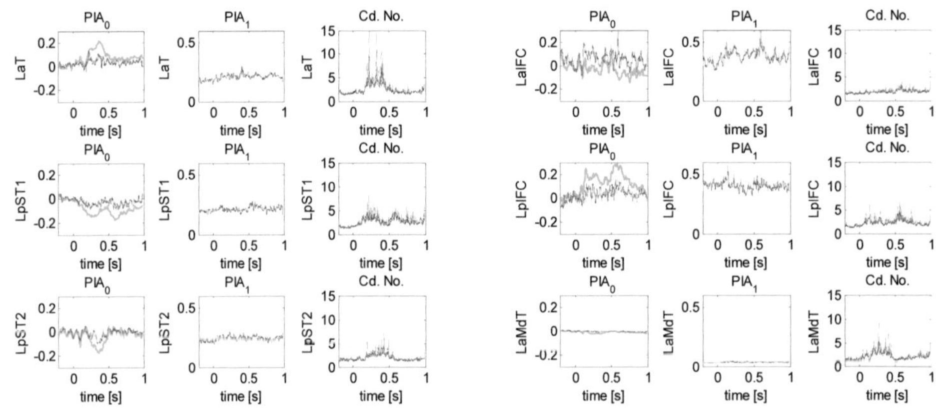

Fig. 7. Phase-interpolated averages of the six dipoles (LaIFC: Dipole 1, LpIFC: Dipole 2, LaMedT: Dipole 4, LaT: Dipole 6, LpST1: Dipole 8, and LpST2: Dipole12). The ROIs are indicated on the vertical axes. The title of each panel indicates the 0th phase-interpolated average (PIA_0), the 1st phase-interpolated average (PIA_1), or the condition number (Cd. No.). Gray lines indicate the conventional averages. Dashed, solid, and dotted lines respectively indicate the *K*=2, 3, 4 cases (mostly overlap).

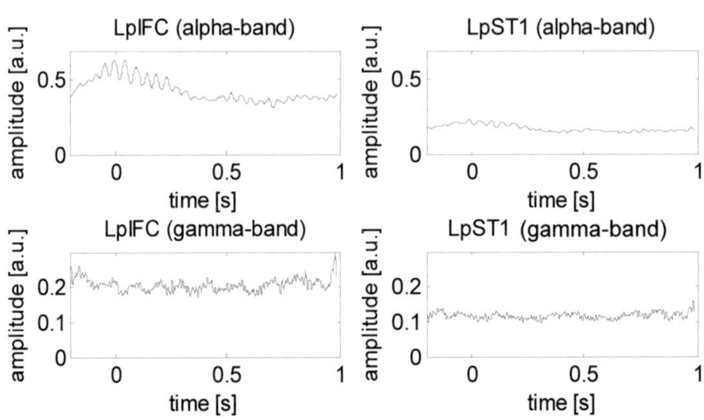

Fig. 8. Frequency-band-limited phase-interpolated averaging. Left-column) 1st phase-interpolated averages of LpIFC (Dipole 3) for the related condition. Right-column) 1st phase-interpolated averages of LpST1 (Dipole 8) for the related condition. Top-row) *I*: Alpha-band limited (8-13 Hz). Bottom-row) *I*: Gamma-band limited (26-52 Hz).

The 1st phase-interpolated averages of the alpha-band-limited LpIFC and LpST1 dipole activities show alpha-band ERD (top-row, Fig 8). On the other hand, those of the gamma-band-limited LpIFC and LpST1 dipole activities show intermittent amplitude increments (bottom-row, Fig 8). These results might be gamma-band ERS. Since gamma-band ERS is generally not much more time-locked than alpha-band ERD, phase-interpolated averaging only vaguely visualizes gamma-band ERS. Thus, although 1st phase-interpolated averages of the wide-frequency-band limited ERF give almost no information, those of the narrow-frequency-band limited ERF are at least useful for extracting alpha-band ERD.

3.3 Phase-compensated averages

Unlike phase-interpolated averaging, phase-compensated averaging generates many auto- and cross-averages. Therefore, an overview of the all averages is extremely important and should be performed first. Furthermore, non-significant averages, in the surrogate test sense, should be masked in the overview. For this purpose, we would recommend using image-like matrix (l-by-m) plots of the root-mean-squares: $\sqrt{\sum_{n\in F}\left|\bar{x}_{l|m}[n]\right|^2}$, where F is a temporal neighbor duration of n (Fig. 9). Although the intensity (white means maximum intensity) is used for the sake of visibility, all the non-significant averages should be displayed in black (minimum intensity). Now, in typical control ERF experiments, the difference between two ERFs, which may be caused by the only different condition out of many common ones, is evaluated. Thus, two conventionally averaged ERFs for enhancing an S/N ratio should basically be similar to each other. In fact, in this ERF experiment, phase-compensated averages of the related and unrelated conditions for N of the alpha band (W: 1-52 Hz) are quite similar in duration F of 100-300 ms (top and middle rows and second column, Fig. 9). Those for the other durations are only slightly different (top and middle rows to the left of the separation line, Fig. 9). This implies that the averages for the F of 100-300 ms are reliable and those for the other durations would merit further investigation. The significances of the differences are checked after the reliabilities of the individual auto- and cross-averages (significance and similarity) are evaluated (bottom row to the left of the separation line, Fig. 9). The significance difference should be valid regardless of whether or not the significances of the two conditional auto- or cross-averages that produce the difference are valid, because these two conditional significance tests are independent of each other. Note that the numbers of surrogates are 1000 for the auto- and cross-averages and 1000 pairs (total 2000) for the differences. If one performs phase-compensate averaging on a single condition ERF recording, ERFs can be randomly divided into two bins for the similarity check.

We cannot deny that the above-mentioned procedure is somewhat paradoxical. Our approach ends up finding a small but significant difference in almost the same two averages. Only the significance of the differences may be important; the significances of the individuals are not so important. On the other hand, we would like to narrow down the number of significant averages. It might be difficult for researchers, in particular, those having a hypothesis bias, to fairly compare a huge number of data on the same basis. Individual researchers should thus decide whether the auto- and cross-averages for N of the beta band should be investigated or not (right-most column, Fig. 9). As an aside, none of the auto- and cross-averages for N of the gamma-band were significant to the individual auto- and cross-averages and their differences. Note that W is always set to 1-52 Hz despite that N changes.

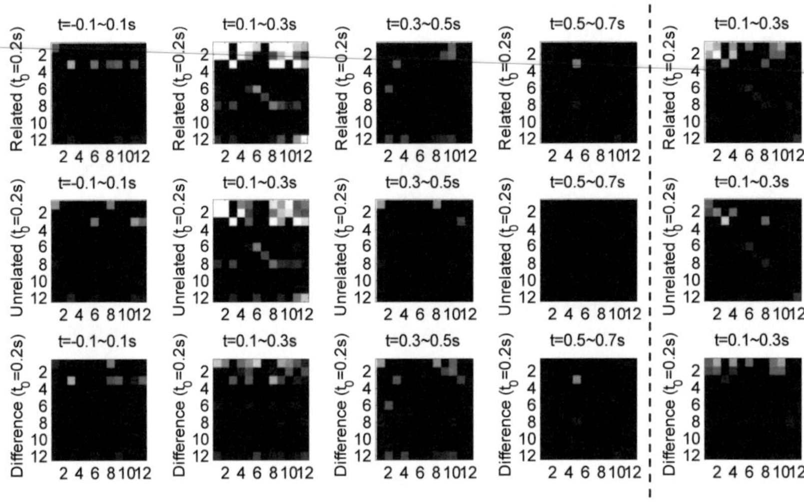

Fig. 9. Root mean squares of phase-compensated averages (*N*: alpha band (left of the dashed vertical line), *N*: beta band (right of the dashed vertical line), *W*: 1-52 Hz, reference time: 200 ms). Top-row) Related condition. Middle row) Unrelated condition. Bottom-row) Difference between related and unrelated conditions. Horizontal axis) Dipole for calculating instantaneous phases. Vertical axis) Dipoles to be filtered. Panel title) Duration *F* for calculating the root mean squares. The gray-scale intensity of each crossover square indicates the root mean squares of its auto- or cross-average (black: not significant).

Next, let us investigate the phase-compensated averages (*N*: alpha-band, *W*: 1-52 Hz) of two dipole pairs: Dipole 1 at LaIFC and Dipole 6 at LaT, and Dipole 3 at LpIFC and Dipole 8 at LpST1 (Fig. 10). This is because these two combinations are directionally brighter and darker (almost in black) in the difference plot (third row and second column panel, Fig. 9). Note that we shall hereafter use the ROI names for dipole numbers.

First, regarding the LaIFC and LaT pair, the auto- and cross-averages (top-left four panels, Fig. 10) and their differences (bottom-left four panels, Fig. 10) for both conditions significantly appear around the reference time (vertical gray lines), but the cross-averages for the unrelated condition (thick lines) are very small. Therefore, the phase-synchronization between LaIFC and LaT might occur especially for the related condition (thin lines) although the local phase-synchronizations within LaIFC and LaT might occur for whatever the condition.

Let us discuss the related condition by inspecting the panels in a row-wise fashion. Suppose the current time is the reference time. The auto-average of LaIFC reaches a significant peak at the current time (no temporal lag), and the cross-average of LaIFC|LaT does so before the current time. Thus, the current phase of LaIFC is up-to-date whereas that of LaT is older. On the other hand, the auto-average of LaT reaches a significant peak at the reference time, and the inverted cross-average (LaT|LaIFC) does so after the current time. Thus, the current phase of LaT is up-to-date whereas that of LaIFC is younger. This row-wise comparison indicates that the phase of LaIFC precedes that of LaT. Therefore, LaT might be drawn to phase synchronization with LaIFC around the reference time. Such temporal comparisons of the peaks are relatively easy to perform when the auto- and cross-averages are all single-peaked.

We should point out that only the auto-average of LaIFC for the unrelated condition consists of significant intermittent bursts, which accordingly yields a significant conditional difference (top-left, bottom-left four panels, Fig. 10). For instance, if one is interested in which dipoles are drawn to phase synchronization with Dipole 1 (at LaIFC) for unrelated condition, the cross-averages between Dipole 1 and Dipole 8 should be subsequently evaluated by consulting the corresponding column of Dipole 1 (Unrelated panels, Fig. 9).

Regarding the LpIFC and LpST1 pair, the auto- and cross-averages (top-right four panels, Fig. 10) and their differences (bottom-right four panels, Fig. 10) for both conditions significantly appear around the reference time (vertical gray lines). There is a consistent tendency in their differences that the auto- and cross-averages of LpIFC and LpST1 for the related condition are greater than those for the unrelated condition just before the reference time and the amplitude relation is inverted just after the reference time (bottom-right four panels, Fig. 10).

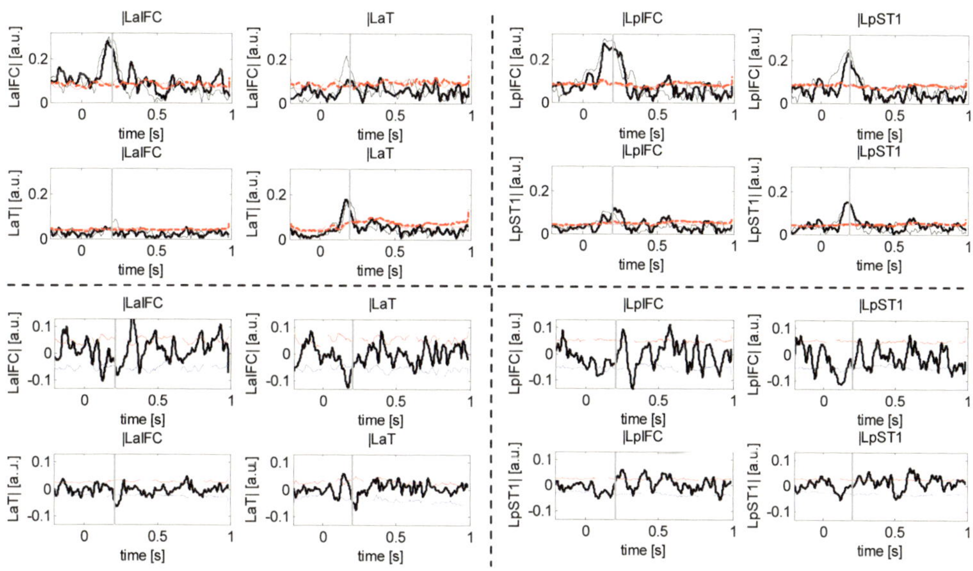

Fig. 10. Phase-compensated averages (*N*: alpha band, *W*: 1-52 Hz, reference time: 200 ms (vertical gray lines)). Top-left four panels) Absolute values of LaIFC×LaT. Bottom-left four panels) Difference of absolute values of LaIFC×LaT. Top-right 4 panels) Absolute values of LpIFC×LpST1. Bottom-right four panels) Difference of absolute values of LpIFC×LpST1. The thin and thick lines in the top eight panels indicate the related and unrelated conditions, respectively. The dashed lines in all panels indicate significance levels.

Let us examine the results for the related condition in more detail. LpIFC might be drawn to phase synchronization with LpST1 for the same reason as the LaIFC and LaT pair. However, for the unrelated condition, the cross-average of LpST1 | LpIFC is double-peaked across the reference time whereas the auto-average of LpST1 has a single peak at the reference time. Therefore, phase-drawing between LpIFC and LpST1 might be bidirectional for the unrelated condition. If one is interested in such double-peaked cross averages, one may wish to investigate the cross averages between Dipole 3 (at LaIFC) and Dipole 12 by consulting the corresponding columns of Dipole 3 (Unrelated and *F* of the 100-300 ms panel, Fig. 9).

3.4 Discussion

We will briefly discuss the actual ERF analyses using the two epoch filters.

In the typical sematic priming ERF, the conventional average for the unrelated condition is larger (in absolute value) than that of the related condition after a certain latency these two averages branch off. In fact, this original study concluded so (Ihara et al, 2007). However, the same is not necessarily true for the phase-compensated averages (Fig. 10). The phase-interpolated averages indicate that the conventional averages might consist of AD and PM and these two might cooperatively act when they have the same polarity (Fig. 7). If there is a gap between the conditional difference between the conventional averages and the phase-compensated averages, the activity that fills in the gap might be PM. In addition, directional relationships between ROIs can be discussed with these two epoch filters. This is the most conspicuously different point from the original study.

Are these two epoch filters able to analyze phase-related phenomena? Phase-interpolated averaging can be used to visualize ERD and ERS without additive activities (Fig. 8). Long-distance directional synchronization between LaIFC and LaT and between LpIFC and LpST1 can be visualized by phase-compensated averaging. In fact, these long-distance directional synchronizations likely happen since LaIFC and LaT are connected by the uncinate fasciculus and LpIFC and LpST1 by the arcuate fasciculus. In contrast, we can only speculate about phase-resetting. When the phase is reset, by which instantaneous phase jumps to a specific phase regardless of the phase just before phase-resetting, the condition number of phase-interpolated averaging could be very large at that moment. In fact, there are spike-like shapes in the condition numbers (Fig. 8). However, it must be noted that the spikes always appear if K ($2K+1$: the number of interpolated ERFs) increases and the condition number cannot detect phase-resetting if the neuronal population in charge of phase-resetting is small. Thus, we cannot say that this spike indicates phase-resetting. There is one other thing we should point out about phase-resetting: recall the difference between using the cosine and sine in the simulation described in section 1.2 (Fig. 1). Conventional averages of various ERF experiments have shapes that are experiment-dependent. According to the phase-interpolated averages (Fig. 9), AD and PM would have similar waveforms and be similar to conventional averages, and hence AD and PM would be time-locked. Therefore, cosine, sine, or their combination has to be determined by something in the case of the simulation. This determination is identical to setting the instantaneous phase to a specific value at a specific time. We wonder if this could be achieved only by resetting the phase. In the case of phase-resetting driven by stimuli, the first phase reset should occur at a very early latency, e.g., before N70 for visual stimuli if N70 is observed.

4. Conclusion

In this chapter, we explained the methodological and practical aspects of two epoch filters. The epoch filters are made possible by giving epochs an order. Since the order is of the instantaneous phases, these filters can be used to analyze phase-related phenomena. If another order is introduced, a different epoch filter can be designed and a different concept can be created accordingly. We hope that new epoch filters besides the ones presented here will be designed.

5. Acknowledgments

The authors thank Mr. Masaaki Nakayama and Mr. Norihiro Takamune of the University of Tokyo for their fruitful comments on the draft version. This work was supported in part by a Grant-in-Aid for Scientific Research (B) (No. 21300102) from the Ministry of Education, Science, Sports and Culture, Japan.

6. References

Başar, E. (1998). *Brain Function and Oscillations II: Integrative Brain Function. Neurophysiology and Cognitive Processes,* Springer, ISBN 978-3540643456, Berlin, Germany

Dornhege, G. del R. Millán, J. Hinterberger, T. McFarland, D.J. & Müller, K.R. (Eds.). (2007). *Toward Brain-computer Interfacing,* The MIT Press, ISBN 978-0-262-04244-4, Cambridge, US

Fujimaki, N.; Hayakawa, T. Nielsen, M. Knosche, T.R. & Miyauchi, S. (2002). An fMRI-constrained MEG Source Analysis with Procedures for Dividing and Grouping Activation. *NeuroImage,* Vol. 17, No. 1, pp. 324–343, ISSN 10538119

Herrmann, C.S. Grigutsch M. & Busch N.A. (2005). EEG Oscillations and Wavelet Analysis, In: *Event-related Potentials. A Methods Handbook.* Handy T.C. (Ed), 229-259, The MIT Press, ISBN 978-0262083331, Cambridge, US

Ihara, A.; Hayakawa, T. Wei, Q. Munetsuna, S. & Fujimaki, N. (2007). Lexical Access and Selection of Contextually Appropriate Meaning for Ambiguous Words. *Neuroimage,* Vol. 38, No. 3, pp. 576-588, ISSN 10538119

Lachaux, J.P.; Rodriguez, E. Le Van Quyen, M. Lutz, A. Martinerie, J. & Varela, R.J. (2000). Studying Single-trials of Phase Synchronous Activity in the Brain, *Intl. J. of Bifurcation and Chaos,* Vol. 10, No.10, pp. 2429-2439, ISSN 0218-1274

Lachaux, J.P.; Rodriguez, E. Martinerie, J. & Varela, F.J. (1999). Measuring Phase Synchrony in Brain Sginals. *Human Brain Mapping,* Vol. 8, No. 4, pp. 194-208, ISSN 1065-9471

Lopes da Silva, F.H. (2006). Event-related Neural Activities: What about Phase ?, In: *Event-related Dynamics of Brain Oscillations,* C. Neuper and W. Klimesch, (Eds.), 3-27, Elsevier, ISBN 978-0-444-52183-5, Amsterdam, The Netherlands

Makeig, S.; Westerfield, Jung, M.T.P. Enghoff, S. Townsend, J. Courchesne, E. & Sejnowski, T.J. (2002). Dynamic Brain Sources of Visual Evoked Responses. *Science,* Vol. 295, pp. 690-694, ISSN 0036-8075

Matani, A & Shigeno, T. (2006). Phase Series Echography with Prior Waveform Distortion for Evaluating Posterior Waveform Distortion, *IEEE Trans. on Ultrasonics, Ferroelectrics, and Frequency Control,* vol. 53, no. 11, pp. 2019-2025, ISSN 0885-3010

Matani, A.; Naruse, Y. Terazono, Y. Fujimaki, N. & Murata, T. (2011). Phase-interpolated Averaging for Analyzing Electroencephalography and Magnetoencephalography Epochs. *IEEE Trans. on Biomedical Engineering,* Vol. 58, No.1, pp. 71-80, ISSN 0018-9294

Matani, A.; Naruse, Y. Terazono, Y. Iwasaki, T. Fujimaki, N. & Murata T. (2010). Phase-compensated Averaging for Analyzing Electroencephalography and Magnetoencephalography Epochs. *IEEE Trans. on Biomedical Engineering,* Vol. 57, No.5, pp. 1117-1123, ISSN 0018-9294

Matsuura, K. & Okabe, Y. (1995). Selective Minimum-norm Solution of the Biomagnetic Inverse Problem. *IEEE Trans. on Biomedical Engineering,* Vol. 42, No. 6, 608–615, ISSN 0018-9294

Mazaheri, A. & Jensen, O. (2006). Posterior α Activity Is Not Phase-reset by Visual Stimuli. *Proc. Natl. Acad. Sci.,* Vol. 103, No. 8, pp. 2948-2952, ISSN 0027-8424

Oppenheim, A.V. & Schafer, R.W. (2007). *Discrete-time Signal Processing (3rd Edition),* Prentice Hall, ISBN 978-0131988422, Upper Saddle River, US

Pfurtscheller, G. (2006). The Cortical Activation Model (CAM), In: *Event-related Dynamics of Brain Oscillations,* C. Neuper and W. Klimesch, (Eds.), 19-27, Elsevier, ISBN 978-0-444-52183-5, Amsterdam, The Netherlands

Rodriguez, E.; George, N. Lachaux, J.P. Renault, B. & Varela, F.J. (1999). Perception's Shadow: Long-distance Synchronization of Human Brain Activity. *Nature,* Vol. 397, pp. 430-433, ISSN 0028-0836

Tallon-Baudry, C. & Bertrand. O. (1999). Oscillatoiry Gamma Activity in Humans and its Role inObject Representation. *Trens in Cognitive Sciences,* Vol. 3. No. 4, pp. 151-162, ISSN 1364-6613

Tallon-Baudry, C.; Bertrand. O. Delpuech, C. & Pernier, J. (1996). Stimulus Specificity of Phase-locked and Non-phase-locked 40 Hz Visual Responses in Human. *J. Neuroscience,* Vol. 16, No. 13, pp. 4240–4249, ISSN 03064522

Part 4

Current State of the Art: Clinical Analyses

9

Clinical MEG Analyses for Children with Intractable Epilepsy

Ayako Ochi, Cristina Y. Go and Hiroshi Otsubo
Division of Neurology, The Hospital for Sick Children
Canada

1. Introduction

Epilepsy is a brain disorder characterized by recurrent and unpredictable interruptions of normal brain function, called epileptic seizures (Fisher et al., 2005). Epilepsy occurs in 1-2% of children (Hauser & Kurland, 1975). Twenty-five percent of children with epilepsy continue to seize despite appropriate medical management and are diagnosed as medically refractory epilepsy (Hauser, 1993). Medically refractory epilepsy is defined as seizures that continue despite at least two appropriate first line anti-epileptic medications at maximally tolerated serum levels for 2 years (Snead, 2001). A subset of patients with medically refractory epilepsy can be surgically treated after anti-epileptic medications fail. Successful control of the seizures can be achieved in children with intractable partial epilepsy by surgical resection of the epileptogenic foci (Duchowny 1995; Wyllie 1998; Snead 2001).

In our institution, magnetoencephalography (MEG) is an essential part of the diagnostic workup in all patients undergoing presurgical evaluation. We introduced the concept of MEG-guided epilepsy surgery (Minassian et el., 1999; Otsubo et al., 1999, 2001a, 2001b; Holowka et al., 2004; Iida et al., 2005; RamachandranNair et al., 2007; Mohamed et al., 2007; Ochi et al., 2008). In patients with intractable partial epilepsy, MEG is a powerful tool for presurgical evaluation to predict an epileptogenic zone (Wheless et al., 1999; Pataraia et al., 2004; Paulini et al., 2007). The epileptogenic zone is a region of cortex that can generate epileptic seizures (Rosenow & Lüders, 2001). By definition, total removal or disconnection of the epileptogenic zone is necessary and sufficient for seizure freedom. In this chapter, we would like to demonstrate our presurgical evaluation, including scalp video-electroencephalography (EEG) monitoring to capture seizures and interictal epileptiform discharges, and clinical MEG studies and analyses to estimate the epileptogenic zone.

2. Scalp video-EEG monitoring

Scalp video-EEG is crucial before MEG analyses. This can be performed over 1 to 5 days using 19 or 25 scalp electrodes placed according to the International 10-20 system (Jasper, 1958). During scalp video-EEG monitoring, seizure semiology, ictal EEG findings and interictal epileptiform discharges are analyzed in detail to determine lateralization and localization of the seizure onset zone and the irritative zone (Rosenow & Lüders, 2001).

Detailed analysis of the scalp video-EEG can predict the approximate epileptogenic zone (Wyllie et al., 1993).
The scalp video-EEG recordings in children often show secondary bilateral synchrony, generalized or multifocal interictal discharges (Wyllie et al., 2007). We have to find (1) consistent leading discharges before these spread to the whole brain, (2) predominant lateralization of multiple independent spike foci, and (3) complexity of spike morphology. Irregular polyspikes/spikes with superimposed fast activity are more epileptogenic than sharp waves with simple and stereotyped morphology. The fast activity is one sign of the epileptogenic zone (Kobayashi et al., 2004; Yamazsaki et al., 2008). Predominantly lateralized or localized interictal spikes during REM sleep also suggest the epileptogenic hemisphere (Samalitano et al., 1991; Ochi et al., 2011). When we analyze MEG data, we always compare the scalp video-EEG and MEG to recognize the characteristics of the interictal spikes, seizure onset zone and seizure semiology for the clinical interpretation of the MEG result.

3. MEG studies and analyses (recording and analysis)

Interictal MEG recordings are performed in patients taking their regular dosage of antiepileptic drugs (AEDs). Most of the time, we have found the occurrence rate of interictal spikes was dramatically reduced by maximum dosage of AEDs when patients undergo MEG as an out-patient procedure. The night prior to MEG, patients are sleep-deprived to accentuate focal interictal epileptiform discharges by sleep (Veldfuizen et al., 1983). If patients can undergo MEG recording during their admission for scalp video-EEG, increase in interictal epileptiform discharges are noted during MEG study because anti-epileptic medications are usually tapered to capture seizures for the video-EEG analysis. In children who are unable to cooperate, we use total intravenous anesthesia with propofol and remifentanil for their MEG and subsequent MRI studies (Fujimoto et al., 2009).
We use a whole-head gradiometer-based Omega system (151 channels, VSM MedTech Ltd., Port Coquitlam, BC, Canada) in a magnetically shielded room. Simultaneous MEG and scalp EEG recordings are performed for at least 30 minutes consisting of 15 two-minute periods of spontaneous data. The sampling rate for data acquisition is 625 Hz. Scalp EEG is simultaneously recorded from 19 electrodes placed according to the International 10-20 system. Head positions are measured at the beginning and end of each two-minute period. For optimal accuracy of co-registration of MEG dipole sources onto MRI, the data set in which patients move their head more than 5 mm, is discarded and not analyzed. MEG dipole source localization has been reported to present 2-3mm error in comparison of somatosensory evoked fields on MEG with intraoperative evoked potentials (Yang et al., 1993). The data with more than 5mm head movement may reach 7-8mm localization error to estimate the dipole source which can be localized in the neighboring gyrus; thus these sets are discarded.
Table 1 shows the process of our MEG analysis.

3.1 Detection and selection of MEG spikes

We visually identify MEG interictal epileptiform discharges – spikes, polyspikes and sharp waves (referred to as spikes) – by reviewing the 151-channel raw MEG wave forms with band pass filter of 10-70 Hz, and cross-reference them with the simultaneous EEG recordings (Fig. 1). Low frequency filter is set relatively high (10Hz) to reduce diffuse slow waves in children with intractable epilepsy and to obtain high signal to noise ratio (Sugiyama et al., 2009).

1. Detection and selection of MEG spikes (Fig. 1)
1) Band pass filter 10-70 Hz
2) Detection of individual MEG spikes with or without simultaneous EEG spikes
3) Placement of a cursor at the earliest spike peak with reasonable magnetic field topography
4) Selection of the spike >1 second apart from previous spikes when continuous spikes occur
2. Calculation of dipole source by single moving dipole analysis
100 ms window (50 msec before and after the cursor, every 1.6 msec, total 63 time points) for sampling rate 625 Hz (Fig. 2)
3. Selection of dipole sources (Fig. 2)
Selection of one dipole source from one spike with following criteria
1) Residual error between measured and calculated magnetic field topographies <30%
2) Dipole moment 50-400 nAm
3) Dipole locations of consecutive 5-6 time points staying within 1 cm on x-, y-, z-axes or within one gyrus
4) Stable strength of dipole moment during consecutive 5-6 time points
5) Dipole with reasonable magnetic field topography with tight "sink and source" pattern and minimum background noise
6) Dipole location in gray matter or gray/white matter junction - with the exception of cortical dysplasia/heterotopia
7) Comparison with simultaneous EEG spike - if dipole location is deep, A) dipole with no simultaneous EEG spike; B) dipole before EEG negative peak
4. Classification of dipoles
1) Cluster, defined as 6 or more dipoles with 1 cm or less between adjacent dipoles
2) Scatter, defined as: A) fewer than 6 dipoles regardless of the distance between dipoles; or B) dipoles with greater than 1 cm between dipoles regardless of number of dipoles

Table 1. MEG analyses

We analyze individual spikes instead of averaged spikes for dipole source localization in order to obtain the extent of possible epileptogenic zone. The spike-averaging methods may result in loss of spatial and temporal information and of details concerning individual spike types (Sato et al., 1991). Spikes superimposed with electrocardiogram (ECG) are excluded for dipole source localization. When polyspikes or repetitive spikes occur (Fig. 1, red cursor), we select the earliest spike peak with reasonable magnetic field topography for dipole source analysis. The zone of the earliest spike and seizure onset zone demonstrate a high correlation that favors a common epileptic generator (Hufnagel et al., 2000). Some interictal spikes can be better visualized by either MEG or EEG, therefore, ideally, selection of interictal spikes should use both methods simultaneously (Iwasaki et al., 2005; Shibasaki et al., 2007). Various technical factors influence MEG and EEG spike detection, including the number of sensors for MEG and the number of channels for EEG, and in particular, the different characteristics of gradiometer vs. magnetometer for MEG. Needless to say, the methods of source analysis and the availability of experts in each institute are very important in the clinical interpretation of MEG data (Shibasaki et al., 2007).

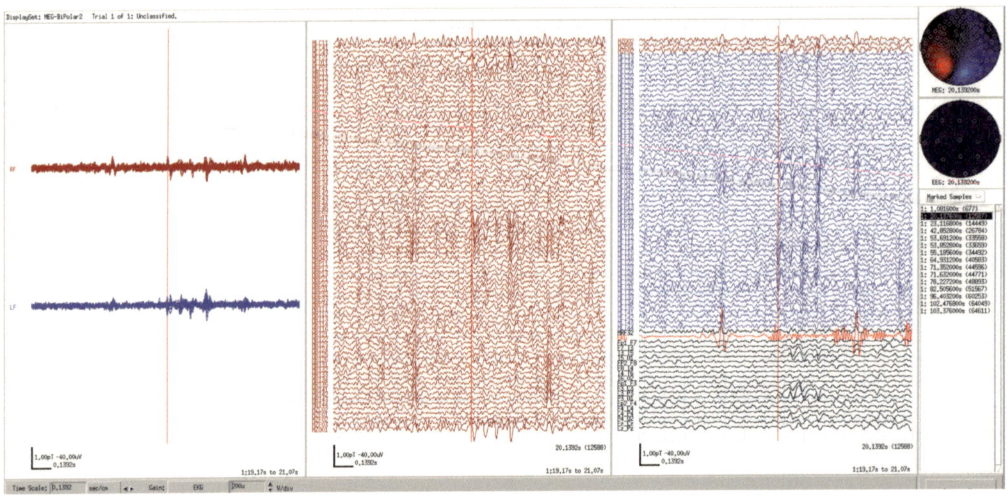

Fig. 1. Detection and selection of MEG spikes. Left panel shows overlaid MEG wave forms over the right hemisphere (brown) and left hemisphere (blue). Middle two panels show raw MEG wave forms of 151 individual coils (right hemisphere, brown; left hemisphere, blue), electrocardiogram (ECG, red) and simultaneous EEG wave forms (black). Right panel shows magnetic field topography (top), EEG field topography (middle), 15 time points of selected spikes during one-set 2-minute recording (bottom). A cursor (red line) is placed at the earliest spike peak in the epoch of four repetitive spikes with magnetic field topography with tight sink and source (top right). Calculation of dipole source is performed 50 msec before and after the cursor (total 100 ms window, each time point every 1.6 msec, total 63 time points).

3.2 Calculation of dipole source by single moving dipole analysis

We apply a single moving dipole analysis with a single-shell, whole-head, individually-created spherical model. Calculation of the dipole source location, strength and orientation that best fits the measured magnetic fields is performed. For each spike, dipole source solutions are examined every 1.6 msec during a 100 msec window (50 ms before and 50 msec after the peak of spikes, total 63 time points) (Fig. 2).

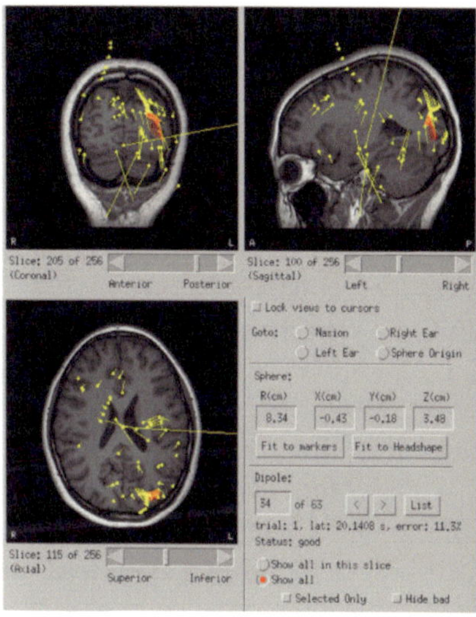

Index	Trial	Sample	Latency(s)	Err.(%)	Good/Bad	Color	Mom(nAm)	xp(cm)	yp(cm)	zp(cm)	decl(deg)	azim(deg)	Label
1	1	12556	20.088	61.58	Bad	Yellow	-19.61	-5.056	-1.139	8.184	54.9	57.5	spike_2.1
2	1	12557	20.0896	60.55	Bad	Yellow	18.12	-5.181	-1.586	8.08	123.7	248.3	spike_2.2
3	1	12558	20.0912	85.8	Bad	Yellow	-13.98	-3.328	4.655	4.116	165.0	55.7	spike_2.3
4	1	12559	20.0928	83.53	Bad	Yellow	16.96	-4.254	3.25	2.585	15.6	189.4	spike_2.4
5	1	12560	20.0944	72.47	Bad	Yellow	-10.5	-7.125	2.009	3.809	174.2	98.9	spike_2.5
6	1	12561	20.096	56.42	Bad	Yellow	10.25	-7.874	1.406	4.544	9.7	312.3	spike_2.6
7	1	12562	20.0976	48.47	Bad	Yellow	10.76	-8.054	1.13	4.896	11.6	322.7	spike_2.7
8	1	12563	20.0992	49.8	Bad	Yellow	10.48	-8.136	0.983	5.177	13.3	328.0	spike_2.8
9	1	12564	20.1008	57.43	Bad	Yellow	-9.51	-8.158	0.9	5.425	165.1	151.4	spike_2.9
10	1	12565	20.1024	80.8	Bad	Yellow	11	0.766	-2.237	9.409	111.9	300.3	spike_2.10
11	1	12566	20.104	72.05	Bad	Yellow	-11.55	1.409	-1.984	9.929	68.7	122.4	spike_2.11
12	1	12567	20.1056	65.78	Bad	Yellow	-11.52	1.957	-1.732	10.35	69.1	124.0	spike_2.12
13	1	12568	20.1072	63.69	Bad	Yellow	-9.25	2.509	-1.432	11.206	70.6	124.9	spike_2.13
14	1	12569	20.1088	65.31	Bad	Yellow	-6.43	2.913	-1.281	12.094	71.3	127.7	spike_2.14
15	1	12570	20.1104	70.82	Bad	Yellow	4.64	3.098	-1.313	12.493	110.2	315.7	spike_2.15
16	1	12571	20.112	79.51	Bad	Yellow	-22.58	-2.595	-0.809	6.444	123.7	225.1	spike_2.16
17	1	12572	20.1136	65.17	Bad	Yellow	-19.38	-2.605	4.94	0.083	61.1	42.8	spike_2.17
18	1	12573	20.1152	58.01	Bad	Yellow	-36.8	-1.179	3.822	1.413	45.3	40.8	spike_2.18
19	1	12574	20.1168	53.78	Bad	Yellow	-50.56	-0.158	3.434	3.3	26.8	1.5	spike_2.19
20	1	12575	20.1184	51.24	Bad	Yellow	-48.68	0.36	3.288	4.854	29.9	305.0	spike_2.20
21	1	12576	20.12	47.91	Bad	Yellow	-37.27	0.249	1.676	7.701	65.0	255.6	spike_2.21
22	1	12577	20.1216	47.2	Bad	Yellow	-37.97	0.126	2.262	7.615	58.8	257.8	spike_2.22
23	1	12578	20.1232	49.28	Bad	Yellow	-39.01	-0.07	2.488	7.402	55.6	259.1	spike_2.23
24	1	12579	20.1248	53.58	Bad	Yellow	47.62	-0.361	2.091	6.621	125.8	83.6	spike_2.24
25	1	12580	20.1264	55.58	Bad	Yellow	151.84	-0.711	1.069	2.855	153.7	278.5	spike_2.25
26	1	12581	20.128	51.52	Bad	Yellow	70.24	-1.964	2.122	1.834	149.1	301.0	spike_2.26
27	1	12582	20.1296	42.62	Bad	Yellow	-45.06	-4.316	2.896	3.665	5.7	253.1	spike_2.27
28	1	12583	20.1312	31.79	Bad	Yellow	-39.53	-5.637	2.868	5.231	18.4	300.2	spike_2.28
29	1	12584	20.1328	23.46	Bad	Yellow	-42.16	-6.144	2.716	5.921	22.5	309.7	spike_2.29
30	1	12585	20.1344	17.57	Good	Red	-46.16	-6.365	2.552	6.285	24.2	318.2	spike_2.30
31	1	12586	20.136	13.63	Good	Red	-49.5	-6.448	2.379	6.497	25.1	326.2	spike_2.31
32	1	12587	20.1376	11.31	Good	Red	-51.03	-6.465	2.195	6.623	26.0	333.6	spike_2.32
33	1	12588	20.1392	10.46	Good	Red	50.02	-6.452	1.99	6.721	153.2	159.1	spike_2.33
34	1	12589	20.1408	11.31	Good	Red	46.26	-6.435	1.744	6.808	152.2	162.1	spike_2.34
35	1	12590	20.1424	14.83	Bad	Yellow	-40.27	-6.419	1.41	6.914	29.0	341.9	spike_2.35
36	1	12591	20.144	22.71	Bad	Yellow	-33.23	-6.391	0.916	7.043	30.9	338.4	spike_2.36
37	1	12592	20.1456	35.77	Bad	Yellow	-26.24	-6.357	0.202	7.151	33.9	333.1	spike_2.37
38	1	12593	20.1472	52.08	Bad	Yellow	-19.5	-6.398	-0.688	7.116	37.0	328.4	spike_2.38
39	1	12594	20.1488	68.75	Bad	Yellow	12.63	-6.849	-1.574	6.58	145.2	144.9	spike_2.39
40	1	12595	20.1504	69.82	Bad	Yellow	12.32	-5.82	4.121	6.692	32.3	4.1	spike_2.40
41	1	12596	20.152	43.08	Bad	Yellow	17.12	-6.716	3.217	6.812	25.0	335.1	spike_2.41
42	1	12597	20.1536	24.45	Bad	Yellow	26.75	-6.744	2.641	6.855	26.8	320.7	spike_2.42
43	1	12598	20.1552	68.76	Bad	Yellow	-978434	-0.43	-0.177	3.484	87.2	328.8	spike_2.43
44	1	12599	20.1568	11.74	Bad	Yellow	48.81	-6.506	1.891	7.008	32.4	311.1	spike_2.44
45	1	12600	20.1584	9.27	Bad	Yellow	55.21	-6.452	1.692	7.11	34.7	309.0	spike_2.45
46	1	12601	20.16	8.03	Bad	Yellow	56.19	-6.46	1.583	7.206	36.4	307.3	spike_2.46
47	1	12602	20.1616	8.28	Bad	Yellow	52.14	-6.525	1.542	7.29	37.7	305.4	spike_2.47
48	1	12603	20.1632	10.48	Bad	Yellow	-44.73	-6.638	1.552	7.357	141.4	123.2	spike_2.48
49	1	12604	20.1648	14.91	Bad	Yellow	-36.04	-6.784	1.593	7.412	140.6	120.9	spike_2.49
50	1	12605	20.1664	21.73	Bad	Yellow	-27.71	-6.945	1.635	7.476	140.0	119.2	spike_2.50
51	1	12606	20.168	31.48	Bad	Yellow	20.49	-7.107	1.629	7.593	40.4	299.1	spike_2.51
52	1	12607	20.1696	45.25	Bad	Yellow	14.41	-7.269	1.535	7.792	40.5	301.7	spike_2.52
53	1	12608	20.1712	78.68	Bad	Yellow	-123.89	0.252	-0.815	2.826	36.2	332.8	spike_2.53
54	1	12609	20.1728	77.27	Bad	Yellow	-18.78	3.058	-3.568	2.316	28.0	19.0	spike_2.54
55	1	12610	20.1744	76.74	Bad	Yellow	12.02	4.197	-3.98	2.6	148.5	216.6	spike_2.55
56	1	12611	20.176	74.38	Bad	Yellow	-10.49	3.72	-3.708	7.705	66.7	210.1	spike_2.56
57	1	12612	20.1776	70.2	Bad	Yellow	-19.54	-1.62	-4.374	5.835	144.1	212.3	spike_2.57
58	1	12613	20.1792	69.54	Bad	Yellow	-16.28	3.813	-2.334	7.453	65.3	220.5	spike_2.58
59	1	12614	20.1808	58.93	Bad	Yellow	-19.07	4.712	-0.837	6.745	43.1	220.5	spike_2.59

Fig. 2. Stability of dipole locations. Left panel shows coronal (left top), sagittal (right top) and axial MRI. Before selection of MEG dipoles by criteria (Table 1), all calculated MEG dipoles in one dataset (two minutes) are shown on transparent MRI. Right table shows information of all MEG dipoles from one spike before selection by the criteria described in Table 1 (latency, residual error, amplitude, x-, y-, z-axes, and angle of moment). To select one dipole from one spike (total 63 time points by sampling rate 625 Hz), dipole locations (red circles on MRI) of consecutive 5-6 time points (right, black highlights on the list) stay within 1cm on x-, y-, z-axes and/or within one gyrus.

3.3 Selection of dipole sources

We select one dipole source from each individual spike with the following criteria; (1) residual error < 30% between measured magnetic field and calculated magnetic field topographies, (2) dipole moment from 50 to 400 nAm, (3) dipole locations of consecutive 5-6 time points (4-8ms) staying within 1cm on x-, y-, z-axes and/or within one gyrus (Fig. 2), (4) stable strength of dipole moment during consecutive 5-6 time points, (5) equivalent current dipole corresponding with tight "sink and source" pattern and minimum background noise on magnetic field topography, (6) dipole source location in gray matter or gray/white matter junction - cortical dysplasia/heterotopia are exceptional (Case 3), (7) Comparison with simultaneous EEG spike - if dipole location is deep, A) dipole with no simultaneous EEG spike or B) dipole before EEG negative peak should be selected.

Our first criterion of residual error (< 30%) is less strict than that of other institutions because we compare measured and calculated magnetic field topography using whole head

151 channels and children tend to present with extratemporal lobe epilepsy and/or multiple foci. We try to detect a small disc of cortex at the onset of interictal spike satisfying our criteria (2) to (7). Strict adherence to the above criteria is needed to select the optimal dipole from non-averaged individual spikes and estimate possible epileptogenic zone by MEG dipole source analysis. It also gives us the most consistent results. If we allow too many exceptions to the criteria, distribution of MEG dipoles would be wider than the possible epileptogenic zone, which includes extensive epileptic network such as irritative zone (Rosenow & Lüders, 2001).

A bundle of pyramidal neuron, which is a small disc of cortex, resembles a dipole source (Gloor, 1985). MEG that was simultaneously recorded with 'intracranial' EEG detected ≥3 cm^2 disc of epileptic cortex in the lateral convexity of brain (Oishi et al., 2002). Scalp EEG can detect 10-20 cm^2 of gyral cortex in patient with temporal lobe epilepsy (Tao et al., 2005). MEG is superior to conventional 19-channel scalp EEG in detecting the beginning of interictal spike in the fissural cortex (Merlet et al., 1997) because the skull is 'transparent' to the magnetic fields for shallow dipole sources (Okada et al., 1999). After an interictal spike at a small area in the fissural cortex spreads to wider area including crown of gyrus, EEG shows negative peak of the spike after the peak of MEG spike (Merlet et al., 1997). Stability of dipole location and moment suggests focal cortical origin of spikes. When focal cortical origin of spikes quickly shows secondarily bilateral synchrony or becomes generalized, the single moving dipole analysis can be applied only to the 1st leading focal cortical spikes. The 2nd and 3rd spikes during an epoch of generalized spike-and-wave complex involve thalamo-cortical network (Meeren et al., 2002).

3.4 Classification of dipole sources

We classify the dipole source locations as follows; (1) A cluster consists of 6 or more dipole sources localized with 1 cm or less between dipoles; (2) Scattered dipole sources consist of either (A) fewer than 6 dipoles sources, or (B) dipole sources localized more than 1 cm apart regardless number. (Iida et al., 2005) MEG dipole clusters suggest the epileptogenic zone requires complete excision (Otsubo et al., 1999; Iida et al., 2005).

4. Case presentations

We will present MEG analyses in three pediatric cases with intractable partial epilepsy demonstrating 1) polyspikes in Rolandic epilepsy, 2) secondary bilateral synchrony in frontal lobe epilepsy, and 3) deep MEG dipoles without simultaneous EEG spikes in parietal lobe epilepsy.

4.1 Polyspikes in Rolandic epilepsy

Pediatric patients with intractable partial epilepsy often present with refractory Rolandic epilepsy that are clinically distinguished from patients with benign Rolandic epilepsy with centro-temporal spikes (Otsubo et al., 2001; Benifla et al., 2009). MEG shows polyspikes in the Rolandic region due to highly epileptogenic focal cortical dysplasia. MEG spike peak appears earlier than EEG spike negative peak in most of cases (Merlet et al., 1997). Especially in cases with the intractable partial epilepsy secondary to the focal cortical dysplasia, MEG dipoles tend to cluster from the earliest spike peak with stable and distinguishable magnetic field topography (see Table 1, 1.3, 3.3-5). This subset of focal cortical dysplasia must have dense epileptic neuronal disk to produce a cluster of MEG dipoles.

Case 1 is an almost 13 year old right-handed girl with intractable Rolandic epilepsy. Her seizures started at 6 ½ years of age, consisting of nocturnal tonic or generalized tonic clonic seizures, at times associated with enuresis. Scalp video EEG at 12 years of age captured 12 seizures, consisting of right arm jerking from sleep, followed by tonic extension of bilateral arms and right leg. Seizures and interictal epileptiform discharges originated from left centro-parietal region. Three-tesla (3T) MRI showed subtle abnormal signal and blurring of grey/white matter in the left mesial Rolandic region. She was on levetiracetam and phenytoin.

MEG was performed at 12 years of age. The steps from a representative analysis of one spike are shown in Figures 3 to 6.

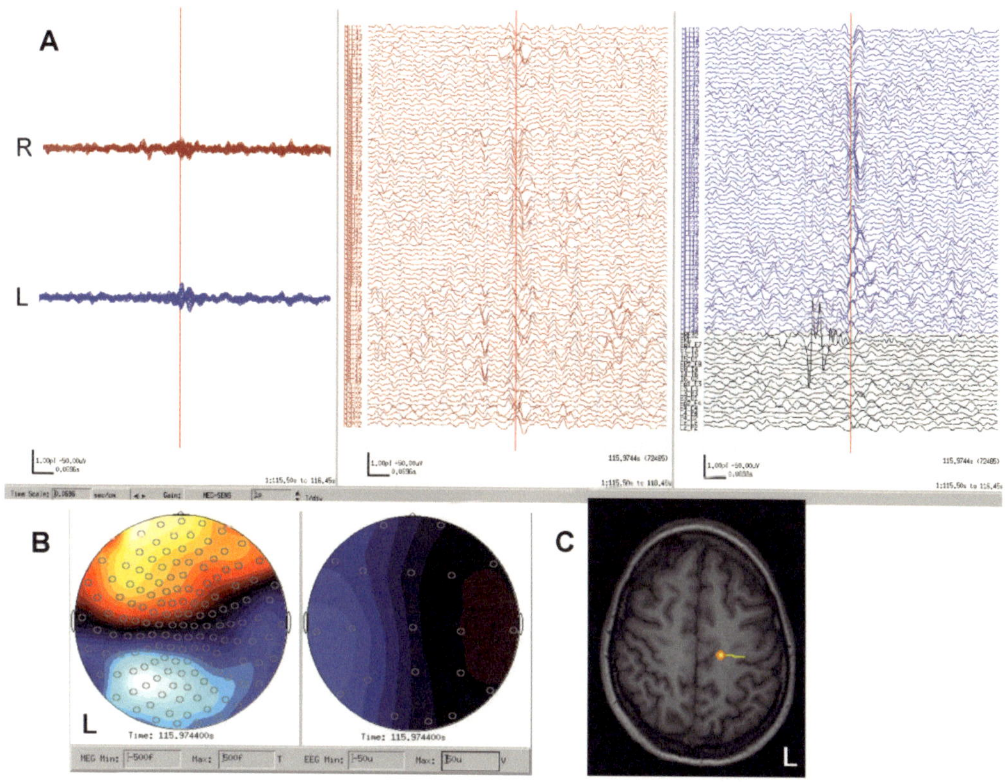

Fig. 3. The first peak of MEG polyspikes. **A**, MEG shows polyspikes. Left side shows two overlaid wave forms (R, right hemisphere; L, left hemisphere) and right side shows individual 151 channels (red channels, right hemisphere; blue channels left hemisphere), ECG and EEG (black channels). The red cursor is placed at the first peak of MEG polyspikes. **B**, magnetic field topography (left, red is sink, blue is source) and EEG topography (right, blue is positive, red is negative) at the first peak (red cursor on MEG wave forms on A). **C**, MEG dipole at the first peak of polyspikes is localized beside a subtle MRI abnormality in the left mesial Rolandic region.

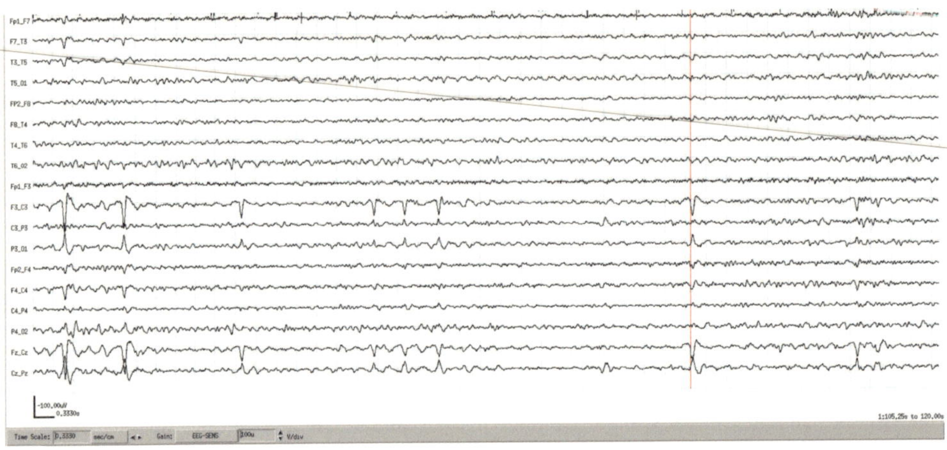

Fig. 4. EEG at the first peak of MEG polyspikes. When MEG shows polyspikes (Fig. 3A), EEG shows simple morphology of spike and wave at C3-P3 and Cz (Fig. 4). The first peak of MEG polyspikes (Fig. 3A, red line) appears before the EEG spike peak (Fig. 4, red line) with 34msec lag.

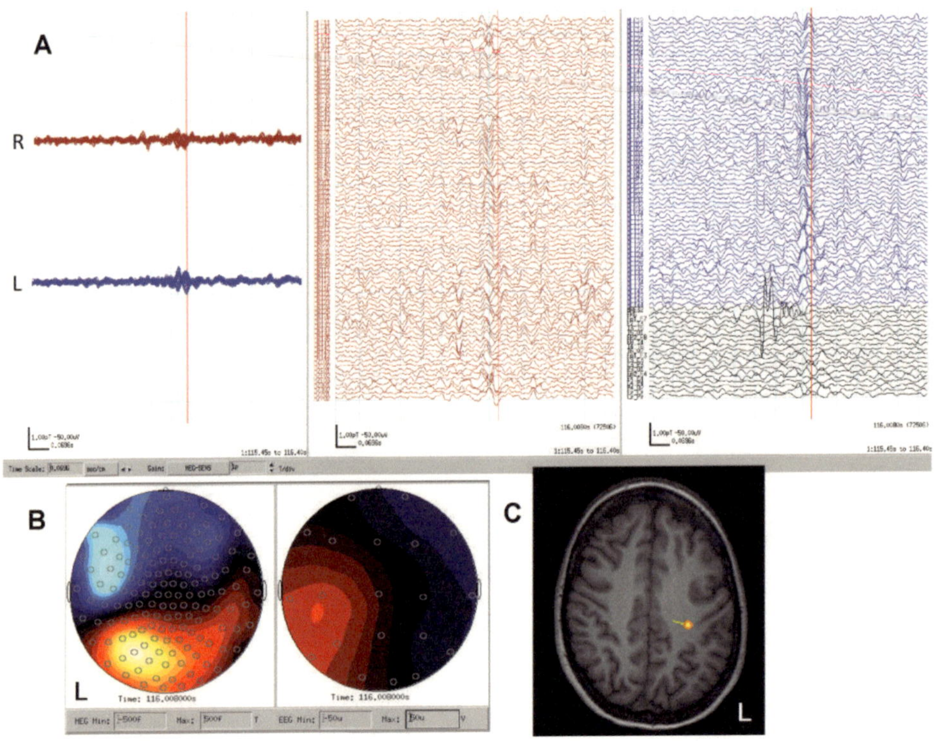

Fig. 5. The second peak of MEG polyspikes. **A**, MEG shows polyspikes. The red cursor is placed on the EEG spike peak which corresponded to the second peak of the MEG polyspikes. **B**, magnetic field topography (left) and EEG topography (right) at the EEG spike peak (red cursor on A). **C**, MEG dipole at the second peak of polyspikes is localized to the left Rolandic region on MRI, lateral to the first peak dipole source (Fig. 3C). It is noted that the dipole orientation and magnetic field topography are in the opposite direction from those of the first dipole (Fig3. C).

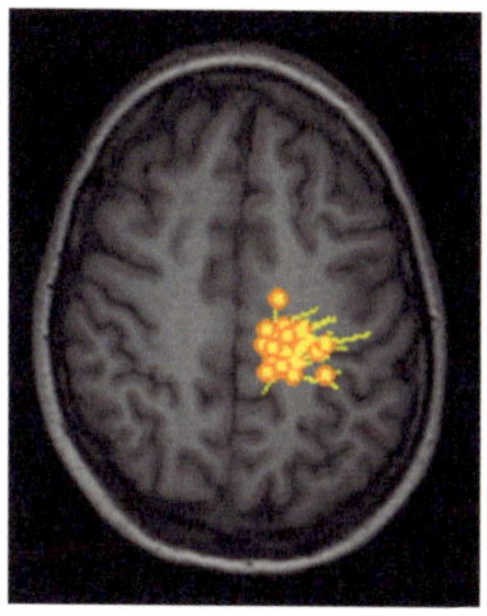

Fig. 6. Cluster of MEG dipoles from one data set. One data set out of 15 two-minute data sets showed a cluster of 26 MEG dipoles fulfilling criteria (see section 3.3) from 43 MEG spikes, which was localized in the left Rolandic region transparently shown on axial MRI.

A total of 203 MEG spikes were detected during 15 two-minute data sets. After dipole calculation from the 203 spikes, 115 MEG dipoles met criteria were selected as the final result. A dense cluster of 109 MEG dipoles was localized in the left mesial to lateral Rolandic region.

Intracranial video-EEG monitoring was performed using subdural grid electrodes over left Rolandic region and depth/strip electrodes toward subtle MRI abnormality in the mesial Rolandic region. Seizure onset zone included both mesial and lateral Rolandic cortices. Mesial Rolandic region started earlier than lateral cortex with a time lag of 300 msec at the beginning of her seizures. Both areas were resected and she has been seizure free for 7 months. She had immediate post-operative right hemiparesis, with almost full recovery of hand and leg motor function 6 weeks after the surgery. Pathology showed focal cortical dysplasia with dysmorphic neurons (type IIa).

4.2 Secondary bilateral synchrony in frontal lobe epilepsy

EEGs often show paroxysmal generalized spike-/polyspike-and-wave complexes in children with intractable partial epilepsy even with focal onset seizures (Wyllie et al, 2007). Frontal lobe epilepsy frequently presents with secondarily bilateral synchronized epileptiform discharges (Akiyama et al., 2011). MEG dipoles can be estimated at the earliest peak of spikes before generalization in the spike complex which should have >1sec interval during continuous spike and waves (see Table 1; 1.3 & 1.4).

Case 2 is an almost 17 year old left handed boy with intractable frontal lobe epilepsy. His generalized tonic clonic seizures started at 6 years of age. Scalp video EEG at the age of 16 years captured 16 seizures, consisting of tonic posturing or single jerking of both arms, right arm more than left. Ictal EEG originated from the left fronto-central and temporal regions. Interictal epileptiform discharges consisted of frequent bursts of generalized polyspike-and-waves with left hemispheric predominance and independent focal spikes over the left fronto-central and temporal regions, indicative of secondary bilateral synchrony originating from left hemisphere. 3T MRI showed abnormal signal within subcortical white matter in the left frontal lobe. Functional MRI (fMRI) showed right hemisphere language predominance. He was on clobazam and valproic acid.

A total of 261 MEG spikes were detected. Ninety MEG dipoles were selected as the final result, consisting of 86 in the left hemisphere and four in the right hemisphere. An extensive cluster of 69 MEG dipoles were localized in the left frontal region (Fig. 9). He underwent

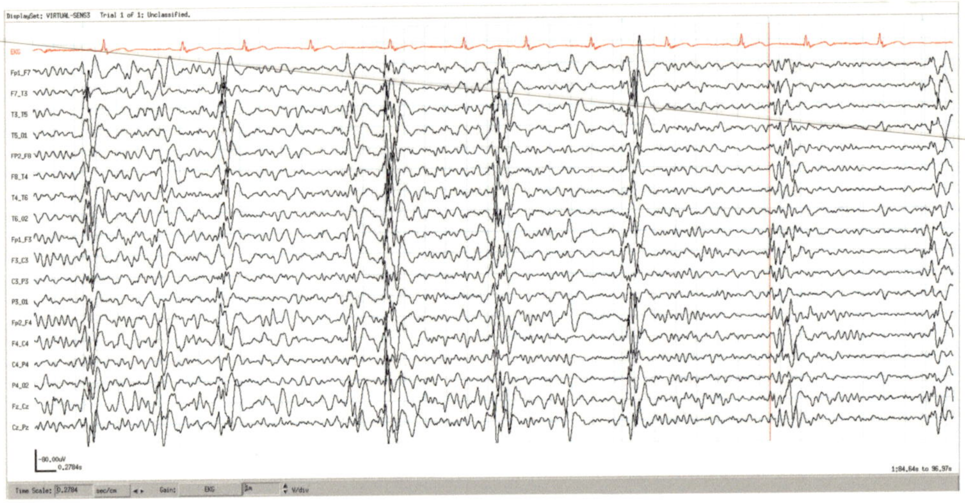

Fig. 7. Frequent generalized polyspike-bursts. EEG shows frequent generalized polyspike-bursts. Red cursor is corresponding to the time point in Fig. 8.

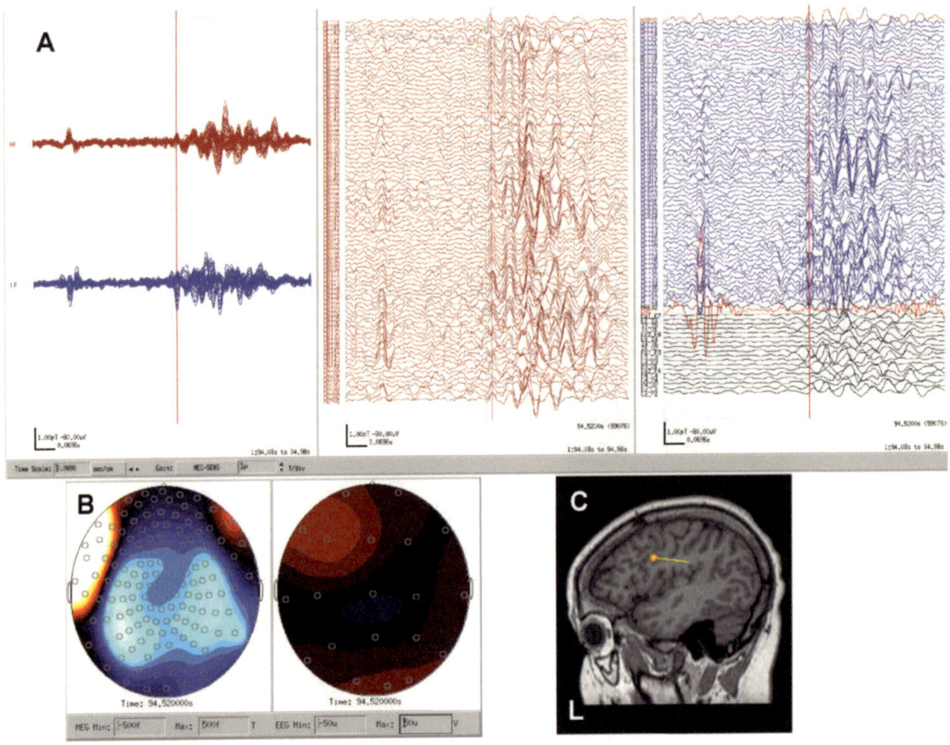

Fig. 8. The earliest component with a reasonable magnetic field topography of generalized polyspike-burst. **A**, The earliest component with a reasonable magnetic field topography of a polyspike-burst is selected (red cursor). **B**, Magnetic field topography shows bilateral "sink and source" pattern with left hemispheric predominance. **C**, Single moving dipole analysis shows an MEG dipole in the left middle frontal gyrus on sagittal MRI.

intracranial video-EEG monitoring using subdural grid electrodes over the left frontal parietal and superior temporal region and three strip electrodes inserted to left frontal pole and left mesial frontal region. Eight seizures were identical, consisting of single spasm followed by brief tonic seizure of right arm originating from left frontal lobe, superior temporal gyrus and inferior parietal region. Left frontal lobectomy and cortical excision of posterior portion of left frontal lobe, superior temporal gyrus and inferior parietal region were performed. Pathology showed microdysgenesis. He has been seizure free for 11 months.

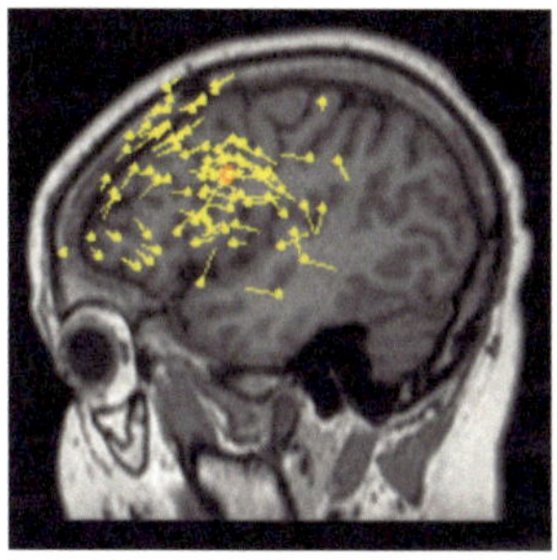

Fig. 9. Total 86 of MEG dipoles in the left hemisphere in Case 2. Sagittal MRI shows a total of 86 MEG dipoles overlaid in the left hemisphere. Sixty-nine dipoles were clustered in the left inferior, middle and superior frontal gyri, anterior to the motor cortex.

4.3 Deep MEG dipoles without simultaneous EEG spikes in parietal lobe epilepsy

The epileptogenic focal cortical dysplasia often involves not only the cortex, but also the gray/white matter junction and even the white matter as heterotopia (Blümcke et al., 2011). When a single MEG dipole with large moment is localized in the deep structure in the brain and shows simultaneous high amplitude EEG spike negative peak, the MEG dipole can be falsely localized by the extensive cortical discharges. The single moving dipole analysis for MEG can only be applied well for the "small" disc of cortical discharges, and not the extensive cortical discharges. If MEG dipoles are deeply localized without EEG spikes, the epileptic neurons in the heterotopia truly exist in the white matter (see Table 1; 3.6 & 3.7).

Case 3 is an 11 year old right-handed boy with intractable partial epilepsy secondary to right temporo-parietal cortical dysplasia. His seizures started at the age of 2.5 years. He was developmentally delayed. His seizures consisted of nocturnal generalized tonic clonic seizures and complex partial seizures (staring, hand and oral automatism). 3T MRI showed abnormally thickened right temporal and parietal cortices, suggestive of cortical dysplasia. Scalp video-EEG at the age of 9 years captured two nocturnal seizures, consisting of tonic clonic seizures with predominant involvement of left arm and face originated from right temporo-parieto-occipital regions. There were frequent interictal epileptiform discharges over the right temporo-parietal regions.

He underwent intracranial video-EEG monitoring using subdural grid electrodes over the right temporal, parietal and occipital region and four depth electrodes inserted to right parietal and right mesial temporal region. Eight seizures started from right temporal parietal occipital regions including subcortical MRI abnormality. Extensive cortical excision of the right parietal including subcortical MRI abnormality, right temporal lobectomy including amygdala and hippocampus were performed. Pathology showed focal cortical dysplasia with neuronal cytomegaly and balloon cells (type IIb). He has been seizure free for three years.

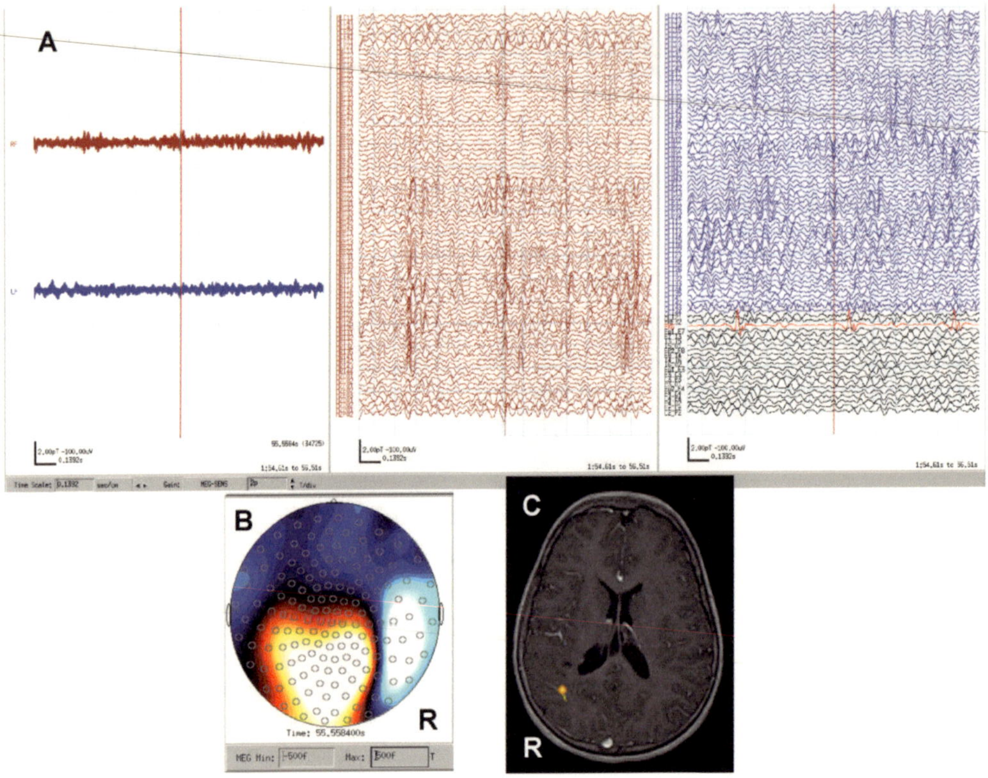

Fig. 10. Deep MEG dipoles without simultaneous EEG spike. **A**, MEG shows a red cursor at right hemispheric MEG spikes. **B**, Magnetic field topography shows tight sink and source at the MEG spike peak. **C**, Single moving dipole analysis shows an MEG dipole in the right temporo-parietal subcortical abnormality on axial MRI.

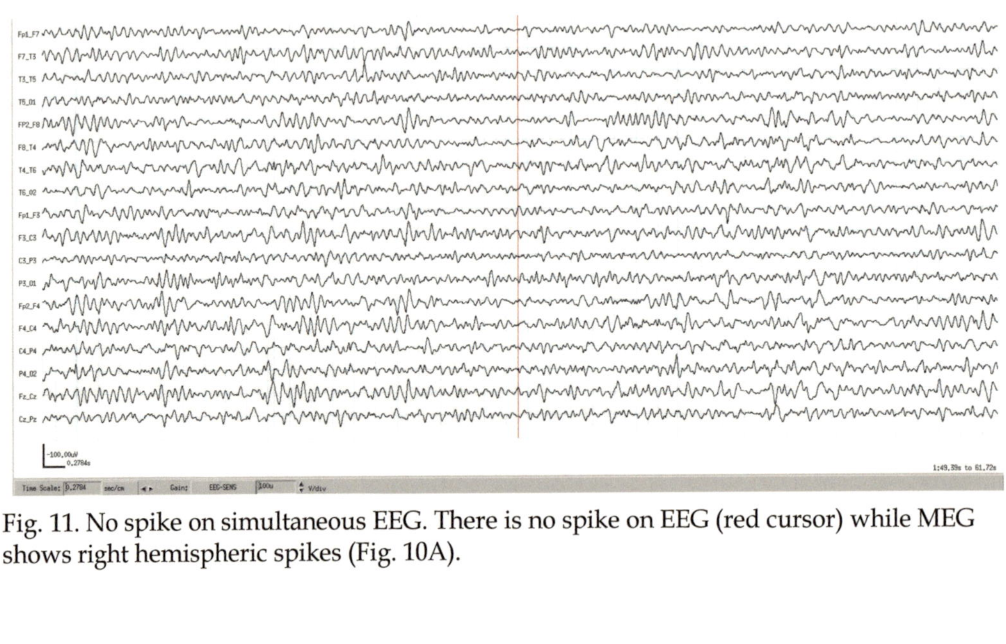

Fig. 11. No spike on simultaneous EEG. There is no spike on EEG (red cursor) while MEG shows right hemispheric spikes (Fig. 10A).

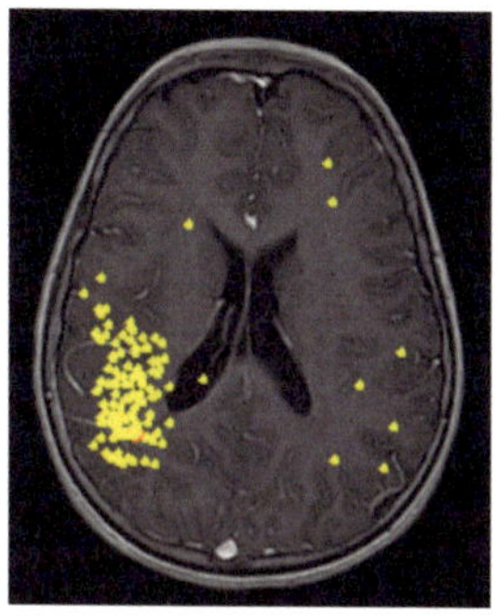

Fig. 12. Total 127 MEG dipoles in Case 3. A total of 127 MEG dipoles are shown on one transparent axial MRI, consisting of 120 over the right hemisphere and 7 in the left hemisphere. Over the right hemisphere, 102 MEG dipoles are clustered in the right temporal and parietal regions. Dipole moments were not shown in this figure.

5. Conclusion

We have described analyses of MEG studies as essential tools in the presurgical evaluation in children with intractable partial epilepsy. Our MEG analyses provide high resolution of temporal and spatial information of intracranial epileptic activities for epilepsy surgery. The cluster of interictal MEG dipoles predicts the epileptogenic zone and this is confirmed by intracranial video-EEG monitoring. MEG is indispensable in guiding the surgical treatment of children with medically intractable partial epilepsy.

6. Acknowledgment

Our particular thanks to the epilepsy team leader, Dr. O. Carter Snead III, and the neurosurgical team leader, Dr. James T. Rutka. We also want to thank our epilepsy surgery team at SickKids, Mr, Rohit Sharma, Ms. Amrita Viljoen, Mr. Bill Chu, Ms. Stephanie Holowka, Dr. Shelly Weiss, Dr. Elizabeth Donner, Dr. Tomoyuki Akiyama, Dr. Elizabeth Pang, Ms. Irene Elliott, Ms. Christine Jursa, Dr. Elysa Widjaja, Dr. Sylvester H. Chuang, Dr. James Drake, Dr. Mary Lou Smith, Dr. Elizabeth Kerr, Ms. Janice Mulligan; without our strong leaders and excellent team members, this work would not be possible.

7. References

Akiyama, T.; Donner, E.J.; Go, C.Y.; Ochi, A.; Snead, O.C. III; Rutka, J.T.; Otsubo, H. (2011). Focal-onset myoclonic seizures and secondary bilateral synchrony. *Epilepsy Res*, Vol. 95, No. 1-2, pp. 168-72

Benifla, M.; Sala, F. Jr.; Jane, J.; Otsubo, H.; Ochi, A.; Drake, J.; Weiss, S.; Donner, E.; Fujimoto, A.; Holowka, S.; Widjaja, E.; Snead, O.C. III; Smith, M.L.; Tamber, M.S.; Rutka, J.T. (2009). Neurosurgical management of intractable rolandic epilepsy in children: role of resection in eloquent cortex. Clinical article. *J Neurosurg Pediatr*, Vol. 4, No. 3, pp. 199-216

Blümcke, I.; Thom, M.; Aronica, E.; Armstrong, D.D.; Vinters, H.V.; Palmini, A.; Jacques, T.S.; Avanzini, G.; Barkovich, A.J.; Battaglia, G.; Becker, A.; Cepeda, C.; Cendes, F.; Colombo, N.; Crino, P.; Cross, J.H.; Delalande, O.; Dubeau, F.; Duncan, J.; Guerrini,

R.; Kahane, P.; Mathern, G.; Najm, I.; Ozkara, C.; Raybaud, C.; Represa, A.; Roper, S.N.; Salamon, N.; Schulze-Bonhage, A.; Tassi, L.; Vezzani, A.; Spreafico, R. (2011). The clinicopathologic spectrum of focal cortical dysplasias: a consensus classification proposed by an ad hoc Task Force of the ILAE Diagnostic Methods Commission. *Epilepsia,* Vol. 52, No. 1, pp. 158-174

Duchowny, M. (1995). Epilepsy surgery in children. *Current Opinion in Neurology,* Vol.8, No. 2, pp. 112-116.

Fisher, R.S.; van Emde Boas, W.; Blume, W.; Elger, C.; Genton, P.; Lee, P.; Engel, J.Jr. (2005). Epileptic seizures and epilepsy: definitions proposed by the International League Against Epilepsy (ILAE) and the International Bureau for Epilepsy (IBE). *Epilepsia,* Vol. 46, No. 4, pp. 470-472

Fujimoto, A.; Ochi, A.; Imai, K.; Chan, D.; Sharma, R.; Viljoen, A.; Chu, B.; Holowka, S.; Kemp, S.M.; Chuang, S.H.; Matsumura, A.; Ayuzawa, S.; Snead, O.C. III; Otsubo, H. (2009). Magnetoencephalography using total intravenous anesthesia in pediatric patients with intractable epilepsy: lesional vs nonlesional epilepsy. *Brain Dev,* Vol. 31, No. 1, pp. 34-41

Gloor, P. (1985). Neuronal generators and the problem of localization in electroencephalography: application of volume conductor theory to electroencephalography. *J Clin Neurophysiol,* Vol. 2, No. 4, pp. 327-354

Hauser, W.A. & Kurland, L.T. (1975). The epidemiology of epilepsy in Rochester, Minnesota, 1935 through 1967. *Epilepsia* Vo. 16, No. 1, pp. 1-66

Hauser, W.A. (1993). The natural history of seizures. In: *The treatment of epilepsy: principles and practices,* Wyllie, E. pp. 165-170, Lea & Febiger, Philadelphia

Hufnagel, A.; Dümpelmann, M.; Zentner, J.; Schijns, O.; Elger CE. (2000). Clinical relevance of quantified intracranial interictal spike activity in presurgical evaluation of epilepsy. *Epilepsia,* Vol.41, No.4, (April 2000), pp. 467-478

Holowka, S.; Otsubo, H.; Iida, K.; Pang, E.; Sharma, R.; Hunjan, A.; Xiang, J.; Snead, O.C.III.; Chuang, N.; Chuang, S.H.; Rutka, J.T. (2004). Three-dimensionally reconstructed magnetic source imaging and neuronavigation in pediatric epilepsy: Technical note. *Neurosurgery,* Vol. 55, pp. E1244-E1248

Iida, K.; Otsubo, H.; Matsumoto, Y.; Ochi, A.; Oishi, M.; Holowka, S.; Pang, E.; Elliott, I.; Weiss, S.K.; Chuang, S.H.; Snead, O.C.III.; Rutka, J.T. (2005). Characterizing magnetic spike sources by using magnetoencephalography-guided neuronavigation in epilepsy surgery in pediatric patients. *J Neurosurg (Pediatrics* 2), Vol. 102, pp. 187-196

Iwasaki, M.; Pestana, E.; Burgess, R.C.; Lüders, H.O.; Shamoto, H.; Nakasato, N. (2005). Detection of epileptiform activity by human interpreters: blinded comparison between electroencephalography and magnetoencephalography. *Epilepsia,* Vol. 46, No. 1, pp. 59-68

Jasper, H.H. (1958). Report of the committee on methods of clinical examination in electroencephalography: 1957. *Electroencephalogr Clin Neurophysiol,* Vol. 10, No. 2, pp. 370-375

Kobayashi, K.; Oka, M.; Akiyama, T.; Inoue, T.; Abiru, K.; Ogino, T.; Yoshinaga, H.; Ohtsuka, Y.; Oka, E. (2004). Very fast rhythmic activity on scalp EEG associated with epileptic spasms. *Epilepsia,* Vol. 45, No. 5, pp. 488-96

Meeren, H.K.; Pijn, J.P.; Van Luijtelaar, E.L.; Coenen, A.M.; Lopes da Silva, F.H. (2002). Cortical focus drives widespread corticothalamic networks during spontaneous absence seizures in rats. *J Neurosci,* Vol. 22, No. 4, pp. 1480-1495

Merlet, I.; Paetau, R.; García-Larrea, L.; Uutela, K.; Granström, M.; Mauguière, F. (1997). Apparent asynchrony between interictal electric and magnetic spikes. *NeuroReport,* Vol. 8, pp. 1071-1076

Minassian, B.A.; Otsubo, H.; Weiss, S.; Elliott, I.; Rutka, J.T.; Snead, O.C.III. (1999). Magnetoencephalographic localization in pediatric epilepsy surgery: Comparison with invasive intracranial electroencephalography. *Ann Neurol,* Vol. 46, pp. 627-633

Mohamed, I.S.; Otsubo, H.; Ochi, A.; Elliott, I.; Donner, E.J.; Chuang, S.H.; Sharma, R.; Holowka, S.; Rutka, J.T.; Snead, O.C.III. (2007). Utility of magnetoencephalography in the evaluation of recurrent seizures after epilepsy surgery. *Epilepsia,* Vol. 48, No. 11, pp. 2150-2159

Ochi, A. & Otsubo, H. (2008). Magnetoencephalography-guided epilepsy surgery for children with intractable focal epilepsy: SickKids experience. *Int J of Psychophysiol,* Vol. 68, No. 2, pp. 104-110

Ochi, A.; Hung, R.; Weiss, S.; Widjaja, E., To, T.; Nawa, Y.; Shima, T., Go, C.; Akiyama, T.; Donner, E.; Drake, J.; Rutka, J.T.; Snead, O.C. III; Otsubo, H. (2011). Lateralized interictal epileptiform discharges during rapid eye movement sleep correlate with epileptogenic hemisphere in children with intractable epilepsy secondary to tuberous sclerosis complex. *Epilepsia,* Article first published online: 29 JUL 2011

Oishi, M.; Otsubo, H.; Kameyama, S.; Morota, N.; Masuda, H.; Kitayama, M.; Tanaka, R. (2002). Epileptic spikes: magnetoencephalography versus simultaneous electrocorticography. *Epilepsia,* Vol. 43, No. 11, pp. 1390-1395

Okada, Y.C.; Lahteenmäki, A.; Xu, C. (1999). Experimental analysis of distortion of magnetoencephalography signals by the skull. *Clin Neurophysiol,* Vol. 110, pp. 230-238

Otsubo, H.; Sharma, R.; Elliott, I.; Holowka, S.; Rutka, J.T.; Snead, O.C.III. (1999). Confirmation of two magnetoencephalographic epileptic foci by invasive monitoring from subdural electrodes in an adolescent with right frontocentral epilepsy. *Epilepsia,* Vol. 40, pp. 608-613

Otsubo, H.; Chitoku, S.; Ochi, A.; Jay, V.; Rutka, J.T.; Smith, M.L.; Elliott, I.; Snead, O.C.III. (2001a). Malignant rolandic-sylvian epilepsy in children: Diagnosis, treatment, and outcome. *Neurology,* Vol. 57, pp. 590-596

Otsubo, H.; Ochi, A.; Elliott, I.; Chuang, S.H.; Rutka, J.T.; Jay, V.; Aung, M.; Sobel, D.F.; Snead, O.C.III. (2001b). MEG predicts epileptic zone in lesional extrahippocampal epilepsy: 12 pediatric surgery cases. *Epilepsia,* Vol. 42, pp. 1523-1530

Pataraia, E.; Simos, P.G.; Castillo, E.M.; Billingsley, R.L.; Sarkari, S.; Wheless, J.W.; Maggio, V.; Maggio, W.; Baumgartner, J.E.; Swank, P.R.; Breier, J.I.; Papanicolaou, A.C. (2004). Does magnetoencephalography add to scalp video-EEG as a diagnostic tool in epilepsy surgery? *Neurology,* Vol. 62, pp. 943-948

Paulini, A.; Fischer, M.; Rampp, S.; Scheler, G.; Hopfengärtner, R.; Kaltenhäuser, M.; Dörfler, A.; Buchfelder, M.; Stefan, H. (2007). Lobar localization information in epilepsy patients: MEG—a useful tool in routine presurgical diagnosis. *Epilepsy Res,* Vol. 76, pp. 124-130

RamachandranNair, R.; Otsubo, H.; Shroff, M.M.; Ochi, A.; Weiss, S.K.; Rutka, J.T.; Snead, O.C. III. (2007). MEG predicts outcome following surgery for intractable epilepsy in children with normal or non-focal MRI findings. *Epilepsia,* Vol. 48, pp. 149-157

Rosenow, F. & Lüders, H. (2001). Presurgical evaluation of epilepsy. *Brain,* Vol. 124, pp. 1683-1700

Sammaritano, M.; Gigli, G.L. & Gotman, J. (1991). Interictal spiking during wakefulness and sleep and the localization of foci in temporal lobe epilepsy. *Neurology,* Vol. 41, pp. 290-297

Sato, S.; Balish, M. & Muratore, R. (1991). Principles of Magnetoencephalography. *J Clin Neurophysiol,* Vol. 8, No. 2, pp. 144-156

Shibasaki, H.; Ikeda, A.; Nagamine, T. (2007). Use of magnetoencephalography in the presurgical evaluation of epilepsy patients. *Clin Neurophysiol,* Vol. 118, No. 7, pp. 1438-1448

Snead, O.C.III. (2001). Surgical treatment of medically refractory epilepsy in childhood. *Brain Dev,* Vol. 23, pp. 199-207

Sugiyama, I.; Imai, K.; Yamaguchi, Y.; Ochi, A.; Akizuki, Y.; Go, C.; Akiyama, T.; Snead, O.C. III; Rutka, J.T.; Drake, J.M.; Widjaja, E.; Chuang, S.H.; Cheyne, D.; Otsubo, H. (2009). Localization of epileptic foci in children with intractable epilepsy secondary to multiple cortical tubers by using synthetic aperture magnetometry kurtosis. *J Neurosurg Pediatr,* Vol. 4, No. 6, pp. 515-522

Tao, J.X.; Ray, A.; Hawes-Ebersole, S.; Ebersole, J.S. (2005). Intracranial EEG substrates of scalp EEG interictal spikes. *Epilepsia,* Vol. 46, No. 5, pp. 669-76

Veldhuizen, R.; Binnie, C.D. & Beintema, D.J. (1983). The effect of sleep deprivation on the EEG in epilepsy. *Electroencephalogr Clin Neurophysiol,* Vol. 55, pp. 505-512.

Wheless, J.W.; Willmore, L.J.; Breier, J.I.; Kataki, M.; Smith, J.R.; King, D.W.; Meador, K.J.; Park, Y.D.; Loring, D.W.; Clifton, G.L.; Baumgartner, J.; Thomas, A.B.; Constantinou, J.E.C.; Papanicolaou, A.C. (1999). A comparison of magnetoencephalography, MRI, and V-EEG in patients evaluated for epilepsy surgery. *Epilepsia,* Vol. 40, pp. 931-941

Wyllie, E.; Chee, M.; Granström, M.L.; DelGiudice, E.; Estes, M.; Comair, Y.; Pizzi, M.; Kotagal, P.; Bourgeois, B.; Lüders, H. (1993). Temporal lobe epilepsy in early childhood. *Epilepsia,* Vol. 34, No. 5, pp. 859-68

Wyllie, E. (1998). Surgical treatment of epilepsy in children. *Pediatric Neurology,* Vol.19, No.3, pp. 179-188

Wyllie, E.; Lachhwani, D.K.; Gupta, A.; Chirla, A.; Cosmo, G.; Worley, S.; Kotagal, P.; Ruggieri, P.; Bingaman, W.E. (2007). Successful surgery for epilepsy due to early brain lesions despite generalized EEG findings. *Neurology,* Vol. 69, No. 4, pp. 389-97

Yamazaki, M.; Chan, D.; Tovar-Spinoza, Z.; Go, C.; Imai, K.; Ochi, A.; Chu, B.; Rutka, J.T.; Drake, J.; Widjaja, E.; Matsuura, M.; Snead, O.C. III; Otsubo, H. (2009) Interictal epileptogenic fast oscillations on neonatal and infantile EEGs in hemimegalencephaly. *Epilepsy Res,* Vol. 83, No. 2-3, pp. 198-206

Yang, T.T.; Gallen, C.C.; Schwartz, B.J.; Bloom, F.E. (1993). Noninvasive somatosensory homunculus mapping in humans by using a large-array biomagnetometer. *Proc Natl Acad Sci USA,* Vol. 90, Vol. 7, pp. 3098-3102

Part 5

Looking Forward: Innovations

10

Helium Circulation System (HCS) for the MEG

Tsunehiro Takeda, Masahiro Okamoto,
Takashi Miyazaki, Naoki Morita and Keishi Katagiri
The University of Tokyo / Frontier Technology Institute Inc.
Japan

1. Introduction

This chapter describes newly developed helium circulation system (HCS) for the magnetoencephalography (MEG) that re-liquefies all the evaporating helium gas using GM (Gifford-Macmahon) cryocoolers operating at 4.2 K. It consumes far less power than conventional systems which cannot be applied for MEGs because of their high noises. Warm helium gas at about 40 K collected high above the surface of the liquid helium in the dewar is used to keep the dewar cold, and cold helium gas just above the liquid helium surface is collected and re-liquefied while still cold. A special transfer tube with multi pipes has been developed to make the system operate efficiently. The system can produce up to 35.5 l/D of liquid helium from the evaporated helium.

A MEG (PR2440 440 CH system, Yokokawa Electric Co. Ltd., Tokyo) with the HCS was used to measure human brain responses for several years without any noise problems. An improved HCS is now operating at Nagoya University, Japan. The noise level is below 10 $fT/Hz^{1/2}$ for 2-40 Hz, below 30 $fT/Hz^{1/2}$ at 1 Hz, and 200 $fT/Hz^{1/2}$ at 60 Hz, which is the power supply frequency. The maintenance cost of the MEG has become less than one-tenth of the previous cost.

2. Requirements for the HCS

MEGs are very expensive to run because of their cooling system. They use about 10 litters per day (l/D) of liquid helium (LHe), and commonly waste all of it by letting it escape into the atmosphere, necessitating the troublesome task of refilling the dewar with LHe once or twice per week, which must be done by a trained technician.

The most common and efficient LHe producing system uses a Collins-type liquefier (Shigi et. al., 1982) . As this system uses very high pressure, it becoms very large and is unsuitable to use for MEGs. Although a cooling system that can achieve LHe temperatures by direct cooling with a small cryocooler has been developed, it is too noisy for MEGs (Kang et. al., 1998). Other small systems that collect the evaporating helium at room temperature and return it to the dewar after liquefaction have also been developed (e.g., TRG-350D, TaiyoNissan Co. Ltd., Tokyo; HRT-K212, Sumitomo Heavy Industries Ltd., Tokyo). They cool the collected evaporated helium to about 40 K using sub-cryocoolers, then to below 4.2 K using the main cryocoolers, and then return the liquefied helium to the cryostat. However, the liquefaction requires much electricity because the evaporated helium approaches room temperature before being cooled and because the specific heat capacity of helium is relatively high. Moreover, they are also still noisy for MEGs. Therefore there had been no cooling system specifically suited to MEGs.

As MEG sensor coils must be placed near to the patient's head to detect their very weak magnetic fields, a liquid nitrogen heat shield, commonly used for Magnetic Resonance Imaging (MRI), cannot be used with MEGs. Hence, LHe is used to cool the dewar as well as the Super conducting Quantum Interference Devices (SQUIDs). In fact, because SQUIDs produce little heat, the LHe is mostly used for the former purpose, which is very inefficient. It would be more efficient to use relatively higher temperature helium gas (HeG) rather than LHe, to cool the dewar (Takeda et. al., 2001, 2005).

In light of all the above serious drawbacks of the existing cooling systems, the requirements of an efficient small cooling system for MEGs to develop are (1) a noise level should be low enough, (2) it need not be refilled the liquid helium frequently, and (3) it should be cheap enough to maintain.

3. Basic idea of the HCS (Takeda et. al., 2008)

The main principle of the HCS is to use relatively warm HeG to counter heat flowing into the dewar from the surroundings, while using the LHe to cool the SQUID. The basic design is outlined in Fig. 1. In the dewar, the HeG near the surface of the LHe will be much colder than the HeG near the top of the dewar. The colder HeG goes through pipe B to the condenser at the second cooling stage where it is liquefied, and then the LHe flows under gravity back to the dewar through pipe A. The outlet of pipe A is near the surface of the

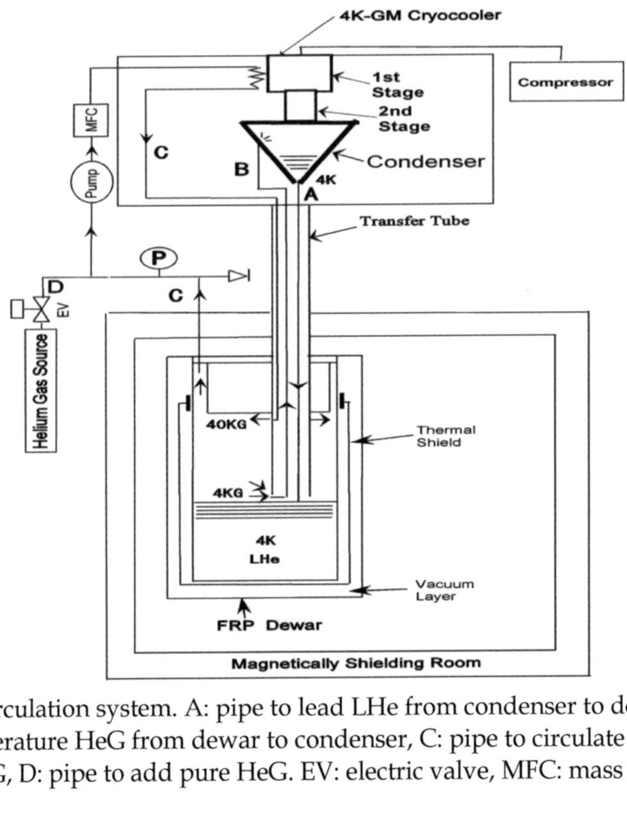

Fig. 1. Helium circulation system. A: pipe to lead LHe from condenser to dewar, B: pipe to lead lower temperature HeG from dewar to condenser, C: pipe to circulate higher temperature HeG, D: pipe to add pure HeG. EV: electric valve, MFC: mass flow controller.

LHe and about 10 mm below the inlet of pipe B. The warmer HeG, which is at about 40 K at the outlet of pipe C, cools the dewar as it passes through its neck. The warmed HeG is led to the first stage of the cryocoolers at a flow rate governed by a small pump and a mass flow controller (MFC). The outlet of pipe C is about 200 mm above the outlet of pipe A. Having the outlet of pipe C high above the LHe ensures that the temperature gradient between the outlet of pipe C and the LHe is relatively small, thus lowering the heat flow into the LHe. If the LHe level drops for some reason, the helium gas from a reservoir can be supplied through pipe D and liquefied, which recovers LHe level.

Since the amount of helium that evaporates, and thus the amount that has to be liquefied, depends on the ambient temperature, a large capacity cryocooler is essential to cope with a wide range of ambient temperature. On the other hand, if the cryocooler liquefies too much helium, the pressure inside the system may drop, causing air to flow into the system. Therefore, our system uses two 1.5W@4.2K GM (Gifford-McMahon) cryocoolers to ensure sufficient cooling capacity and, under feedback control from the pressure in the dewar, a 3 W heater attached to the condenser to prevent overcooling.

The transfer tube is shown in Fig. 2. The transfer tube is attached to the dewar such that a vacuum separating pipes A, B and C, which are concentric, is a continuum of the vacuum in the wall of the cold chamber shown on the far left. The vacuum also separates pipe C from the ambient air. The connection flange (E) allows thermometers to be replaced.

The shield shown in section figure D is made of a thick copper pipe and protects against incoming thermal radiation. It is connected to the first stage of the cryocoolers by flexible copper wires. The copper wires and the flange with bellows enable the transfer tube to be set up through a hole in the wall of the magnetically shielded room (MSR). The heat flowing from the surroundings to the LHe through the transfer tube was estimated to be lower than 0.2 W/m.

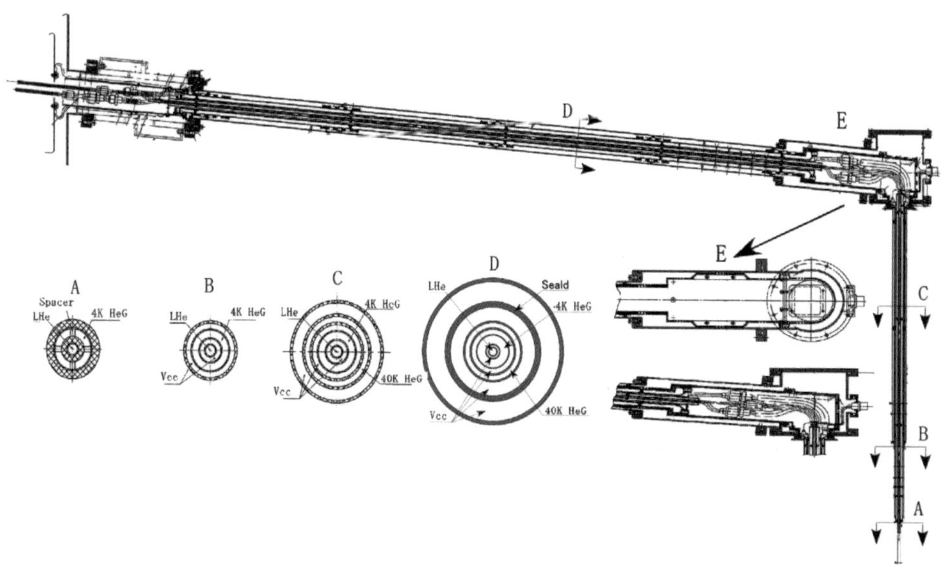

Fig. 2. Transfer tube consisting of seven concentric pipes. A, B, C, D are cross sections of TT at the indicated places. E is the structure of the elbow connecting the horizontal and vertical parts of TT. The lengths of the horizontal and vertical parts are about 2 and 1 m, respectively, and their diameters are 76 and 38 mm, respectively.

4. Performance of the HCS with an experimental Dewar (Takeda et. al., 2008)

Fig. 3 shows how the temperature in different parts of the system changed during the first two and a half days after the system was started up. It also shows the change in the level of the LHe in the dewar. At start up, HeG at room temperature was filled to the system and it was automatically admitted into the system through pipe D according to the temperature drop and helium liquefaction under pressure feedback control. About 5 hours after start up, TA, the temperature of the first stage of the cryocoolers, had decreased from room temperature to 4.2 K, and about 13 hours after start up, T1, the temperature of pipe C just after the first stage of the cryocoolers, had decreased to 40 K. The temperatures at elbows of the TT (Ce, Be, Ae) stabilized at about 22 hours after start up. Though the temperatures at Be and Ae fluctuated in an interesting manner, it is beyond the scope of this report, but its analysis using computer simulation will be discussed elsewhere.
The LHe in the dewar started to increase about 24 hours after start up. As there was a 14-mm gap between the bottom of the LHe level meter and the bottom of the dewar, LHe had started to accumulate about two hours previous. The level reached the height of the inlet of HeG (the inlet of pipe B) about 34 cm above the bottom of the level meter at about 27 hours after start up, and blocked the path of the HeG to the condenser, stopping further increase in the LHe. The level of LHe, however, fluctuated for about 4 hours when the LHe first came into contact with TT due to heat flow from TT. LHe increased at a rate of about 5.5 l/D on average (the diameter of the dewar was250 mm). After the heater on the condenser was

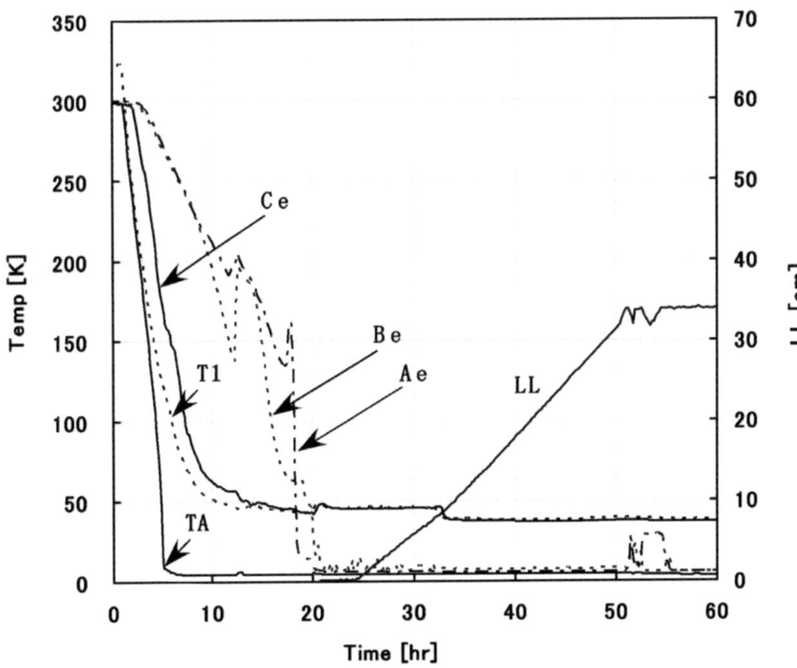

Fig. 3. Typical data showing temperature change, from start up, at different locations of the system, and the LHe level in the dewar. TA: temperature at the second stage of the cryocooler, T1: temperature of the pipe C just after the first stage of the cryocooler, Ce, Be, Ae are temperatures of the pipes C, B, A at the elbow part of the TT. LL: level of LHe.

turned on about 55 hours from start up to keep the pressure of the HeG at about 1 kPa (101 kPa in absolute pressure), the LHe level remained stable.

In the set up used to measure the performance of the system, there was an additional heater at the bottom of the dewar which was used to measure the residual capacity of the cryocoolers to maintain the level of the LHe. The capacity was found to be 1.1 W. When the TT was not attached to the dewar, about 35.5 l/D of helium evaporated from the dewar, estimated by supplying 1.1 W of heat to the LHe. In the real situation, some more heat would be flowing from the inserted TT. Therefore, it was confirmed that at least 35.5 l/D of LHe could be re-liquefied in the experimental system. This amount is adequate for nearly all the existing MEG systems, which require about 10 l/D.

Fig. 4a and 4b shows vibration, measured by a vibrometer (Showa Sokki Inc., Model-2403) on the top plate of the dewar before and after the cryocoolers were turned on. As the operation of GM cryocoolers were very stable, measurements were taken on only several occasions and the figure is representative. The amplitude of the noise doubled when the cooler was turned on but was still only about 1 $\mu m_{p\text{-}p}$, which is quiet enough to measure magnetic fields of the brain by MEG.

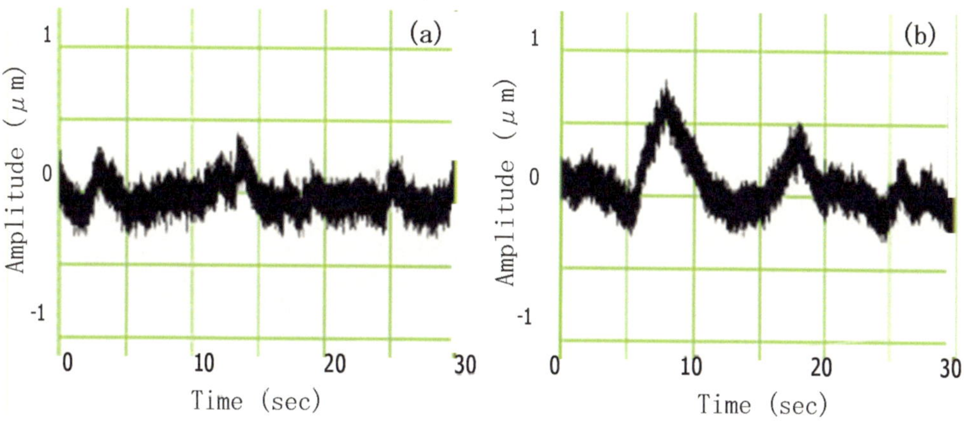

Fig. 4. Vibration on the top plate of the dewar when the cryocoolers were (a) not in operation and (b) in operation.

5. Performance of the HCS with an experimental MEG (Takeda et. al., 2009)

Fig. 5 is a photograph of the setup of the HCS on an operation MEG (PR2440 440 CH system, Yokokawa Electric Co. Ltd., Tokyo; Takeda et. Al., 2004). In the MEG, sensors are located at 300 points over a head and seventy of them are vector sensors. They are distributed roughly equal and mean distance between the sensors are about 20 mm. The total sensor number is 440. All the vector sensors are made by axial type gradiometers. Sensors for Z direction (the axial direction) are two oppositely wound circles and the sensors for X and Y direction are two oppositely wound squares. The areas of the squares are smaller by some 10 %, but the gain is tuned to make the output voltage to be comparable. The system noise is lower than $9fT/\sqrt{Hz}$ and a bit better than common MEG systems. EEG can be measured simultaneously up to 64 CH. There are also 64 external input lines which enables flexible trigger set up.

A special dewar is developed which has a long insert to prevent invading heat from outside of the dewar. The insert is divided into two and has narrow gap to let the helium gas, whose temperature is about 40 K, flow through the gap and the neck tube of the dewar getting rid of the heat invading into the dewar.

The magnetically shielded room (Daido Plant Industries Co., Ltd.) has three permalloy layers with 2 mm thick each and 5 mm thick aluminum layer. Its inner size is 3000 x 3920 x 2900 (width x depth x height). The shielding factors are 60 dB at o.1Hz, 82 dB at 1Hz and 100 dB at 10 Hz. There is a hole 400 x 600 (width x height) with a long sleeve that enables image projection through it.

We put the TT through a magnetically shielded room (MSR) wall and firmly fixed it to the MSR to reduce vibration generated by the GM cryocoolers. The hole of 100 mm diameter that lets the TT penetrate the MSR is covered by a permalloy box (PB) to reduce invasion of magnetic noise into the MSR from the environment. It was confirmed that the hole did not add any detectable magnetic noise.

The cryocoolers are attached to the base of a cold chamber, which is placed on a mount made of aluminium frame shown at the right. The TT is connected to the cold chamber with a welded bellows, which considerably reduces the transfer of vibrations generated by the GM cryocoolers to the TT. The cryocoolers are covered with a small and simple MSR to reduce magnetic and acoustic noise. Acoustic noise on the top plate of the dewar in the MSR, measured using a sound level meter (Yokokawa, LY20), was 34.7 dB. This is small enough for MEG measurements.

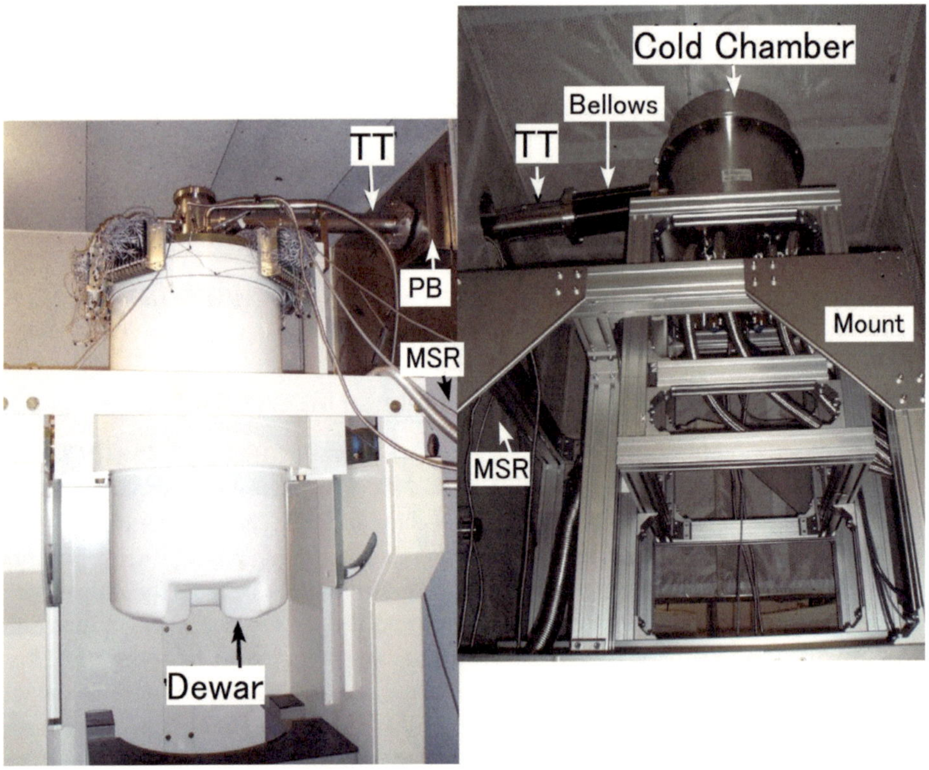

Fig. 5. Setup of HCS on MEG with 440 CH.

5.1 Helium circulation

Fig. 6 shows how the temperatures in different parts of the HCS changed during the first 3 days after HCS operation was started. As the MEG has 440 channels (CH) of SQUIDs, which is the largest number of sensor channels in the world, its dewar has a large heat capacity. Though we could fill up the experimental dewar whose container volume was 5.6 l in 2 days starting from room temperature helium gas in the dewar as described in reference 3, it was estimated that we need to cool the system over two weeks to make liquid helium from the helium gas in the dewar by gradually cooling it with the GM cryocoolers. Thus, we decided to transfer LHe to the dewar on the third day.

Fig. 6a depicts the temperature change at various points in the HCS, where 1 - denotes the temperature at the second stage of the GM cryocooler, 2 - denotes the temperature of its first stage, 3 - denotes the temperature of pipe C in Fig. 1 after the refiner, 4 - denotes the temperature at pipe A near the condenser, and 5 - denotes the temperature of pipe B near the condenser. The figure shows that the temperature 1 dropped to about 5 K after 2.5 h from start up, and temperatures 2 and 3 dropped similarly to about 50 K after 9 h from start

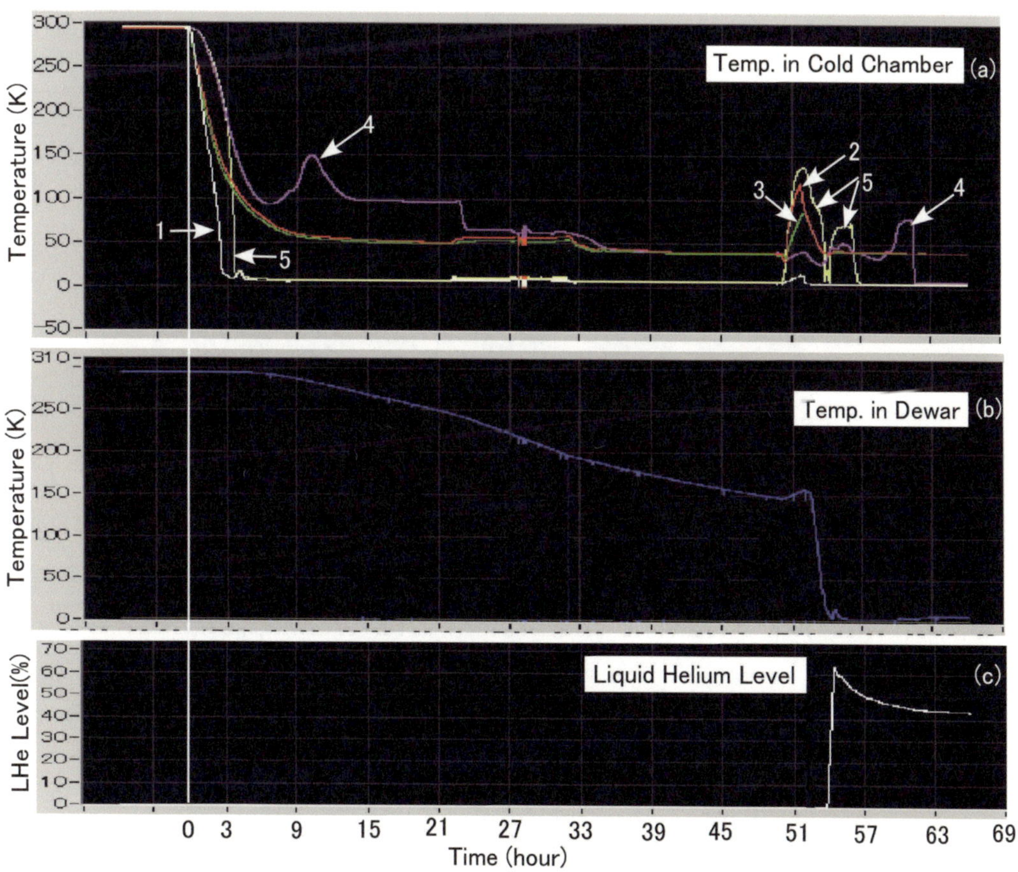

Fig. 6. Temperature change at various points in HCS from start up of HCS for 3 days (a); 1: at second stage of cryocooler, 2: at first stage of cryocooler, 3: at pipe C in Fig. 1 near cryocooler, 4: at pipe A, 5: at pipe B; (b) temperature change in the dewar, and (c) change of liquid helium level in dewar.

up. The temperatures 4 and 5 also descended similarly for 3 h after start up. While 5 continued to descend for one more hour after that time and dropped to about 5 K, 4 started to ascend from about 100 K at 6 h from start up to about 150 K at 10 h from start up. This is probably caused by warm helium gas sucked from the dewar through pipe B. Temperature 4 suddenly dropped from about 100 K to about 60 K at 22 h from start up, when we estimated partial liquidation started in the condenser. Temperatures 2, 3 and 4 gradually decreased as the dewar became cool, as shown in Fig. 6b.

Interesting temperature changes occurred after liquid helium was transferred at 50 h from start up. The flow of relatively warm helium gas from the dewar pushed up the temperatures at 2, 3 and 5 from 50 to 53 h, when cooling of the dewar finished and liquid helium began to accumulate in the dewar. The lower panel shows the liquid helium level in the dewar and indicates accumulation of LHe was completed in about 0.5 h, after which it decreased rapidly for 9 h to cool the dewar. Temperature 4 increased slightly and then suddenly dropped from about 70 K to 4 K at about 61 h after start up, which indicates helium liquidation continuously maintained and circulation of helium began at that time.

In the experimental setup used to measure the performance of the HCS before its installation, there was an additional heater at the bottom of the experimental dewar, which was used to measure the residual capacity of the cryocoolers to maintain the level of the

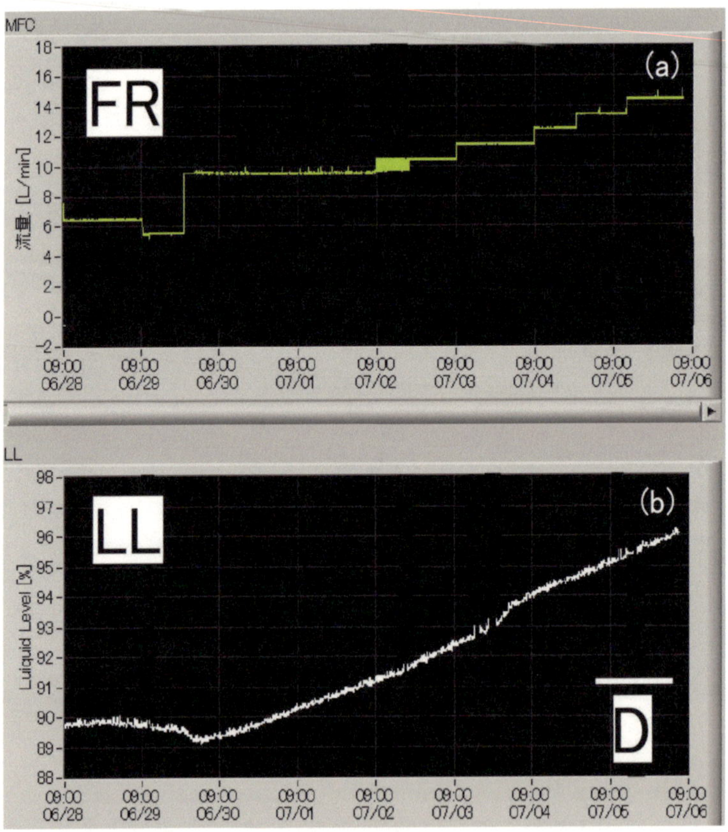

Fig. 7. Flow rate (FR) of the 40 K helium gas was changed for 8 days (a), and resulted in the change of liquid helium level (LL) in the dewar (b).

LHe. This capacity was found to be 1.1 W. When the TT was not attached to the dewar, about 35.5 l/D of helium evaporated from the dewar, as estimated by supplying 1.1 W of heat to the LHe. Therefore, it was confirmed that at least 35.5 l/D of LHe could be re-liquefied in the experimental system. This amount is adequate for nearly all the existing MEG systems, which require about 10 l/D.

In the real situation, more heat would be flowing from the inserted TT into the dewar. Fig. 7 shows the change of LHe level in the dewar (Fig. 7b) according to the change of HeG flow rate at the neck tube of the dewar (Fig. 7a). This means that the helium level decreased when the flow rate was below 6 l/min and increased when the flow was over 10 l/min. As the time constant of the change of the liquid helium level (LL) is very long, the dependence of the LL on helium gas flow rate (FR) is not clear from Fig. 3b. Later, it was determined by several supplemental experiments that 7 l/min is about the minimum flow rate to maintain the liquid helium level for this system. It was also estimated that the HCS can increase the LHe by 2.1 l/D at most in this system.

After the dewar is filled with LHe, we need not add any LHe to the dewar for one year during normal operation. As the GM cryocoolers require regular maintenance once a year, the cryocoolers were warmed up to 300 K by heaters attached to the condenser (with a capacity of 3 W) and on two refiners (each with a capacity of 200 W) for about 10 h. The temperature was kept at about 300 K by controlling the heater with a computer (Fig. 8a). As heat was added to the HCS, the liquid helium evaporated completely in 2 days, as shown in Fig. 8c. The temperature of the dewar began to increase half a day after the final evaporation of the liquid helium. It took about 3 days to warm up the dewar to room temperature (Fig. 8b).

Vacuum pumping of the dewar's vacuum layer was done from the fifth to eighth day for about 3 days. The maintenance was performed during the sixth day, and the liquid helium transfer was done on the eighth day (Fig. 8c).

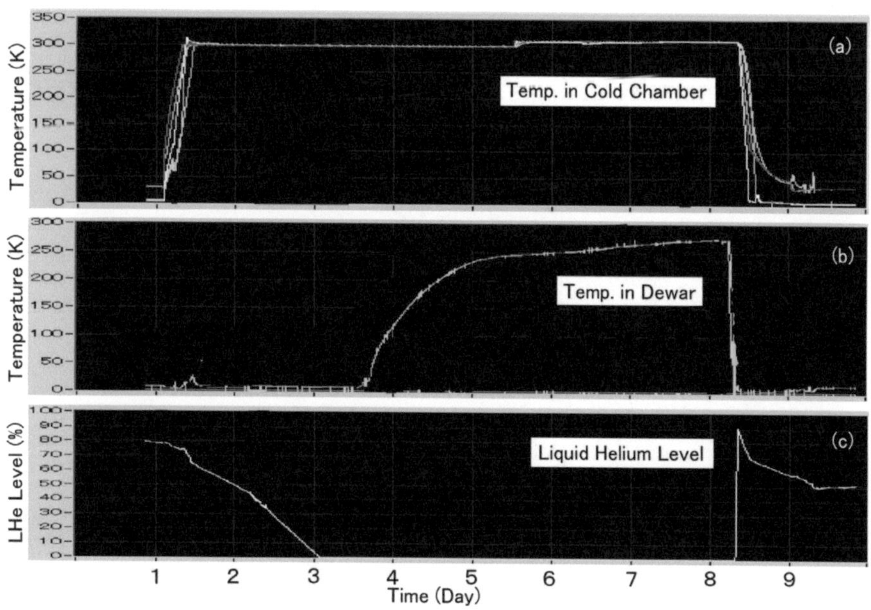

Fig. 8. Temperature change at various points in HCS during cryocooler maintenance for 8 days (a), temperature change in the dewar (b), and change of liquid helium level (c).

5.2 Noise reduction

Fig. 9a shows the locations of 14 representative CH (closed dots) of the 440 CH MEG sensors spread almost evenly over the head, viewed from above the head with the sensor locations projected onto a horizontal plane. The up direction is the direction of the subject's forehead. Because the data from those 14 channels indicate the general characteristics of the noise in all the MEG sensors, these channels' data will be used in the following paragraphs.

Fig. 9b depicts the temporal wave of magnetic noise measured by the MEG, where the noise added by the installation of the HCS is removed as much as possible. Although most channels show acceptable noise levels, several channels, such as channels 96 and 384, have a bit larger (apparently 50 Hz) power line noise, which will be suppressed in the near future by further improvements.

Fig. 10a depicts the amplitude spectrum of magnetic noise measured by the MEG before the HCS was installed. The noise levels are roughly below 10 $fT/Hz^{1/2}$ for 2-1000 Hz, similar to that in common MEGs. The amplitude spectrum has a typical 1/f noise pattern below 2 Hz. It is below 35 $fT/Hz^{1/2}$ at 1 Hz and 170 $fT/Hz^{1/2}$ at 50 Hz, which is the power supply frequency.

Fig. 10b depicts the amplitude spectrum of magnetic noise measured just after the HCS was installed. It shows noise of about 200 $fT/Hz^{1/2}$ at 1 Hz, which was apparently produced by the vibration of the TT driven by the GM cryocoolers. The GM cryocoolers produce a strong 1 Hz vibration when the compressed helium gas expands adiabatically in the cryocoolers. The amplitude spectrum also has a very large noise spectrum at other frequencies, especially at the higher harmonics of 1 Hz and 50 Hz.

To reduce the noise levels, thick plates were placed between the aluminium frames where the cryocoolers are mounted to act as stiffeners. Fig. 10c shows the amplitude spectrum of magnetic noise measured after the modification of the cryocooler stage. The magnitude of the amplitude spectrum at 1 Hz was reduced considerably, to about 100 $fT/Hz^{1/2}$. However,

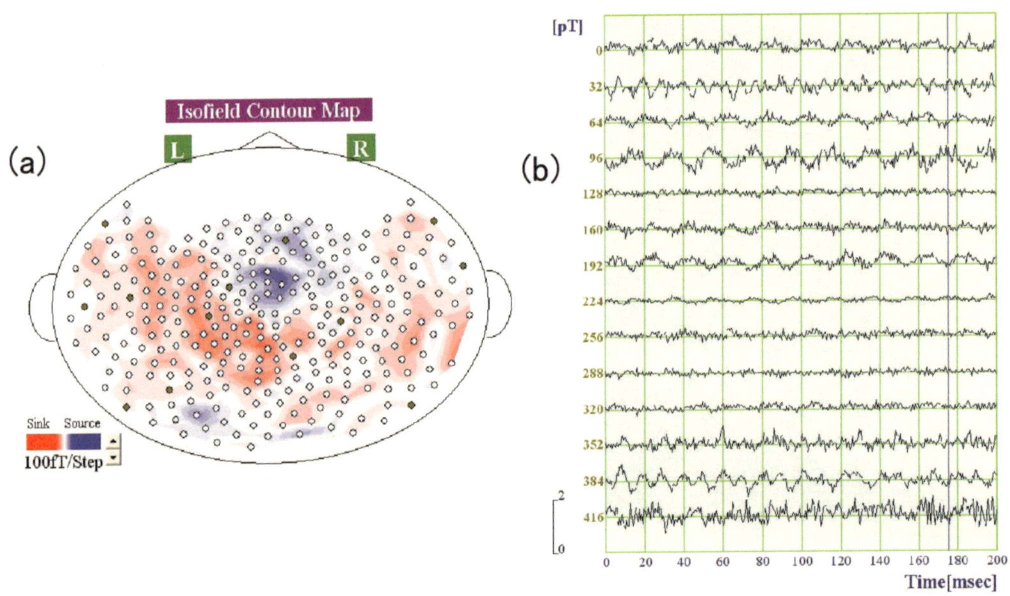

Fig. 9. The location of selected 14 CH sensor channels (a), and their typical noise (b).

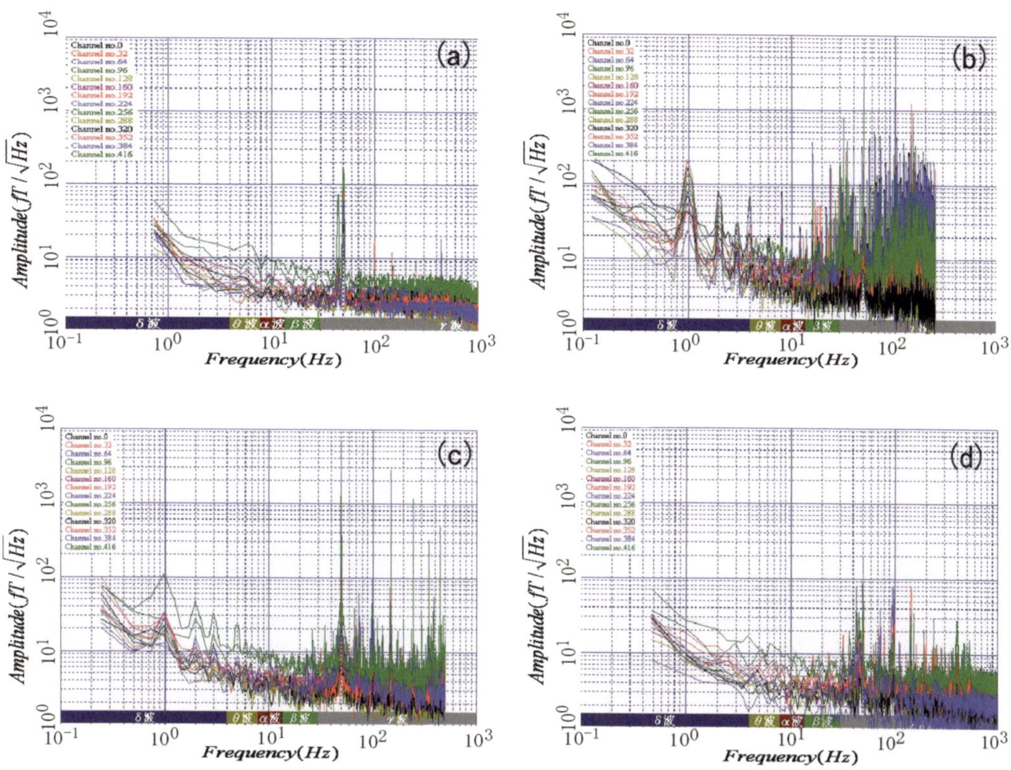

Fig. 10. Noise amplitude spectra of the selected 28 channels of the system, (a) before HCS installation, (b) just after HCS installation, (c) after stiffness increase of the HCS mount, and (d) after grounding improvements.

there remained considerable noise caused by the HCS, especially at 50 Hz and its higher harmonics. The noise amplitude at 50 Hz was about 7 $pT/Hz^{1/2}$, which was more than ten times of that in Fig. 10a.

Various improvements were made to reduce the noise added by the HCS. As the details of those measures are not in the scope of this paper, they are not explained here. The most effective measure was to reduce current leak from the power supplier to the TT by various methods in the electrical grounding of the MEG and the HCS. Fig. 10d depicts the amplitude spectrum of magnetic noise measured after the improvements. The noise level at 1 Hz is reduced to less than 30 $fT/Hz^{1/2}$, which is a bit smaller than that in Fig. 10a. The noise level at 50 Hz is reduced to 200 $fT/Hz^{1/2}$, which is still a little bit bigger than before HCS installation. There are also slight noise increases in the range of 30-50 Hz and at the higher harmonics of 50 Hz.

Though there are small noise increases, it can be said that noise level is roughly the same as before the HCS installation. As it is common to use a band pass filter of 1-40 Hz in the MEG measurement to get rid of power supply noise, which is very difficult to eliminate completely, the remaining noise has virtually no negative effect. Fig. 10a shows the noise level after the band pass filter was applied (a 6th-order Butterworth filter with a 1-40 Hz band). There could be found no prominent noise there. Fig. 10b shows the amplitude

spectrum of the remaining noise. It clearly shows that there remains virtually no influence from the noise produced by the HCS after the band pass filter is applied.
Acoustic noise in the hollow of the dewar, measured using a sound level meter (Yokokawa Ltd., DT-805), was 34.7 dB while the cryocoolers were running. There is a hole (300 mm x 250 mm; width x height) in our MSR to allow visual image projection through the hole by a liquid crystal projector, and the acoustic noise level could be lowered to 33.0 dB if this hole was closed. This sound noise level is small enough for MEG measurements.

6. Control system of the HCS

Fig. 11 shows schematic gas flow (a) and control diagram (b) of the HCS. Evaporated helium gas in the dewar is absorbed to the condenser and liquefied. It then drops to the dewar by the gravity.
The controller of the HCS uses compact Field Point (cFP-2020 : National Instrument) and the software is based on LabVIEW Real-Time. The cFP has three RS-232C ports and one RS-485 port. External module has 8 CH A/D (cFP-AI-110) and two 8 CH relay modules (cFP-RLY-421).

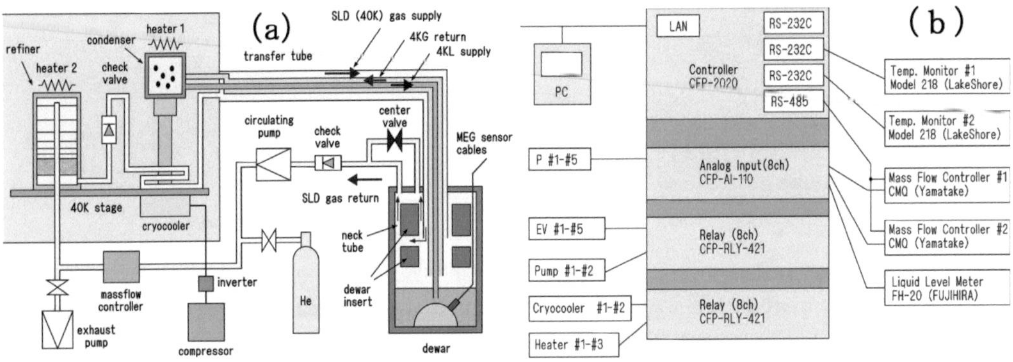

Fig. 11. Block diagram of the gas flow in the HCS (a), and the control interfaces of various control elements in the system (b). P: pressure gauge, EV: electromagnetic valve.

Fig. 12a shows the gas flow control system which has several electric valves, mass flow controller and several pressure gauges. Fig. 12b shows the temperature monitors, liquid helium level meter and PC for the control of gas flow system and monitoring of the whole HCS.

7. Installation the HCS to a commercialized MEG

The most serious problem remained to be improved was that the HCS had a TT insert tube with diameter of 3/2 inches. As all the existing MEGs have 1/2 inch insert hole to refill liquid helium, extensive redesign or reconstruction of MEGs was required to use the developed HCS. Hence, we have tried to reduce the diameter of the TT insert tube to 1/2 inch to avoid the requirement. Though it was very hard to reduce the diameter of the multi-pipe TT insert tube to 1/3, we managed to achieve the goal. Once we have succeeded to develop a TT with standard insert tube diameter of 1/2 inch, there is no need to modify the MEG per see. So we could easily install the HCS on a commercialised MEG produced from Yokokawa Electric Corporation Inc. (PQ1160C) as shown in Fig. 13.

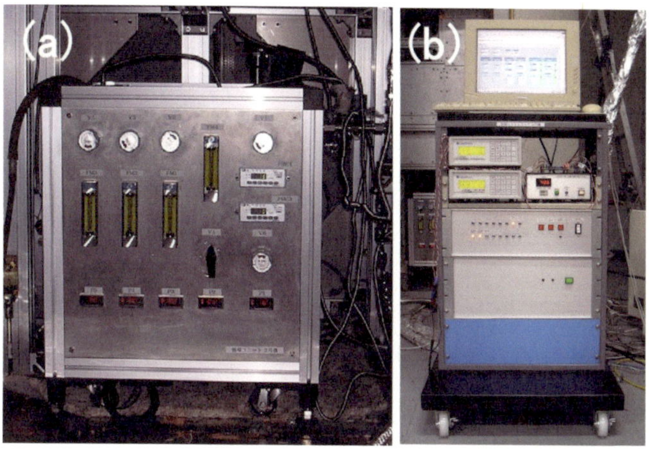

Fig. 12. Hardware of the gas control system of the HCS (a), and computer to control the gas flow together with temperature minitors and Liquid helium level meter (b).

As the MEG has been installed in a magnetically shielded room (MSR) about a year ago without any plan to add a HCS to it, there isn't any proper hole to let through the TT just behind or left/right side of the MEG, which enables to use simple straight pipe TT same as

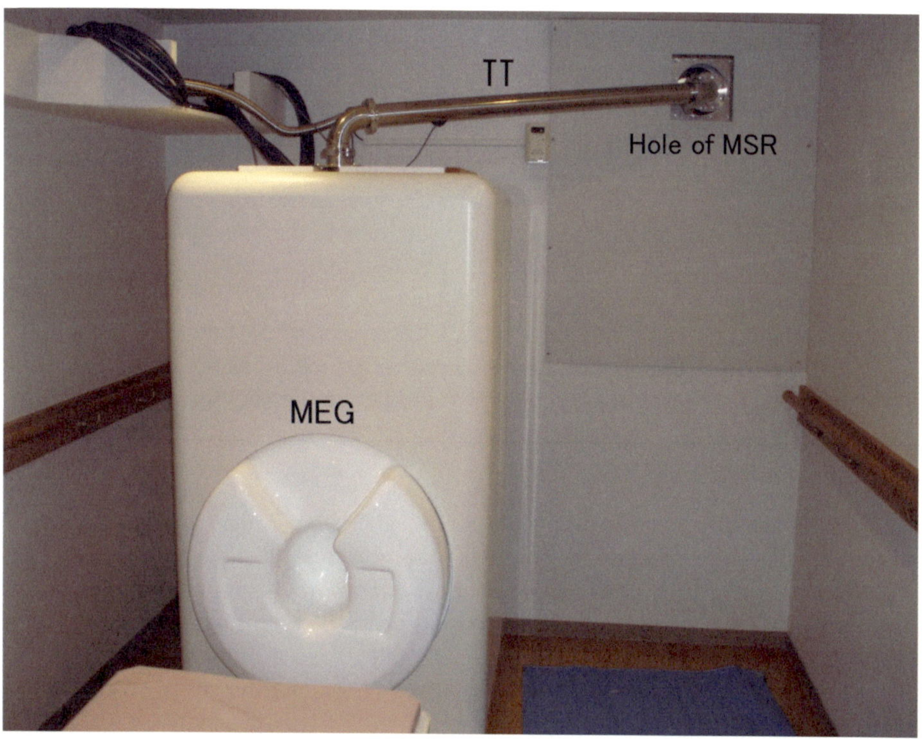

Fig. 13. Multi-pipe TT of the HCS installed on the commercialized MEG (PQ1160C, Yokokawa Electric Cor. Inc., Japan). As the TT has 1/2 inch insert tube, there was no need to modify the MEG to install the HCS. TT is twisted twice to use the ventilation hole located upper light to get through the MSR. It is tilted 5 degrees to get the LHe drop to the dewar.

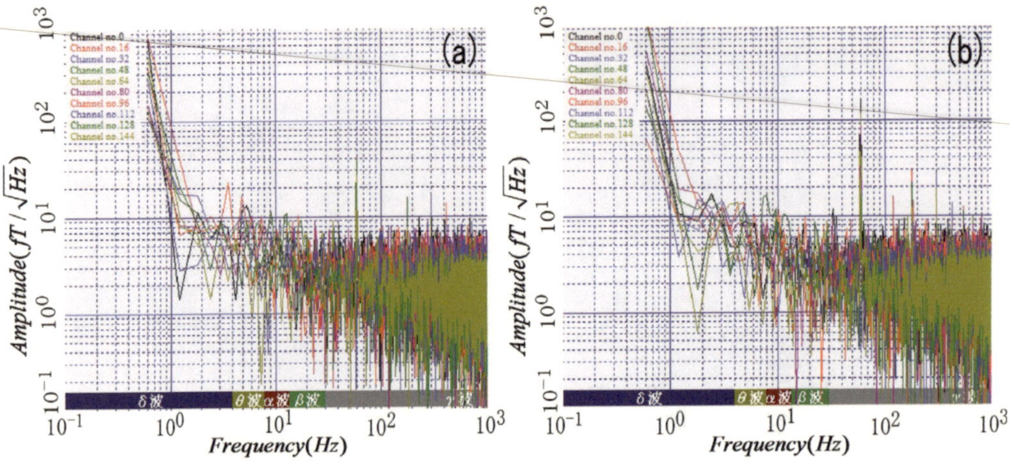

Fig. 14. Noise amplitude spectra of the selected 10 channels of the system (Yokokawa, PQ1160C); (a) before HCS installation, (b) after instalation. There isn't any noticable difference. Instalation of the HCS is successful.

used in an experimental MEG at the University of Tokyo. It was rather difficult to make a suitable hole through the existing MSR, because it requires extensive modification of the MSR. We planned to utilize the ventilation hole located right upper in the MSR, whose diameter was 170 mm. To use the hole, we designed a new TT with reduced diameter of 60.5 mm from 76.3 mm used for the experimental MEG. We also vented the TT twice to use the hole as shown in Fig. 5. The TT is tilted about 5 degrees to let the LHe flow by the gravity.

It took about a week to install the HCS on the MEG in May, 2011. HCS can increase the LHe by about 3 litters per day and add no extra noticeable noise in the MEG noise recording. As the compressor of the cryocooler is located another room next to the MEG room and cryocooler is located outside of the MEG room, there is no noticeable additional acoustic noise.

Fig. 14 shows noise amplitudes of the MEG (Yokokawa, PQ1160C) at the Nagoya University before (a) and after (b) the installation of the HCS. There is no noticeable noise difference in the two measurements. So, it can be said the installation of the HCS has no negative effect on the MEG measurements and eliminate necessity of liquid helium transfer for at least a year.

8. Discussion and future HCS

MEGs would be cheaper to run if high-Tc SQUIDs, cooled by liquid nitrogen, could be used. Unfortunately, high-Tc SQUIDs are currently too noisy, so costly LHe systems must be used. The develloped HCS would reduce the cost to run MEGs because almost none of the He, a rare material, is allowed to escape into the atmosphere, eliminating the hazardous task of replacing lost LHe, which requires trained personnel. Also, although helium itself is not a major pollutant, because our system consumes less energy, it is indirectly more environmentally friendly.

Since we wanted to do maintenance including vacuum pumping of the dewar, we warmed up the dewar completely. However, the vacuum level of the dewar could be sustained low enough for several years. Thus, we could skip vacuum pumping, and can perform the maintenance by just warming up the cryocoolers. We will warm the cryocoolers overnight, replace wearing parts of the GM cryocoolers the next day, cool the cryocoolers down overnight during the following night, and resume circulation on the third day. From Fig. 4 data, it is estimated that about 60 % of the liquid helium in the dewar is lost into the atmosphere for 48 h. Hence, about 40 l of liquid helium and about 48 h of time are necessary for the maintenance.

In the experimental MEG at the University of Tokyo, the magnetic noise level between 2 and 40 Hz is below 10 $fT/Hz^{1/2}$, which is about the same as the noise level before the HCS is installed. Although the noise level at 50 Hz was about 170 $fT/Hz^{1/2}$ before the HCS installation, the noise level of 200 $fT/Hz^{1/2}$ at 50 Hz is a little bit bigger after HCS installation. There is also a slight noise increase in the range of 40-50 Hz and at the higher harmonics of 50 Hz. However, the noise level of the Nagoya university is roughly same between before and after the installation of the HCS (Fig. 14). So, it can be said, the HCS has no bad influence for the commercialized MEGs.

The acoustic noise level was 34.7 dB at the center of the head hole in the MEG dewar in the MSR. The noise level is about the same as before the installation and quiet enough to perform ordinary MEG measurement.

Our system can produce at least 35.5 l of LHe per day from the evaporated helium with two 1.5W at 4.2K GM cryocoolers (Takeda et. al., 2008). The total cooling capacity of the system was estimated to be about 2.4 W. We are still improving our system and hope to be able to produce 10 l/D of LHe using only one 1.5 W GM cryocooler in the near future.

Though we designed our HCS for MEGs, the HCS, with its advantages, can be used for other devices in the field of cryogenics. Several low temperature physical property measurement devices, which measure magnetic or electrical properties at low temperatures by cooling materials with liquid helium, could serve as promising applications. We are now developing HCSs suitable for such purposes.

9. Summary

We have developed a helium circulation system that uses two 1.5 W at 4.2 K GM cryocoolers and has dual helium streams; one to collect evaporated HeG immediately and return it as liquefied helium to the Dewar, and the second to use higher temperature HeG (approximately 40 K) to cool the Dewar. We installed this mechanism on an experimental MEG system with 440 CH measurement SQUIDs (Yokokawa PR2440) and operated it for three and a half years. We also installed a new model on a real commercialized MEG system (Yokokawa PQ1160C) at the Nagoya University and operated it for five months.

It has been confirmed that magnetic and acoustic noises added by installing the HCSs have no problem for MEG measurements.

The HCS can increase the level of liquid helium by at least 3 l per day with the Yokokawa PQ1160C. Without needing to perform Dewar pumping, regular cryocooler maintenance can be done in 2 full days, losing approximately 40 l of liquid helium in the process. The maintenance cost (electricity charges and cryocooler maintenance fee) of the MEG has been reduced to be less than one-tenth of the previous cost (liquid helium and maintenance fees).

10. References

Ackermann RA, Herd KG, Chen WE (1999). Advanced cryocooler cooling for MRI system, *Cryocooler*, Vol. 10, pp. 857-67.

Kang Y et. al. (1998). Cryocooled SQUID system, *The Journal of Japan Biomagnetism and Bioelectromagnetics Society,* Vol. 11 No. 1, pp. 15-16 (in Japanese).

Shigi T et. al. (1982). Handbook of cryogenics, in Japanese translated from VDI: LEHRGANGSHANDBUCH KRYOTECNIK by Klipping G et. al., Uchida Rokakuhoshinsya, pp. 135-136.

Takeda T, Takae T (2001). A liquid helium circulation system for biomagnetometers, *Biomag 2000,* pp. 951-952.

Takeda T, Owaki T, Haruta Y, Uehara G (2004). Characteristics of a 440ch MEG system with vector sensors, *Biomag 2004,* pp. 640-641.

Takeda T, Horinouchi H (2005). A liquid helium circulation system for MEG, *Transactions of the Cryogenics Engineering Conference-CEC,* Vol. 51, pp. 427-432.

Takeda T, Okamoto M, Atsuda K, Katagiri K (2008). An efficient helium circulation system with small GM cryocoolers, *Cryogenics* Vol. 48, pp. 6-11.

Takeda T, Okamoto M, Atsuda K, Katagiri K (2009). Performance of a Helium Circulation System for a MEG, *Cryogenics,* Vol. 49, pp. 144-150.

Takeda T, Okamoto M, Miyazaki T, Katagiri K (2011). Performance of the Helium Circulation System on a Commercialized MEG, *Transactions of the Cryogenics Engineering Conference-CEC,* Vol. 57, in print.

Wang C (2001). Helium liquefaction with a 4K pulse tube cryocooler, *Cryogenics,* Vol. 41, pp. 491-496.

11

Accessing and Processing MEG Signals in Real-Time: Emerging Applications and Enabling Technologies

Stephen Foldes[1,2], Wei Wang[1,2,3], Jennifer Collinger[1,4], Xin Li[5], Jinyin Zhang[2,5], Gustavo Sudre[2], Anto Bagić[2,6] and Douglas J. Weber[1,2,3]
[1]*Department of Physical Medicine and Rehabilitation, University of Pittsburgh*
[2]*Center for the Neural Basis of Cognition, Carnegie Mellon University*
[3]*Department of Bioengineering, University of Pittsburgh*
[4]*Human Engineering Research Laboratories, VA Pittsburgh Healthcare System*
[5]*Department of Electrical and Computer Engineering, Carnegie Mellon University*
[6]*Department of Neurology, University of Pittsburgh*
USA

1. Introduction

Magnetoencephalography (MEG) offers great temporal resolution; however, traditional MEG studies have only exploited this advantage during offline analysis. With the advancement of computing capabilities, the ability to process and analyze MEG data during an experiment, and even in real-time is now a reality. Online MEG processing opens new opportunities for basic research and clinical applications. For example, by providing real-time feedback a subject could learn to modify their neural activity patterns. This real-time neurofeedback training may be useful in rehabilitation, for example to promote neuroplasticity to strengthen or retrain motor-cortical activity after central nervous system damage due to conditions such as stroke or spinal cord injury. Online MEG analysis could also be used for advancing neuroscience research by allowing for adaptive paradigms that could identify which stimuli are most effective, or to determine if more data needs to be collected to fulfill analysis criteria. However, online MEG presents a number of challenges, including managing the complexities of the data acquisition, addressing noise contamination, and dealing with the processing requirements of data analysis methods. This chapter introduces the concept of online MEG and discusses current research efforts to address its challenges while presenting some novel applications to advance basic and clinical research.

Processing of brain activity in real-time is not a new concept. Observing the complex dynamics of the brain on a millisecond scale has provided great insight into how the brain works in healthy individuals and those with neurological disorders. To date, most real-time analysis of brain activity has been with electroencephalography (EEG) using electrodes placed on the scalp. Because EEG is non-invasive and poses essentially no risk of injury, it can be performed on healthy individuals and patients. However, the spatial resolution and effective bandwidth of EEG are limited, because electrical signals passing through the skull and scalp are greatly attenuated, particularly at frequencies above 50 Hz (Nunez & Ramesh Srinivasan 2005). Intracranial EEG, commonly referred to as electrocorticography (ECoG) alleviates this issue of tissue attenuation by placing electrodes beneath the skull closer to the brain. ECoG is used routinely in the diagnosis and treatment of patients with intractable epilepsy (Leuthardt, Schalk, Wolpaw, Ojemann, & Moran, 2004). Cranial surgery is required to place ECoG electrodes and therefore its utility for many research, and even clinical, investigations is limited. MEG provides a safe, non-invasive alternative capable of capturing the high temporal resolution dynamics of the brain activity. However, the magnetic fields generated by neural activity are extremely small and require complex hardware and software to collect. By averaging across many events, traditional MEG analysis improves the signal-to-noise ratio to better emphasize spatial and temporal characteristics. Yet, by averaging across trials, MEG loses its ability for accessing neural activity in real-time and therefore limits the application of this sophisticated technology.

One area where real-time MEG (rtMEG) is being used is the development of brain machine interface (BMI) applications, which require analysis of brain activity in real-time. Most BMI applications are focused on using an individual's brain activity to directly control the actions of a device. It has been demonstrated that a delay longer than 200 ms between a person's movement intention and a device's reaction is noticeable and can be distracting and lead to degraded task performance (Lauer et al. 2000; Welford 1968). This 200 ms delay is considered the maximum time a system can use for collecting and processing the neural data and for driving the device. For these reasons, this chapter considers a system delay less than 200 ms to be "real-time".

The majority of BMI systems have utilized EEG because it is noninvasive, the equipment is readily available, and the standard signal processing algorithms can be implemented easily in real-time (Mason, Bashashati, Fatourechi, Navarro, & Birch, 2007). EEG-BMI systems have been used successfully to control devices with a few degrees of freedom (Wolpaw & McFarland 2004; McFarland et al. 2010). However, for complex device control a system must be able to localize multiple separable sources of neural activity with high spatial and temporal resolution.

An alternative non-invasive method of assessing brain activity that does not rely on electromagnetics is "real-time fMRI" (rtfMRI) (DeCharms 2008). First established in 1995, rtfMRI combines the high spatial resolution found with recording the hemodynamic response (i.e. Blood-Oxygen-Level Dependence – BOLD) with advanced computational ability for reconstruction (Cox et al. 1995). Real-time fMRI is a valuable tool that can be used for many of the applications discussed in this chapter including many of the adaptive paradigms. However, the temporal resolution of rtfMRI is limited by the biological signals being recorded; the hemodynamic response. The hemodynamic response inherently has dynamics that change only on the order of multiple seconds. This fundamental limitation to the temporal resolution means rtfMRI neurofeedback systems have delays on the order of several seconds, which would be very noticeable to the participant. In addition, the hemodynamic changes recorded with fMRI are not direct measurements of neural activity as are the magnetic fields recorded with MEG. The high spatial resolution is a great advantage to fMRI, but the hemodynamic timing limits the applications rtfMRI can be used for.

While other neural recording technologies have utility across a range of applications, this chapter focuses on MEG for real-time analysis of neural activity with high spatial and temporal resolutions. This chapter covers some of the current and potential applications of rtMEG. Benefits of online analysis of MEG data range from real-time monitoring of data integrity and experiment validity, to clinical neurofeedback paradigms for the rehabilitation of central nervous system injuries and disorders. Also discussed are some of the remaining challenges that occur with real-time analysis of high throughput data as well as some potential solutions that can be applied.

2. Applications for online MEG

2.1 Basic neuroscience research

The ability to access and process MEG data in real-time opens up many new opportunities for basic neuroscience research. Applications as simple as having real-time visualization of neural data would be useful for assessing data quality during an experiment. Commercial MEG systems display the raw, and even filtered, magnetic signals in real-time, but it is difficult for operators to interpret 200-300 channels of data quickly during a scanning session. Often MEG operators are interested in particular features of the data, such as specific frequency bands or sources of activity in specific anatomic areas. Real-time spectral analysis, source-localization and visualization tools would be very beneficial. Visualization can be straightforward, such as displaying the power spectra for individual channels (see section 4.2), or complex such as projecting the MEG data into source space to display neural activity mapped onto the space of the cerebral cortex (see section 4.3). By watching neural characteristics, such as the frequency content in time, and changes in source localization, experimenters can quickly determine if the paradigm needs to be changed or if more data needs to be collected.

A powerful use for rtMEG is in running adaptive paradigms where the experiment progression is determined by the neural data that was collected (MacKay 1992; Chaloner & Verdinelli 1995). Adaptive paradigms can use outcomes from prior trials (e.g. neural responses to specific stimulus classes) to determine what the next stimulus should be. For example, neural activity can be analyzed during an experiment to determine if a task is too easy or too hard for eliciting the required neural activity. In a memory task, for example, experimenters might be able to adjust the difficulty of the paradigm to elicit activity in a particular brain area.

Real-time data analysis is also useful to quickly determine if sufficient amounts of data have been collected for a given stimulus. One common example is localization of motor or sensory cortices where a large number of trials (>100) are typically recorded to ensure that sufficient data is available for offline analysis. Limiting the number of trials can reduce the scan time for each stimulus and ensure sufficient data was collected thereby making the most of the time in the scanner.

Analyzing MEG data during an experiment can also be used to rapidly determine if a subject's brain activity fits a certain criteria for a study. For example, subjects could be screened for their ability to modulate neural activity during a given paradigm. By analyzing this data in real-time, the amount of time spent on unnecessary data collection and offline data analysis can be reduced. This can allow experimenters to quickly determine whether the experimental paradigms should proceed or if different paradigms should be performed.

2.2 Applications of real-time MEG in neurology and neurosurgery

MEG's most established clinical use is for providing non-redundant localizing information for epilepsy patients being considered for surgical treatment (Bagic et al. 2011; Bagic et al. 2009; Burgess, Funke, et al. 2011; Stefan et al. 2011). MEG has also received increasing acceptance as a superb non-invasive tool for localizing eloquent cortices in presurgical functional brain mapping in patients with tumors and other operable lesions (Burgess, Barkley, et al. 2011). Further efforts of the MEG community are focused on establishing new clinical indications where dementia (Zamrini et al. 2011), traumatic brain injury (TBI) (Huang et al. 2009; Maruta et al. 2010) and autism (Roberts et al. 2011; Roberts et al. 2010) are considered current front runners among many other neurologic and psychiatric disorders that are being studied (Stufflebeam et al. 2009; C. Stam 2010). These clinical applications have been developed with the idea that MEG data must be processed offline. However, by assessing MEG data during a patient session, many useful tools and new clinical techniques can be developed.

One of the most appealing uses of online MEG analysis would be to provide instant results to clinicians. For clinicians who regularly spend many hours analyzing complex epilepsy cases (Bagic et al. 2011; Burgess, Funke, et al. 2011), having a software package that can process data online and provide at least preliminary localizing information by the time a patient walks out of the magnetically shielded room would be invaluable. However, at least initially, more stereotypical and less labor-intensive clinical applications, such as presurgical functional brain mapping (PFBM) using MEG evoked fields (MEFs) (Burgess, Barkley, et al. 2011), are more likely to be amenable to this type of application. Even if these analysis methods are not automated and would initially require the interaction of an expert operator, they would still provide invaluable time-saving and could directly increase efficiency and quality of patient care. This is especially the case in urgent situations leading to a surgical intervention, when the timeliness of a clinical decision is critical. With quick analysis methods that could begin while a patient is still in the MEG scanner, ideally, neural imaging reports could be sent directly to the operating neurosurgeons' planning workstations so patients could have a seamless transition from the MEG room to the operating table. Furthermore, neurosurgeons or other collaborating physicians could request additional data as needed while the patient is still in the MEG scanner.

Another very valuable clinical application for online MEG would be to provide MEG clinicians feedback on the quality and quantity of the data that has been collected. By evaluating the MEG data online the clinician could receive instant feedback on when enough data have been collected for mapping a particular functional modality, such as motor or language mapping. Similarly, software could provide indications to the clinician if the data collected were not sufficient for mapping and additional data are needed. This would help ensure that the amount and quality of collected data was sufficient to render an accurate clinical diagnosis. Of course, making rtMEG accessible and accepted by clinicians will require a collaborative effort between the signal processing community to develop automated systems and the clinical experts to guide and validate the development of the specific technology.

2.3 MEG for BMI technology research and development

While unsuitable for portable BMI applications, MEG can play an important role in BMI research and development as it offers a non-invasive, whole-head, and reasonably high-resolution brain interface with real-time capability. For instance, MEG can be used as an approximate surrogate for invasive technologies that place electrodes directly on the brain surface. Several studies have suggested that MEG might share similar spatial and temporal characteristics as direct cortical surface recording (i.e. ECoG) in terms of source localization accuracy and capability to resolve cortical activity represented by amplitudes of different frequency bands (Dalal et al. 2008; Korvenoja et al. 2006; Gharib et al. 1995). It was also demonstrated that movement-related information could be decoded accurately from MEG signals (Georgopoulos et al. 2005; Waldert et al. 2008; Wang, Sudre, et al. 2010). Figure 1 shows the time-frequency responses of a contralateral MEG sensor (a gradiometer) when a participant performed simple center-out wrist movements (Wang, Sudre, et al. 2010). There is a clear decrease in power for the low frequency sensorimotor rhythm (10-30 Hz) and a distinct increase in power for the high-gamma band (60-200 Hz) during movement. These changes in low and high frequency bands are in agreement with previous MEG (Waldert et al. 2008) and ECoG studies (Leuthardt et al. 2004; K. J. Miller et al. 2007; Wang et al. 2009). In addition, Wang et al. (Wang, Sudre, et al. 2010) demonstrated that high-gamma band activity captured by MEG showed directional modulation similar to what was observed previously using invasive recordings in humans (ECoG) (Leuthardt et al. 2004) and non-human primates (local field potentials) (Heldman et al. 2006) and has been used for BMI control.

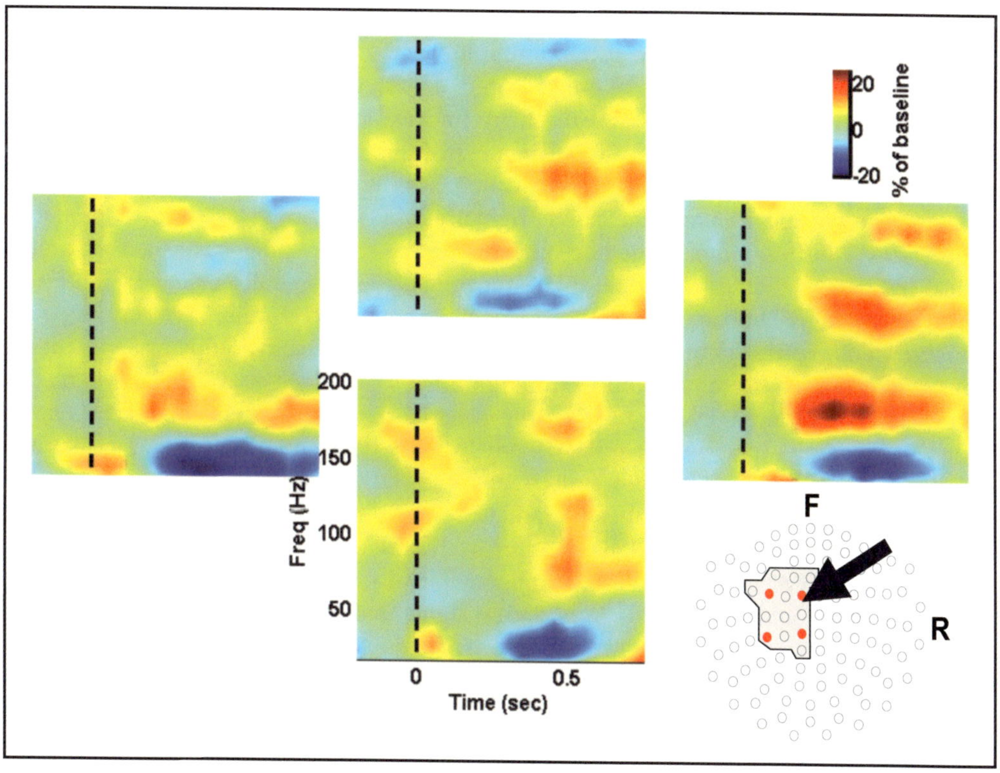

Fig. 1. Spectrograms of MEG signals recorded from one gradiometer (marked by the black arrow) during overt wrist movement. A total of 84 trials were aligned at target onset (time = 0) and averaged. The color indicates the percent change in spectral power from baseline. The arrangement of the four spectrograms corresponds to the four directions of wrist movements performed: up, down, left and right. The low frequency band shows a decreased power during movement in all directions while the high frequency band shows increased power during movement with directional preference for movement to the right. Inset: The red dots represent four MEG sensor locations (of the 102) whose high frequency band showed directional preference to contralateral wrist movement ($p<0.05$).

Recently, Mellinger et al. demonstrated that real-time MEG processing could provide control over a computer cursor in one-dimension with the individuals modulating their sensorimotor rhythms (mu and beta frequency bands) using imagined hand and feet movements (Mellinger et al. 2007). In this study, 3 out of 6 able-bodied participants achieved reliable cursor control (accuracy around 90%) with less than 45 minutes of training. More recent pseudo-real-time studies have shown that by using more advanced decoding algorithms only 5 minutes of initial open-loop data is needed to achieve reliable one dimensional device control using hand-related sensorimotor rhythms (Foldes et al. 2011). Limiting the amount of time spent collecting initial data means more time can be devoted to performing neurofeedback training tasks.

The non-invasive nature of MEG and its recording capability, as demonstrated in the above examples, support the utility of MEG for investigating basic neuroscience questions and piloting engineering solutions for BMI research and development. Using MEG, BMI studies can be conducted with large numbers of participants including both able-bodied individuals and individuals with disabilities (e.g. spinal cord injury, degenerative neurological disorders, stroke and etc.), while posing minimum risks to study participants. Important neurophysiology questions can be investigated across multitudes of subjects to better determine the cortical substrates and plasticity for BMI control. For example, what is the most dominant type of movement information in human primary motor cortex; abstract movement information (e.g. movement direction; (Georgopoulos et al. 1986)) or detailed somatotopy representation as established originally by Penfield and colleagues (Penfield & Boldrey 1937)? Furthermore, while non-human primate studies have suggested that motor cortical neurons encoding individual finger movements are generally mixed in anatomical location (Schieber & Hibbard 1993), several recent human ECoG studies have suggested that in human motor cortex there might exist at least some level of somatotopy or separation in finger representation for movements of different fingers (Kubanek et al. 2009). Such matters are further complicated by potential cortical reorganizations induced by corticospinal lesions in the individuals who would benefit from BMI technology (Cramer et al. 2005; Kokotilo et al. 2009). These questions about motor cortical representation of movement and its potential difference between able-bodied subjects and patients with chronic disabilities, are fundamental scientific questions of critical clinical importance for the research and development of BMI systems. MEG, complementary to other invasive and non-invasive neural recording tools, can provide important insights that can effectively guide the design specifications for implantable neural interface electrodes and neural decoding algorithms. Furthermore, real-time MEG provides a safe test-bed for researchers to investigate various neural decoder training paradigms, such as action observation-based neural decoder training paradigms (Tkach et al. 2008; Velliste et al. 2008) and co-adaptive paradigms where a neural decoder is frequently updated in parallel to potential cortical adaption during BMI training and operation (D. M. Taylor et al. 2002).

MEG can also play a direct role in pre-surgical planning and patient training for invasive or minimally invasive BMI systems. For one, MEG can be used to localize cortical areas that are significantly modulated by intended movement direction, and intracranial electrodes can then be implanted at those cortical sites (Wang, Sudre, et al. 2010). Accurate localization is important particularly in individuals who may have cortical reorganization secondary to injury (e.g. spinal cord injury, stroke, and amputation). Also, implantable electrode arrays typically cover only a small cortical area making accurate pre-surgical localization of the targeted implantation site critical. For example, intracortical microelectrode arrays typically cover only a small area of cortex (4×4mm^2 (Hochberg et al. 2006)) and high density ECoG grids (Wang et al. 2009) may cover an area only slightly larger (15×15mm^2). Another direct role for rtMEG is in pre-surgical training of patients who are scheduled to have electrodes implanted for BMI applications. Using rtMEG analysis, participants could practice BMI control with MEG as a surrogate for invasive technology. This training would orient patients to BMI operation and could potentially improve cortical activity modulation, thus improving performance with the implanted BMI. In summary, MEG and especially rtMEG, offers many opportunities for supporting and advancing BMI research and development.

2.4 Neurofeedback therapies for physical rehabilitation

Neurofeedback can be used to help individuals learn to modulate their own brain activity volitionally (Angelakis et al. 2007; Heinrich et al. 2007) and has been applied to many clinical conditions such as epilepsy, anxiety, and even attention deficit hyperactivity disorder (ADHD) using EEG (Angelakis et al. 2007; Heinrich et al. 2007; Monderer et al. 2002; Sterman & Egner 2006; Patrick & Friel 2007). Generally, individuals are provided visual, auditory, or tactical feedback of their neural activity, which allows them to volitionally control their brain activity. Real-time MEG has the capabilities of providing high quality neural signals for neurofeedback training, leveraging the advantages of MEG over other non-invasive brain recording technologies such as EEG or rtfMRI. In addition, rtMEG can be applied to an emerging area of neurofeedback therapy for motor impairment rehabilitation.

Many traditional physical rehabilitation methods strive to improve motor function using strategies that rely on patients having at least some residual muscle strength. However, when there is little or no residual motor function (e.g. after stroke and incomplete spinal cord injury) a therapy using motor-related signals collected directly from the brain may be a better option. By providing feedback of cortical activity, neuroplasticity can be induced which could potentially impart therapeutic benefits on sensorimotor function. BMI training paradigms have been used to induce motor-related neuroplasticity by providing direct neural feedback of individual's brain activity (Gage et al. 2005; Nijboer et al. 2008; Hochberg et al. 2006; Helms Tillery et al. 2003; Buch et al. 2008; Mellinger et al. 2007).

Some work has been done directly with individuals with paralysis as a proof-of-concept for using MEG as rehabilitation therapy. Buch et al. demonstrated that MEG could be used to allow individuals with chronic and complete hand paralysis due to stroke to control a one-dimensional computer cursor and a hand orthosis by modulating their sensorimotor rhythms (Buch et al. 2008). The combination of neurofeedback and physical practice may have additive rehabilitative effects, although this remains to be fully investigated. In Buch et al., 2008, individuals with complete paralysis achieved an average success rate of 72% during a BMI-controlled 'grasping' task. Six out of the 8 participants significantly improved their quality of brain-control across multiple sessions (13-22 sessions) demonstrating the possibility of neuroplasticity. However, in this group of 8 participants no significant improvement in hand-function was observed, which is not surprising since all had cortical lesions resulting in complete paralysis. Performing similar studies on participants with incomplete hand paralysis and using more advanced data processing methods designed specifically to encourage neuroplasticity may result in more improved motor function. In particular, the feedback in this study was updated with a 300 ms delay, which would be noticeable to participants (Lauer et al. 2000; Welford 1968). This long delay between the participant's brain activity and the corresponding feedback could result in limited neuroplasticity based on Hebbian plasticity mechanisms where tighter temporal coupling results in better plasticity (Muralidharan et al. 2011; Cooper & Donald 2005; Florian 2007; Caporale & Dan 2008). Being able to access and process neural data at a fast rate is critical for achieving a tight coupling in time with the feedback needed to achieve a stronger therapeutic effect. The fast processing necessary for strong neuroplasticity can be achieved with real-time MEG (Sudre et al. 2011). Furthermore, using advanced neural decoders that adapt over time to encourage stronger and more spatially localized activity could be used to improve the neuroplasticity effectiveness.

3. Challenges of online MEG

3.1 System considerations

Whole-head MEG systems contain up to 306 sensors that can be sampled at high rates (typically ≥1000 Hz). Unlike EEG, which has fewer channels and typically lower sampling rate, the high data throughput of MEG data requires more complex data collection hardware and software. For example, MEG machines utilize multiple Digital Signal Processors (DSPs) working in parallel each of which manages the data from a set of sensors. Using multiple small processing units in parallel complicates direct access to the raw data. In the standard workflow, MEG signals are recorded directly to a hard disk and analyzed offline without concern for accessing and processing data at a fast rate (see figure 2). In order to analyze the data as it is collected, special software is needed to access the data stream at a low level before it is stored in data files.

As a typical example, the Elekta Neuromag systems have a dedicated computer that receives, synchronizes, and stores the sensor data received from the DSP units. The compiled data is typically transferred in large 'chunks' of about 1 s duration. Such a long delay is unacceptable for real-time applications that operate on neural data at a millisecond scale. It is possible to adjust the speed and manner at which data chunks are transmitted and to directly access the data stream to allow for real-time MEG processing. Some real-time MEG software tools have been created to access the raw data of various MEG machines. One particular software interface has been developed for the Elekta Neuromag and CTF/VSM MedTech systems and is available in the open-source toolbox "FieldTrip" (Oostenveld et al. 2011; Sudre et al. 2011). This software copies small data segments directly from the data stream and puts them into a separate data buffer that can be accessed by other software running real-time applications. These systems copy the raw data leaving the original data stream intact to ensure the standard data saving occurs as it would normally. The buffer can be hosted on the acquisition computer itself or can even be run on a separate computer via a network connection (i.e. TCP/IP protocol) allowing for customizable network architectures. The buffer is shared across a network connection and can be accessed by other computers running analysis software specifically tailored for the real-time applications. Figure 2 illustrates the typical setup for a real-time neurofeedback system.

Tools for working with the rtMEG data buffer, such as routines to write and read from it, are freely available and designed to be straight-forward for researchers to incorporate customized scripts. Specifically, scripts to read from the buffer in Matlab and C are available, as well as functions to use the buffer as a source module in BCI2000 (Schalk et al. 2004). This real-time software has been used with a 306-channel Elekta Neuromag system to demonstrate some basic neurofeedback and source imaging applications as a proof-of-concept (Sudre et al. 2011). In particular, weighted and cortically constrained minimum-norm estimation (WMNE) was applied in real-time with average delays of 44±17 ms (forward head model and source imaging kernel were calculated ahead of time). Results from this online study compared favorably with the results from using standard offline processing methods. A major contribution to the differences between the online and offline results was found to be head movement, but this may be rectified with real-time motion correction (see section 4.1).

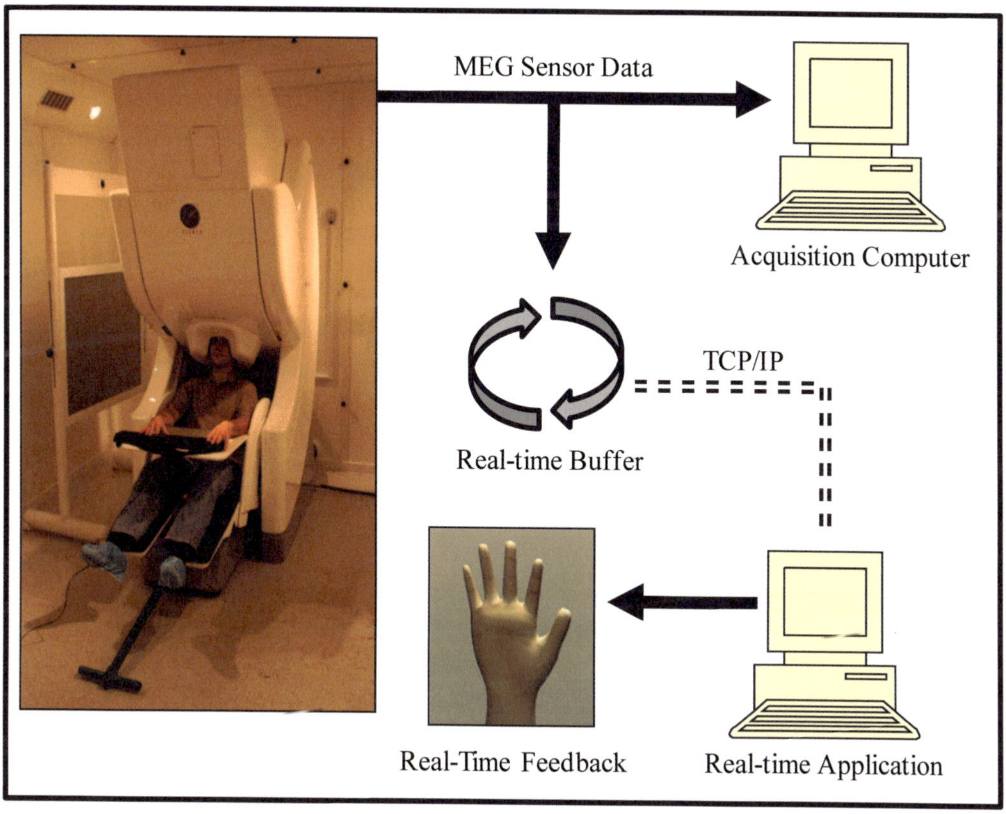

Fig. 2. Example system diagram for real-time MEG using rtMEG software and the Elekta Neuromag system. After sensor data is collected and synchronized, it is sent to the acquisition computer and the real-time buffer. The real-time buffer, which can be hosted on any computer, can be accessed via TCP/IP network connection by computers running real-time analysis software. The real-time application computer can process the neural data and provide real-time feedback to the subject and/or experimenter.

3.2 Artifacts and noise

Magnetic fields measured by SQUIDs (superconducting quantum interference devices) contain both the signals associated with neural activity and the noise and artifacts from various sources. The magnetic fields resulting from neural activity are extremely weak (typically 50-500 fT), about 8-9 orders of magnitude smaller than the geomagnetic field generated by the earth and 1-2 orders of magnitude smaller than the magnetic fields generated with eye movement (Hamalainen et al. 1993). Because the magnetic fields resulting from neural activity are inherently small relative to many noise and artifacts, MEG can have a low signal-to-noise ratio. The appropriate detection and removal of noise and artifacts is especially critical for rtMEG analysis where offline techniques, such as averaging across repeated trials are not available for improving the signal-to-noise ratio.

In general, the noise and artifacts observed in MEG recordings can be classified into four broad categories.

- *Environment-induced*: There are many magnetic sources in the surrounding environment that generate noise and artifacts in MEG measurements. These environment-related noise/artifact sources include, 60 or 50 Hz power lines, electric appliances, moving equipment such as elevators and hospital beds, and geomagnetic field generated by the earth.
- *Device-induced*: Both the SQUIDs and the electronic circuits of MEG systems can also introduce noise and artifacts. For example, the electronic circuits (e.g. amplifier, analog-to-digital converter, etc.) in MEG systems generate thermal noise, shot noise, and flicker noise. In addition, a large magnetic signal can temporally saturate the electronic circuit, resulting in one or multiple bad channels that contain large artifacts over a short time period (e.g. spurious interference in time domain).
- *Biologic-induced*: Subjects can also add noise and artifacts that contaminate MEG signals. For instance, a subject may have dental fillings or braces that interfere with the magnetic fields generated by their brain. Furthermore, periodic heart beats, muscle activity (i.e. electromyographic), and eye blinking generate electromagnetic fields adding unwanted components to MEG signals.
- *Experiment-induced*: Many clinical and neuroscience paradigms may themselves introduce noise and artifacts to MEG. Consider the example where a subject is instructed to perform a movement task in response to a cue. In this case, the corresponding muscle activity and movement can generate electromagnetic fields causing artifacts. These artifacts would be highly correlated with the movement cue and may be mistaken for task-related modulation in neural activity.

In practice, a small noise or artifact can drastically distort the MEG signals and eventually produce misleading conclusions after data analysis. Careful experimental design is a critical first step for mitigating artifact contamination in rtMEG, similar to the case of traditional offline analysis. For example, subjects with metallic dental fillings and braces should be excluded from research studies and subjects should be instructed to avoid unnecessary eye and body movement during the experiment. However, many sources of artifacts cannot be avoided, such as those caused by involuntary physiological behavior (e.g. heart beats and eye blinks) and in studies that require subjects to perform movements. In addition, it is important that the subjects are in a natural state and do not intentionally try to control their normal physiological behavior which could induce unwanted neural activity (Ochoa & Polich 2000).

To combat artifacts and noise, two complementary problems must be addressed: (1) noise/artifact detection, and (2) noise/artifact removal. Often noise and artifacts are not easy to detect because their time and frequency characteristics are not always predictable (e.g. head and eye movements). Even after a noise/artifact is detected, appropriately removing them from the MEG signals is another challenging task. In many situations the neural signals and noise/artifacts overlap in both time domain and frequency domain. In these cases, advanced signal processing algorithms are required to accurately remove the noise and artifacts to improve the signal-to-noise ratio.

Real-time MEG poses a number of additional challenges for both experiment design and data analysis. In particular, noise/artifact removal methods must process data quickly (i.e. high throughput) and maintain low latencies for rtMEG applications. To maintain high throughput, noise/artifact removal must be implemented with low computational complexity for fast processing. To minimize latency, the signal processing algorithms should generate results using only short time windows. For these reasons, special consideration is needed for addressing noise and artifacts in rtMEG.

4. Real-time analysis methods and solutions

4.1 Noise detection and suppression

Real-time MEG analysis poses a number of challenges for noise/artifact removal due to the unique requirements of high throughput and low latency. These requirements play an important role in designing the appropriate algorithms for noise/artifact reduction in rtMEG. However, while many techniques used to address noise and artifacts in offline MEG studies are directly valid for rtMEG other techniques need to be adapted for real-time use. In general, noise/artifact removal techniques fall into two broad categories: hardware-based methods and software-based methods, as summarized in Figure 3.

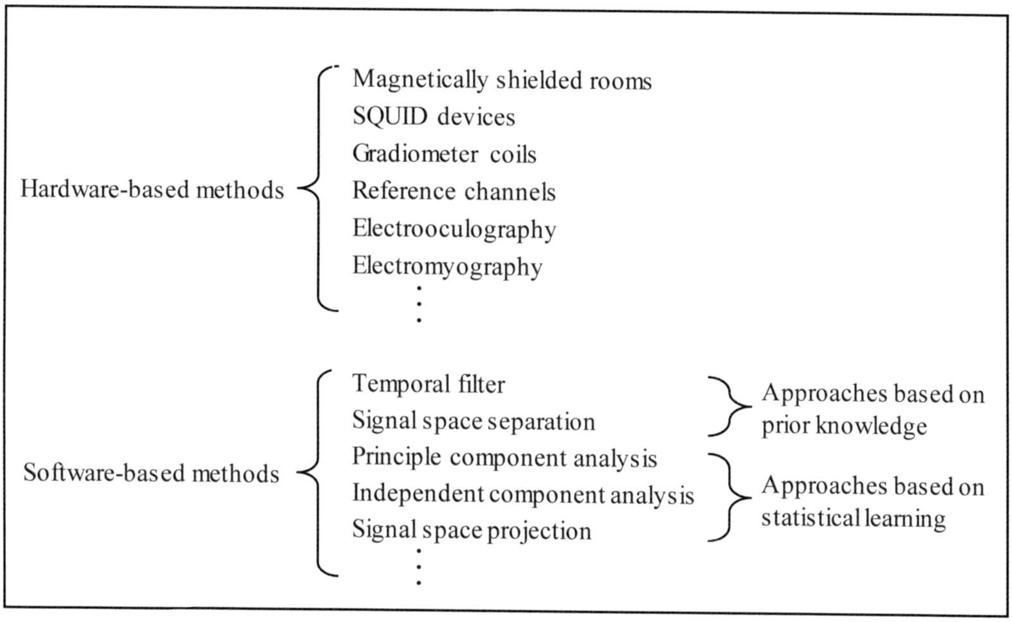

Fig. 3. A list of some existing methods for noise reduction and artifact removal of MEG.

Hardware-based methods rely on specific devices and instruments to reduce MEG noise and artifacts. For instance, magnetically shielded rooms have been designed to reduce environmental interference (Kelha et al. 1982; Zimmerman 1977), SQUIDs have been used to detect weak magnetic field and achieve improved signal-to-noise ratio (Clarke & Braginski 2006a; Clarke & Braginski 2006b), and gradiometer coils have been used to measure local gradients of the MEG signals by effectively suppressing the "common-mode" noise caused by external sources (Hamalainen et al. 1993). Adding a reference channel is another important hardware-based method. Instead of recording brain signals, a reference channel captures the interference which can be used to remove artifacts and noise from the MEG signals (Vrba & S. E. Robinson 2001; Hansen et al. 2010). Additionally, electrooculography (EOG) and electromyography (EMG) can be recorded simultaneously during MEG measurement and used to detect possible artifact contamination due to eye or body movements (Fatourechi et al. 2007).

Complementary to hardware-based methods, software-based techniques have also been developed to further increase the signal-to-noise ratio. These software-based techniques offer superior flexibility and are cheap to implement. Hence, they are often integrated into the data analysis flow of many practical MEG applications. Many software based noise removal methods are already appropriate for use in real-time and others can be adjusted to work in real-time applications. These software methods typically fit into two categories: approaches that require a priori information and those that use statistical characteristics of the measured MEG data.

Temporal filtering aims to remove the noise and artifacts based on their frequency-domain characteristics. Temporal filtering assumes that the noise/artifacts and the neural signals occupy different frequency bands. Hence, the noise and artifacts can be removed by filtering out the signals within an appropriately selected frequency band. For example, power line noise occurs at 60 (or 50) Hz and can be attenuated by applying a notch filter. Many temporal filters are computationally simple and can be run easily in real-time. The temporal filter method, however, will fail to work if the noise/artifacts and the neural signals are too close to each other in the frequency domain. For rtMEG applications, causality and latency must be taken into account during filter design. First, the output of the filter can only depend on the current and past inputs, meaning that non-causal filters are not applicable in real-time applications. Second, the filter-induced delays must be minimized. Taking N-tap finite impulse response (FIR) filter as an example, the delay is proportional to the filter order. In order to reduce the delay, the filter order should be minimized while simultaneously maintaining the preferred frequency response.

Different from temporal filters, signal space separation (SSS) is a spatial filter technique that is derived from quasi-static Maxwell's equations (S. Taulu et al. 2005; S. Taulu & Simola 2006). The key idea of SSS is to derive two different subspaces that correspond to brain signals and external interference respectively. By reconstructing the signals for these two subspaces based on measured MEG data, SSS can successfully separate the noise and artifacts from the MEG signals generated by human brain. However, extending SSS to real-time applications is not trivial. As a spatial filter technique, SSS is sensitive to the "bad channels" that contain large non-magnetic interference (e.g. saturated electronic circuits). Spurious interference is often observed for these bad channels (shown in Figure 4) and can distort SSS results. Traditionally, bad channels are detected and removed using statistical analysis of the recorded MEG data over large time windows on the order of a few seconds. This approach results in artifact removal that reacts slowly which can have a detrimental effect in rtMEG applications. To address this issue, a robust SSS (rSSS) algorithm has been developed to extend the conventional SSS algorithm to real-time applications (Guo et al. 2010). The key idea is to apply robust regression to dynamically detect and attenuate corrupted signals in real-time. In addition, a specially designed numerical solver was been developed to minimize the computational cost of rSSS to be suitable for real-time applications.

The aforementioned temporal and spatial filter methods rely on prior knowledge about the MEG signals (e.g. noise frequency and signal subspaces). A number of other software-based techniques attempt to detect and remove noise and artifacts by statistically modeling their characteristics from the measured data. Three common approaches are: principal component analysis (PCA) (Guimaraes et al. 2007; J. W. Kelly et al. 2011), independent component analysis (ICA)(J. W. Kelly et al. 2011; Hyvärinen & Erkki Oja 2000; Vigário et al. 2000; Choi et al. 2005), and signal space projection (SSP) (Uusitalo & Ilmoniemi 1997; Tesche et al. 1995).

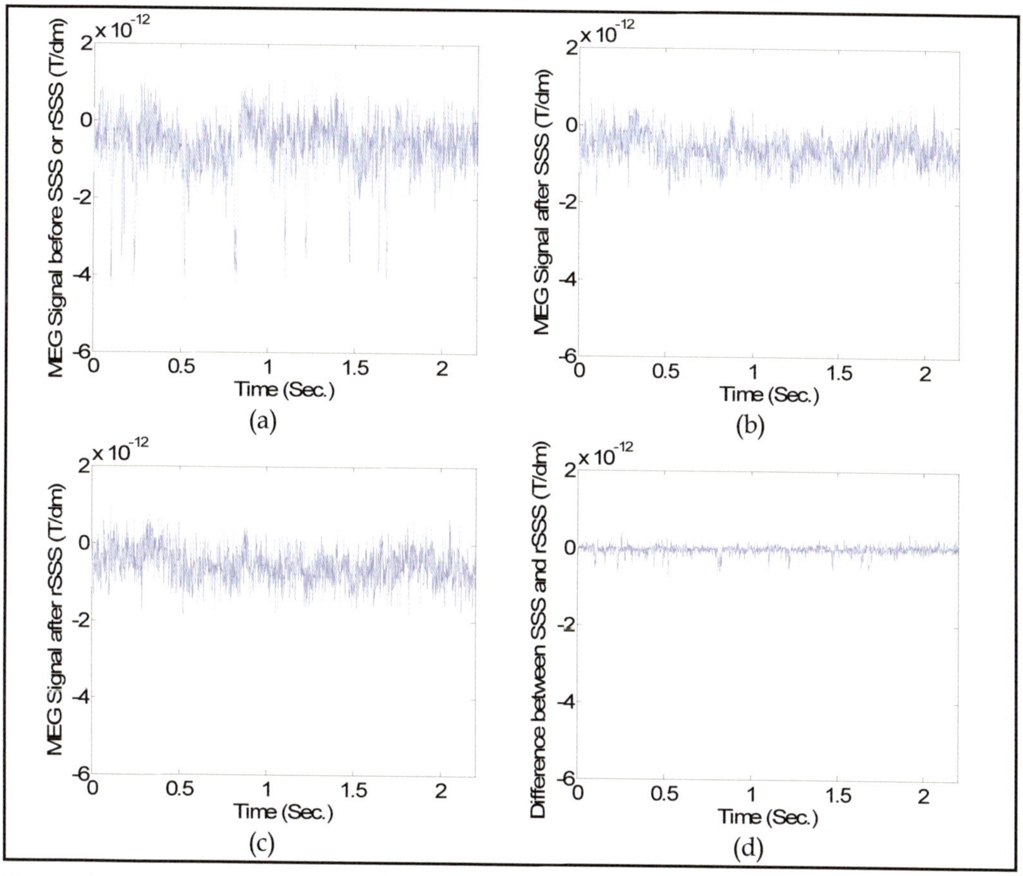

Fig. 4. a) Recorded MEG data contain interference where the MEG channel is sporadically saturated. b) SSS is applied to attenuate noise and artifacts in real-time. c) rSSS is applied to attenuate noise and artifacts in real-time. d) Because SSS cannot automatically handle bad channels in real-time, its results vary from the rSSS results mainly when spurious interference occurs

PCA applies eigenvalue decomposition to the covariance matrix calculated from measured data. It uses the resulting eigenvectors to transform the MEG signals to a new coordinate frame where the transformed signals are uncorrelated. Ideally, in the transformed signal space some of the principal components capture the neural signals of interest, while other components represent the sources of noise and artifacts and should be removed (Guimaraes et al. 2007; Fatourechi et al. 2007; Choi et al. 2005). ICA extends PCA and aims to find the signal space where all transformed signals are mutually independent (J. W. Kelly et al. 2011; Hyvärinen & Erkki Oja 2000; Vigário et al. 2000; Choi et al. 2005). As such, ICA offers an alternative way to separate the sources of noise/artifacts from the recorded MEG signals. Finally, SSP applies the idea of signal space decomposition that is similar to SSS, but instead uses statistical characteristic of the measured signals to determine the two subspaces associated with the MEG signals and the unwanted noise/artifacts respectively. Once these subspaces are determined, SSP projects the MEG data onto the signal subspace, thereby removing the components belonging to the noise subspace. All of these statistical methods (i.e. PCA, ICA, and SSP) often require a large amount of measured data for characterization. For the applications where preliminary characterization data are limited, these methods may fail to work or specific modifications are required to improve their accuracy and stability. When rtMEG is considered, these statistical methods can be directly applied to real-time signals as linear weights. However, since the generation of these weights relies on preliminary data that were collected before an rtMEG paradigm, updating the statistical characterization (i.e. the linear weights) may be needed if the signals are not stationary. If the signals are not stationary, adaptive algorithms (He et al. 2004; Selvan & R. Srinivasan 1999) may be useful to dynamically track the signal/noise characteristics over time. Introducing these adaptive algorithms may increase the computational cost and result in system delays.

In summary, many of the standard noise and artifact suppression methods are applicable to rtMEG. Most hardware-based methods and simple software-based methods (e.g. temporal filtering) can be implemented readily in real-time, while the more complicated software-based methods require adaptation (e.g. rSSS) or separate data collection (e.g. ICA). All of the discussed noise/artifact detection and removal methods have unique design trade-offs that must be carefully explored for each real-time experimental paradigm.

4.2 Real-time spectral analysis

Spectral analysis is performed to study the modulation of specific frequency bands contained in a recorded signal. The dynamical properties of neural networks in the brain give rise to 'rhythms' or oscillations in several distinct frequency bands, which are often studied offline or in real-time (Nunez & Ramesh Srinivasan 2005; Wolpaw et al. 2002). For example, mu (8-13 Hz) and beta (12-30 Hz) rhythms are typically associated with motor cortex activation during movement and can be used in BMI systems to control devices in real-time (Pfurtscheller & Lopes da Silva 1999; Waldert et al. 2008).

In a typical offline MEG analysis scenario, data are time-locked to a particular event, such as a stimulus onset, and then the frequency content is extracted and averaged across similar repeated events. Trial averaging improves the signal-to-noise ratio in offline analysis, but is typically not possible in rtMEG applications. For example, controlling a prosthesis in real-time requires that control signals be generated continuously (i.e. within a single trial). Figure 5 illustrates an example of a single trial of MEG data that was analyzed in a real-time manner. Shown are the time-varying spectral representations from one MEG sensor over the contralateral sensorimotor area during hand grasp. The frequency content was determined using autoregressive filters on a sliding 300 ms window of data shifted every 50 ms to produce the time-frequency plots. In addition to the example of real-time spectral analysis (left figure), the spectrograms of 10 trials were averaged together demonstrating a distinct and more stable suppression of the mu and beta bands during movement. In rtMEG applications that are not restricted to using only the latest data, averaging each trial with the previous trials can be used to produce a spectral estimate that improves as the experiment progresses. This is useful, for example, when experimenters want to observe the frequency changes as a study is occurring.

If an experimenter wants to analyze brain signals in real-time, special consideration is needed when picking the analysis method. In traditional MEG analysis many minutes of data are available for characterizing events, but in rtMEG only a few milliseconds may be available. For example, in a BMI application it may be desirable to perform a spectral analysis on short duration time windows (e.g. <500 ms). The duration of the spectral analysis window is an important parameter to consider when doing any real-time signal processing. For example, with a short duration analysis window the spectral estimate can be updated quickly resulting in faster neural feedback but potentially limiting the frequency resolution, because there are simply not enough time points to estimate the power spectrum. Conversely, with a longer duration analysis window, a higher frequency resolution is possible, yet the resulting frequency information will not update as quickly and can produce delays in the neurofeedback. This timing-frequency resolution tradeoff is not unique to MEG spectral analysis and has led to the development of different spectral estimation methods. Some of the most commonly used methods are short-time Fast Fourier Transform (FFT), AutoRegressive (AR) filters, wavelets, and band-pass frequency filters (Kay & Marple 1981). Band-pass filters require the design of filters, which have trade-offs to consider such as ringing and roll-off rate that can limit frequency resolution. Fast Fourier Transform is a common spectral estimation method that is easy to use, but works best with long time segments of data. With short analysis windows, FFT has a tendency to result in erratic spectral estimations across adjacent frequencies. AR filters, such as Maximum Entropy Method (MEM), attempt to solve the erratic estimation issue of FFT by effectively smoothing changes in the power spectrum for a more stable estimate (Kay & Marple 1981; E. A. Robinson 1982). This frequency smoothing effect produces accurate estimates of broadband signals, such as gamma frequencies in motor related activity (Bashashati et al. 2007), but poor estimates of narrowband signals. Wavelets are used to help remove the timing-frequency resolution trade-offs for signals with specific and known characteristics. Typically, wavelets are used to encourage higher frequency resolution in the lower frequency bands while preserving higher temporal resolution in the higher frequency bands. However, this leads to poor timing resolution in the low frequencies and poor frequency resolution in the high frequencies added to the fact that wavelets need to be designed for specific signal waveforms.

Due to the large number of channels and high sampling rate found with MEG, performing spectral analysis quickly and often, such as in a real-time application, can be computationally expensive. Thus for rtMEG, the method for spectral estimation and rate at which the analysis is performed need to be chosen based on the computational resources available. For example, if neurofeedback needs to be updated every 50 ms from the power spectrum of over 200 channels sampled around 1000 Hz, the power spectrum method can only afford at most 0.25 ms per channel (though many software packages allow for parallel processing). With numerous signals and limited time for processing, choosing estimation methods that are computationally intensive, such as AR filters, may not be possible.

One method for decreasing the computational requirements of spectral estimation in real-time is to decrease the number of sensors evaluated. This can be done simply by picking a sensor type (e.g. longitudinal gradiometers) or by selecting a region of interest. The sensor locations could be predetermined based on neuroanatomy or using source localization methods based on specific data from the paradigm.

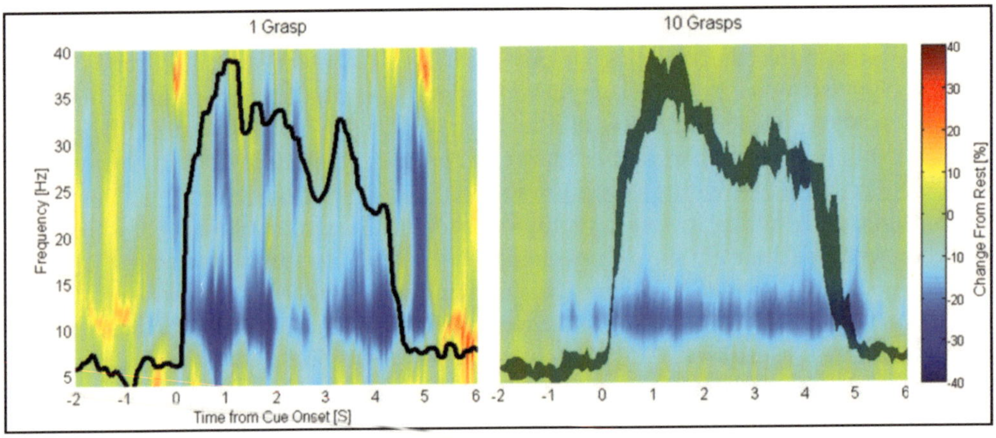

Fig. 5. Spectral analysis of hand grasp from a contralateral sensorimotor sensor using different amounts of data for estimating the spectrum. Shown is the modulation depth in time calculated as the percent change in power during grasping relative to the power during hand rest. In black is the interquartile range for the muscle activity (EMG is processed and standardized to fit the figure). A decrease in the mu and beta frequency bands (dark blue) is seen preceding and during muscle activity. With more trials used to estimate the frequency content the estimate becomes more stable. Yet, in the real-time case (left panel) modulation due to hand grasp can be accurately detected

4.3 Real-time source imaging

One of the major advantages of MEG is the good spatial resolution and wide coverage of the head. Combining these advantages allows for imaging of the relevant sources of neural activity in the brain. By applying source localization online the experimenter can get immediate feedback of the subject's brain activity in source space. This information can be used to determine if a subject/patient has the expected brain activity and which additional evaluations should be performed next. In addition, a considerable change in the source location could indicate the subject is no longer performing the task, has become desensitized to the task, or their mind is simply wandering and a break is needed.

Many source imaging techniques can be applied in a straight forward manner for real-time MEG applications. In particular, beamformers, such as synthetic aperture magnetometry (SAM), produce sensor-weight matrices which, when applied to the MEG sensor signals as a spatial filter, produce source images (Brookes et al. 2004). These spatial filter weights can be calculated offline before an experiment using previously recorded data and then applied online, during an experiment. Though the calculation of a leadfield matrix from a generic or subject specific head models can take considerable computational time, the final inverse transform is just a linear weighting of the MEG sensors which takes a negligible amount of computation to apply in real-time. This technique was demonstrated by Sudre et al. to perform source localization of ongoing brain activity (i.e. alpha waves during eye opening and closing) in real-time (Sudre et al. 2011).

Spatial filters from source imaging can also be combined with spectral analysis. For example, dynamic imaging of coherent sources (DICS) method performs beamforming with consideration to the frequency domain which can then be applied to the spectral estimates in real-time (Timmermann et al. 2001; Gross et al. 2001). This frequency-focused source imaging technique combined with real-time spectral estimation can be used to increase the signal-to-noise ratio and help accentuate brain activity associated with attempted movement in sensorimotor frequency bands thereby improving neurofeedback for rehabilitation.

5. Real-time feedback systems

The real-time capability of MEG makes it possible for software programs to acquire instantaneous MEG signals and provide feedback to a subject on-the-fly with minimum lag and high update rate (Sudre et al. 2011). Many neural signal processing algorithms and software packages developed previously for other neurophysiological signals, such as EEG, ECoG, local field potentials, and neuronal firing rates, can be adapted to work with real-time MEG signals. In order to provide real-time feedback, MEG signals (or any neural signals) are typically processed in multiple stages (see figure 6). First, signal conditioning is typically applied to neural signals, such as band-pass filtering, removal of line noise and artifacts (see section 4.1 above), and spatial filtering/beamforming (see section 4.3 above). Second, signal processing algorithms are used for real-time feature extraction, most commonly time-frequency analysis in various frequency bands (see section 4.2 above) (Degenhart et al. 2011; Schalk et al. 2004). Finally, decoding algorithms transform neural signal features into control signals for feedback, such as moving a computer cursor, a robotic/prosthetic arm, or other devices.

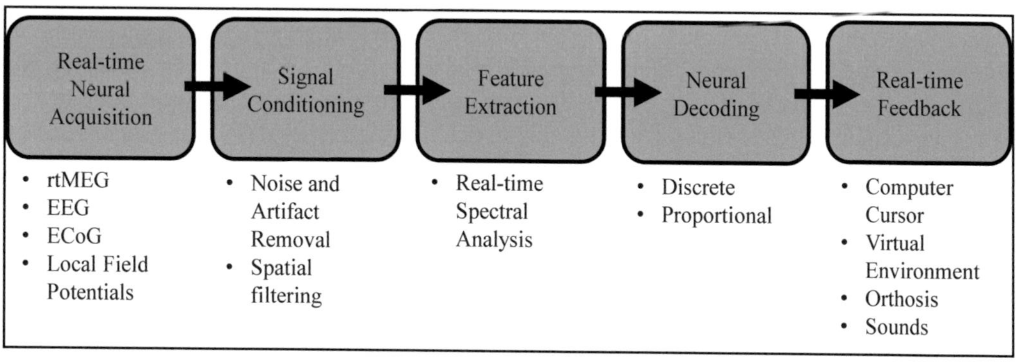

Fig. 6. Standard processing flow diagram for real-time neurofeedback. Listed are examples of methods possible during each step

Most studies using neural feedback have used decoding algorithms that take a signal classification approach where certain behavioral parameters are used to generate discrete outputs (e.g. decoding neural activity associated with the imagined movement of the right hand and left hand to change a feedback between two states) (Mason et al. 2007). These discrete decoding methods can be implemented in real-time MEG and are valuable for some neurofeedback applications. In addition, proportional neural decoding algorithms that can generate continuous, time-varying control signals can also be done with rtMEG (Mellinger et al. 2007) and may be more suitable for applications such as BMI. Many neural decoding algorithms have been used for real-time BMI control, including population vector algorithm (Georgopoulos et al. 2005; Georgopoulos et al. 1986; D. M. Taylor et al. 2002), optimal linear estimator/multivariable linear regression (Salinas & Abbott 1994; Foldes & D. M. Taylor 2011; Wang et al. 2007), and Kalman filters (Malik et al. 2011; Wu et al. 2006).

At the final stage, the decoded neural signals are used to control various external devices and generate real-time feedback, which can be visual, auditory, tactile, or proprioceptive. These methods are already being piloted with rtMEG to control simple devices such as computer cursors and hand orthoses (Buch et al. 2008) (see section 2.1 above). Using a combination of visual, tactile and proprioceptive feedback of an orthosis or similar device could improve task performance and perhaps promote plasticity for rehabilitation applications. Providing sensory feedback directly to participants by artificially stimulating the peripheral or central nervous system to promote plastic changes in neural function in the brain is a BMI technology currently under development (Wang, Collinger, et al. 2010). However, neural stimulation can introduce additional artifacts that could distort MEG recordings. In many cases the stimulus artifacts could be removed in real-time by ignoring MEG data during stimulation periods or using artifact removal methods (see section 4.1). Yet in other cases, for example stimulation of the cortex directly, removing stimulus artifacts from MEG signals would be particularly challenging.

Advanced ways to display visual feedback are being increasingly used for BMI applications (Marathe et al. 2008). Paradigms using virtual reality models of a human are useful particularly for neurofeedback applications because they can induce a sense of ownership over the virtual body (Bailenson et al. 2003; Stanney et al. 2003) and it was observed that when participants empathize with the virtual person they perform tasks better (Friedman 2001). Furthermore, compared to abstract cursor movement, movement of a virtual arm is likely to evoke much stronger activity in the premotor and motor cortices for observation-based BMI training (Tkach et al. 2008). Paradigms using interactive games are also valuable for improving BMI control by minimizing both boredom and frustration by adjusting the difficulty of the games. Using games for feedback helps participants work harder and remain engaged while still enjoying the experience (Csikszentmihalyi 1991). This is critical to motivate human subjects for repetitive neurofeedback tasks regardless whether the goal is to achieve robust brain control of assistive devices or to promote functional recovery after nervous system injuries.

There are a number of real-time software packages for neural signal processing, neural decoding, controlling assistive devices, and rendering feedback. "BCI2000" is a successful example of real-time software that was developed for BMI (Schalk et al. 2004) and adapted to work with rtMEG toolboxes for Elekta Neuromag and CTF systems (Mellinger et al. 2007; Sudre et al. 2011). Another example is "Craniux" which is written in LabVIEW engineering programming environment (National Instruments, TX, USA) (Degenhart et al. 2011). The Craniux software package takes advantage of the advanced signal processing, real-time data visualization, and distributed processing capabilities offered by the LabVIEW environment. It can operate either in conjunction with BCI2000 or as a stand-alone package for real-time MEG, ECoG, or EEG. Similar to BCI2000, it has a modular architecture for signal recording, signal processing and decoding, and experiment paradigm control. Furthermore, Craniux offers a variety of display options for real-time spectral analysis, neural decoding algorithm parameters, and visualization of neural command signals including a virtual environment and avatar with fully articulated arms and hands as well as real-time Flash-based games (Adobe Systems Incorporated) that keep participants engaged in the neurofeedback task.

6. Conclusions

MEG is an exciting tool for analyzing neural activity in the brain at high temporal and spatial resolution. Using software that can access, manage, and process the high throughput available with MEG can open up many new opportunities for researchers, engineers, and clinicians. Accessing MEG data during an experiment could enable new paradigms employing neurofeedback and improve existing neuroscience and clinical paradigms by relaying processed data to the experimenters while a participant is still in the scanner. Freely distributed tools have been developed to help experimenters tap into the complex data stream of MEG to access data in real-time. Utilizing the real-time noise and artifact removal algorithms being developed and leveraging the analysis methods used in BMI research, rtMEG can become a valuable instrument for many clinical and neuroscience studies. Of course there are many more opportunities for rtMEG developments by signal processing engineers, neuroscientists, and clinicians.

7. References

Angelakis, E. et al., 2007. EEG neurofeedback: a brief overview and an example of peak alpha frequency training for cognitive enhancement in the elderly. *The Clinical Neuropsychologist*, 21(1), pp.110–129.

Bagic, A.I., Funke, M.E. & Ebersole, J., 2009. American Clinical MEG Society (ACMEGS) position statement: the value of magnetoencephalography (MEG)/magnetic source imaging (MSI) in noninvasive presurgical evaluation of patients with medically intractable localization-related epilepsy. *Journal of clinical neurophysiology*, 26(4), pp.290-3.

Bagic, A.I. et al., 2011. American Clinical MEG Society (ACMEGS) Clinical Practice Guideline (CPG) #1 (ACMEGS CPG#1): Recording And Analysis Of Spontaneous Cerebral Activity. *Journal of clinical neurophysiology*, 28, pp.348-354.

Bailenson, J.N. et al., 2003. Interpersonal distance in immersive virtual environments. *Personality and Social Psychology Bulletin*, 29(7), p.819.

Bashashati, A. et al., 2007. A survey of signal processing algorithms in brain-computer interfaces based on electrical brain signals. *Journal of neural engineering*, 4(2), pp.R32-57.

Brookes, M.J. et al., 2004. A general linear model for MEG beamformer imaging. *NeuroImage*, 23(3), pp.936-46.

Buch, E. et al., 2008. Think to move: a neuromagnetic brain-computer interface (BCI) system for chronic stroke. *Stroke*, 39(3), pp.910-7.

Burgess, R., Barkley, G. & Bagic, A.I., 2011. Turning a new page in clinical MEG: Practicing according to the 1st Clinical Practice Guidelines (CPGs). *Journal of clinical neurophysiology*, 28, pp.336-340.

Burgess, R., Funke, M.E., et al., 2011. American Clinical MEG Society (ACMEGS) Clinical Practice Guideline (CPG) #2 (ACMEGS CPG#2): Presurgical Functional Brain

Mapping (PFBM) Using MEG Evoked Fields (MEFs). *Journal of clinical neurophysiology*, 28, pp.355-361.

Caporale, N. & Dan, Y., 2008. Spike timing-dependent plasticity: a Hebbian learning rule. *Annu. Rev. Neurosci.*, 31, pp.25–46.

Chaloner, K. & Verdinelli, I., 1995. Bayesian experimental design: A review. *Statistical Science*, pp.273–304.

Choi, S. et al., 2005. Blind source separation and independent component analysis: A review. *Neural Information Processing-Letters and Reviews*, 6(1), pp.1–57.

Clarke, J. & Braginski, A., 2006a. *The SQUID Handbook: Vol. 1: Fundamentals and Technology of SQUIDs and SQUID Systems*, Weinheim, Germany: Wiley-VCH.

Clarke, J. & Braginski, A., 2006b. *The SQUID Handbook: Volume II: Applications of SQUIDs and SQUID Systems*, Wiley-VCH.

Cooper, S.J. & Donald, O., 2005. Hebb's synapse and learning rule: a history and commentary. *Neuroscience & Biobehavioral Reviews*, 28(8), pp.851–874.

Cox, R.W., Jesmanowicz, A. & Hyde, J.S., 1995. Real-time functional magnetic resonance imaging. *Magnetic resonance in medicine*, 33(2), pp.230-6.

Cramer, S.C. et al., 2005. Brain motor system function after chronic, complete spinal cord injury. *Brain*, 128(12), pp.2941-50.

Csikszentmihalyi, M., 1991. *Flow: The psychology of optimal experience: Steps toward enhancing the quality of life*, Harper Collins Publishers.

Dalal, S.S. et al., 2008. Five-dimensional neuroimaging: localization of the time-frequency dynamics of cortical activity. *NeuroImage*, 40(4), pp.1686-700.

DeCharms, R.C., 2008. Applications of real-time fMRI. *Nature Reviews Neuroscience*, 9(9), pp.720-9.

Degenhart, A.D. et al., 2011. Craniux: A LabVIEW-Based Modular Software Framework for Brain-Machine Interface Research. *Computational intelligence and neuroscience*, 2011, p.363565.

Fatourechi, M. et al., 2007. EMG and EOG artifacts in brain computer interface systems: A survey. *Clinical neurophysiology*, 118(3), pp.480-94.

Florian, R.V., 2007. Reinforcement learning through modulation of spike-timing-dependent synaptic plasticity. *Neural Computation*, 19(6), pp.1468–1502.

Foldes, S.T. & Taylor, D.M., 2011. Offline comparison of spatial filters for two-dimensional movement control with noninvasive field potentials. *Journal of neural engineering*, 8(4), p.046022.

Foldes, S.T. et al., 2011. Stability of MEG for Real-Time Neurofeedback. *Conference Proceedings of the International Conference of IEEE Engineering in Medicine and Biology Society*, In Press.

Friedman, Y., 2001. Navigating the world of alternative medicine. *AJN The American Journal of Nursing*, 101(3), p.87.

Gage, G.J. et al., 2005. Naive coadaptive cortical control. *Journal of neural engineering*, 2(2), pp.52-63.

Georgopoulos, A.P. et al., 2005. Magnetoencephalographic signals predict movement trajectory in space. *Experimental brain research*, 167(1), pp.132-5.

Georgopoulos, A.P., Schwartz, A.B. & Kettner, R.E., 1986. Neuronal population coding of movement direction. *Science*, 233(4771), p.1416.

Gharib, S. et al., 1995. MEG and ECoG localization accuracy test. *Electroencephalography and Clinical Neurophysiology*, 94(2), pp.109–114.

Gross, J. et al., 2001. Dynamic Studying human imaging neural brain of cohereni interactions in the. *Proceedings of the National Academy of Sciences of the United States of America*, 98(2), pp.694-699.

Guimaraes, M.P. et al., 2007. Single-trial classification of MEG recordings. *IEEE Transactions on Biomedical Engineering*, 54(3), pp.436-43.

Guo, C. et al., 2010. Real-time robust signal space separation for magnetoencephalography. *IEEE Transactions on Biomedical Engineering*, 57(8), pp.1856-66.

Hamalainen, M. et al., 1993. Magnetoencephalography—theory, instrumentation, and applications to noninvasive studies of the working human brain. *Reviews of modern Physics*, 65(2), p.413.

Hansen, P.C., Kringelbach, M.L. & Salmelin, R., 2010. *MEG: An introduction to methods*, Oxford Univ Press.

He, P., Wilson, G. & Russell, C., 2004. Removal of ocular artifacts from electro-encephalogram by adaptive filtering. *Medical and Biological Engineering and Computing*, 42(3), pp.407–412.

Heinrich, H., Gevensleben, H. & Strehl, U., 2007. Annotation: Neurofeedback–train your brain to train behaviour. *Journal of Child Psychology and Psychiatry*, 48(1), pp.3–16.

Heldman, D.A. et al., 2006. Local Field Potential Spectral Tuning in Motor Cortex During Reaching. *IEEE Transactions on Neural and Rehabilitation Systems Engineering*, 14(2), pp.180-183.

Helms Tillery, S., Taylor, D.M. & Schwartz, A.B., 2003. Training in cortical control of neuroprosthetic devices improves signal extraction from small neuronal ensembles. *Reviews in the Neurosciences*, 14(1-2), pp.107–120.

Hochberg, L.R. et al., 2006. Neuronal ensemble control of prosthetic devices by a human with tetraplegia. *Nature*, 442(7099), pp.164-71.

Huang, M.X. et al., 2009. Integrated imaging approach with MEG and DTI to detect mild traumatic brain injury in military and civilian patients. *Journal of Neurotrauma*, 26(8), pp.1213–1226.

Hyvärinen, A. & Oja, Erkki, 2000. Independent Component Analysis: Algorithms and Applications. *Neural Networks*, 13(4-5), pp.411-430.

Kay, S.M. & Marple, S.L., 1981. Spectrum Analysis-A Modern Perspective. *Proceedings of the IEEE*, 69(11), pp.1380-1419.

Kelha, V. et al., 1982. Design, construction, and performance of a large-volume magnetic shield. *IEEE Transactions on Magnetics*, 18(1), pp.260–270.

Kelly, J.W. et al., 2011. Fully Automated Reduction of Ocular Artifacts in High-Dimensional Neural Data. *IEEE Transactions on Biomedical Engineering*, 58(3), pp.598-606.

Kokotilo, K.J., Eng, J.J. & Curt, A., 2009. Reorganization and preservation of motor control of the brain in spinal cord injury: a systematic review. *Journal of neurotrauma*, 26(11), pp.2113-26.

Korvenoja, A. et al., 2006. Sensorimotor Cortex Localization: Comparison of Purpose: Methods: Results: Conclusion: *World Health*, 241(1), pp.213-222.

Kubanek, J. et al., 2009. Decoding flexion of individual fingers using electrocorticographic signals in humans. *Journal of neural engineering*, 6(6), p.066001.

Lauer, R.T. et al., 2000. Applications of cortical signals to neuroprosthetic control: a critical review. *IEEE transactions on rehabilitation engineering*, 8(2), pp.205-8.

Leuthardt, E.C. et al., 2004. A brain-computer interface using electrocorticographic signals in humans. *Journal of neural engineering*, 1(2), pp.63-71.

MacKay, D.J.C., 1992. Information-Based Objective Functions for Active Data Selection. *Neural Computation*, 4(4), pp.590-604.

Malik, W.Q. et al., 2011. Efficient decoding with steady-state Kalman filter in neural interface systems. *IEEE Transactions on Neural and Rehabilitation Systems Engineering*, 19(1), pp.25-34.

Marathe, A.R., Carey, H.L. & Taylor, D.M., 2008. Virtual reality hardware and graphic display options for brain-machine interfaces. *Journal of neuroscience methods*, 167(1), pp.2-14.

Maruta, J. et al., 2010. A unified science of concussion. *Annals of the New York Academy of Sciences*, 1208(1), pp.58–66.

Mason, S.G. et al., 2007. A comprehensive survey of brain interface technology designs. *Annals of biomedical engineering*, 35(2), pp.137-69.

McFarland, D.J., Sarnacki, W. a & Wolpaw, J.R., 2010. Electroencephalographic (EEG) control of three-dimensional movement. *Journal of neural engineering*, 7(3), p.036007.

Mellinger, J. et al., 2007. An MEG-based brain-computer interface (BCI). *NeuroImage*, 36(3), pp.581-93.

Miller, K.J. et al., 2007. Spectral changes in cortical surface potentials during motor movement. *The Journal of neuroscience*, 27(9), pp.2424-32.

Monderer, R.S., Harrison, D.M. & Haut, S.R., 2002. Neurofeedback and epilepsy. *Epilepsy & Behavior*, 3(3), pp.214–218.

Muralidharan, A., Chae, J. & Taylor, D.M., 2011. Early detection of hand movements from electroencephalograms for stroke therapy applications. *Journal of neural engineering*, 8(4), p.046003.

Nijboer, F. et al., 2008. An auditory brain-computer interface (BCI). *Journal of neuroscience methods*, 167(1), pp.43–50.

Nunez, P.L. & Srinivasan, Ramesh, 2005. *Electric Fields of the Brain: The Neurophysics of EEG, 2nd Edition*, Oxford University Press, USA.

Ochoa, C.J. & Polich, J., 2000. P300 and blink instructions. *Clinical Neurophysiology*, 111(1), pp.93–98.

Oostenveld, R. et al., 2011. FieldTrip: Open source software for advanced analysis of MEG, EEG, and invasive electrophysiological data. *Computational intelligence and neuroscience*, 2011, p.156869.

Patrick, N. & Friel, B., 2007. EEG biofeedback in the treatment of attention deficit/hyperactivity disorder. *Alternative medicine review*, 12(2), pp.146–151.

Penfield, W. & Boldrey, E., 1937. Somatic motor and sensory representation in the cerebral cortex of man as studied by electrical stimulation. *Brain*, 60(4), p.389.

Pfurtscheller, G. & Lopes da Silva, F.H., 1999. Event-related EEG/MEG synchronization and desynchronization: basic principles. *Clinical neurophysiology*, 110(11), pp.1842-57.

Roberts, T.P.L. et al., 2011. Auditory magnetic mismatch field latency: a biomarker for language impairment in autism. *Biological Psychiatry*, 70(3), pp.263-9.

Roberts, T.P.L. et al., 2010. MEG detection of delayed auditory evoked responses in autism spectrum disorders: towards an imaging biomarker for autism. *Autism Research*, 3(1), pp.8–18.

Robinson, E.A., 1982. Historical Perspective of Spectrum Estimation. *Proceedings of the IEEE*, 7(9), pp.885-907.

Salinas, E. & Abbott, L., 1994. Vector reconstruction from firing rates. *Journal of Computational Neuroscience*, 1(1), pp.89–107.

Schalk, G. et al., 2004. BCI2000: a general-purpose brain-computer interface (BCI) system. *IEEE Transactions on Biomedical Engineering*, 51(6), pp.1034–1043.

Schieber, M.H. & Hibbard, L.S., 1993. How somatotopic is the motor cortex hand area? *Science*, 261(5120), p.489.

Selvan, S. & Srinivasan, R., 1999. Removal of ocular artifacts from EEG using an efficient neural network based adaptive filtering technique. *IEEE Signal Processing Letters*, 6(12), pp.330–332.

Stam, C., 2010. Use of magnetoencephalography (MEG) to study functional brain networks in neurodegenerative disorders. *Journal of the neurological sciences*, 289(1-2), pp.128–134.

Stanney, K.M. et al., 2003. Identification of metaphors for virtual environment training systems. *Ergonomics*, 1(3), pp.197–219.

Stefan, H., Rampp, S. & Knowlton, R., 2011. Magnetoencephalography adds to the surgical evaluation process. *Epilepsy & Behavior*, 20(2), pp.172–177.

Sterman, M.B. & Egner, T., 2006. Foundation and practice of neurofeedback for the treatment of epilepsy. *Applied psychophysiology and biofeedback*, 31(1), pp.21–35.

Stufflebeam, S.M., Tanaka, N. & Ahlfors, S.P., 2009. Clinical applications of magnetoencephalography. *Human brain mapping*, 30(6), pp.1813-23.

Sudre, G.P. et al., 2011. rtMEG: A Real-Time Software Interface for Magnetoencephalography. *Computational intelligence and neuroscience*, 2011, p.327953.

Taulu, S. & Simola, J., 2006. Spatiotemporal signal space separation method for rejecting nearby interference in MEG measurements. *Physics in Medicine and Biology*, 51, p.1759.

Taulu, S., Simola, J. & Kajola, M., 2005. Applications of the signal space separation method. *IEEE Transactions on Signal Processing*, 53(9), pp.3359-3372.

Taylor, D.M., Tillery, S.I.H. & Schwartz, A.B., 2002. Direct cortical control of 3D neuroprosthetic devices. *Science*, 296(5574), pp.1829-32.

Tesche, C.D. et al., 1995. Signal-space projections of MEG data characterize both distributed and well-localized neuronal sources. *Electroencephalography and clinical neurophysiology*, 95(3), pp.189-200.

Timmermann, L. et al., 2001. Dynamic imaging of coherent sources: Studying neural interactions in the human brain. *Proceedings of the National Academy of Sciences of the United States of America*, 98(2).

Tkach, D., Reimer, J. & Hatsopoulos, N.G., 2008. Observation-based learning for brain-machine interfaces. *Current opinion in neurobiology*, 18(6), pp.589–594.

Uusitalo, M. a & Ilmoniemi, R.J., 1997. Signal-space projection method for separating MEG or EEG into components. *Medical and Biological Engineering and Computing*, 35(2), pp.135-40.

Velliste, M. et al., 2008. Cortical control of a prosthetic arm for self-feeding. *Nature*, 453(7198), pp.1098–1101.

Vigário, R. et al., 2000. Independent component approach to the analysis of EEG and MEG recordings. *IEEE Transactions on Biomedical Engineering*, 47(5), pp.589–593.

Vrba, J. & Robinson, S.E., 2001. Signal processing in magnetoencephalography. *Methods San Diego Calif*, 25(2), pp.249–271.

Waldert, S. et al., 2008. Hand movement direction decoded from MEG and EEG. *The Journal of neuroscience*, 28(4), pp.1000-8.

Wang, W. et al., 2007. Motor cortical representation of position and velocity during reaching. *Journal of neurophysiology*, 97(6), p.4258.

Wang, W., Collinger, J.L., et al., 2010. Neural interface technology for rehabilitation: exploiting and promoting neuroplasticity. *Physical medicine and rehabilitation clinics of North America*, 21(1), pp.157-78.

Wang, W. et al., 2009. Human motor cortical activity recorded with Micro-ECoG electrodes, during individual finger movements. *Conference Proceedings of the International Conference of IEEE Engineering in Medicine and Biology Society*, pp.586-9.

Wang, W., Sudre, G.P., et al., 2010. Decoding and cortical source localization for intended movement direction with MEG. *Journal of neurophysiology*, 104(5), pp.2451-61.

Welford, A.T., 1968. *Fundamentals of skill.*, Methuen.

Wolpaw, J.R. & McFarland, D.J., 2004. Control of a two-dimensional movement signal by a noninvasive brain-computer interface in humans. *Proceedings of the National Academy of Sciences of the United States of America*, 101(51), pp.17849-54.

Wolpaw, J.R. et al., 2002. Brain-computer interfaces for communication and control. *Clinical neurophysiology*, 113(6), pp.767-91.

Wu, W. et al., 2006. Bayesian population decoding of motor cortical activity using a Kalman filter. *Neural Computation*, 18(1), pp.80–118.

Zamrini, E. et al., 2011. Magnetoencephalography as a putative biomarker for Alzheimer's disease. *International journal of Alzheimer's disease*, 2011, p.280289.

Zimmerman, J.E., 1977. SQUID instruments and shielding for low-level magnetic measurements. *Journal of Applied Physics*, 48(2), pp.702–710.

12

Non-Conscious Brain Processes Revealed by Magnetoencephalography (MEG)

Peter Walla
*University of Newcastle, School of Psychology,
Centre for Brain and Mental Health Research
Australia*

1. Introduction

Information processing in the human brain can happen fully conscious or in total absence of consciousness. Despite being far away from understanding consciousness in terms of being a subjective phenomenon based on neural activity we can at least imagine what it means to be consciously aware of a sensory perception or knowledge or ourselves. At the very moment we know that we know and what we know, the respective knowledge is consciously processed and can be verbally expressed, but what about information processing in the absence of consciousness? Can non-conscious information processing do the same just without consciousness? It is difficult to imagine what kind of information processing happens below the level of consciousness and what it actually means. What does non-conscious information look like? What does non-conscious information represent and what can it do? These are important questions to be answered in order to better understand consciousness itself. Among others a recent review reports about unconscious high-level processing in the human brain (van Gaal et al., 2011). In this review, the authors summarise scientific evidence to support the idea that decision making, an apparently conscious process, as well as other parts of highly sophisticated human behaviour can happen automatically without conscious control. This is exactly in line with the spirit of this book chapter that is written to support this notion with neuroimaging data collected via magnetoencephalography (MEG).

For those who trust the well known iceberg analogy related to Sigmund Freud's work about the human spirit the above mentioned questions must be very exciting, because according to this analogy non-conscious (in Freud's terminology pre- and unconscious) information processing accounts for more than 80% of all information processing. This highlights the importance and the dominance of brain functions that happen in the absence of consciousness.

According to my own view, the function of the brain is to produce controlled behaviour, besides managing basic body functions. The brain produces behaviour by processing information in three major steps. Step 1 is to process sensory input from outside and inside the body. In step 2 cognition- and emotion-related aspects of a stimulus are processed to make decisions. Finally, in step three the output of cognition and emotion is translated into motor programs that are then executed to elicit motor action which equals behaviour, at least in the view of a neurobiologist. Step 2 and to some extent perhaps step 1 contain information that can be processed either in the absence of or with full consciousness, whereas motor-related information always stays unconscious.

After all, it seems obvious that a better understanding of non-conscious information processing, especially related to cognition and emotion (step 2), leads to a better understanding and to a more accurate prediction of human behaviour. This is in contrast to focusing only on explicit measures, which just look at the tip of the iceberg.

The major goal of this chapter is to provide an overview of MEG-work about non-conscious brain processes. Traditional approaches to investigate human behaviour utilised questionnaires to acquire qualitative data and also behavioural experiments were conducted. Both strategies are limited in measuring non-conscious information processing, although some behavioural measures are able to tackle some aspects of it. Anyway, after the advent of neuroimaging techniques it turned out that neural activity measures are most adequate to demonstrate non-conscious brain processes, some of them even in the absence of any conscious behavioural consequence at the very moment of testing. One of the best examples was published by Rugg et al. (1998). In that study it was shown that repeated words that were incorrectly judged as new (so called misses) elicit different brain activity than new words that were correctly judged as new (so called correct rejections). In both cases the explicit responses were exactly the same ("I haven't seen this word"), but objective measures (brain activities) told another story. First, such discrepancy raised a number of specific questions. Now, we do have a general answer. Our brain knows more than it admits. The MEG has proved to provide access to some of that hidden knowledge. We only begin to understand to what extent and how information processing outside consciousness actually guides human behaviour. With its excellent temporal resolution in the range of milliseconds and its localisation capacities the MEG is a highly appreciated tool (see Hari et al., 2010) to access and describe non-conscious functions. Sensory-related, motor-related as well as emotion- and cognition-related information processing have been described. Although a certain gap between non-conscious information processing and actual behaviour has yet to be bridged, we learn to accept how unaware we are of most decisions that are made in our brains to guide our behaviour. We do not know everything that our brain knows.

This chapter has a further goal. As a matter of fact, various different terms are currently being used to describe the non-conscious character of some brain processes. Unfortunately, these terms (e.g. preconscious, subconscious, unconscious, non-conscious) are used interchangeably and thus produce considerable confusion. As a consequence of that, this chapter is also written to propose a simple model about non-conscious information processing in the human brain. This model is not an attempt to modify existing views of other areas (especially psychoanalysis), but it shall help to provide clarification in the field of cognitive and affective neuroscience. The model defines anything not conscious as non-conscious and it distinguishes only between unconscious and subconscious (both are non-conscious). Unconscious refers to information that can never become conscious, whereas subconscious refers to information that can be processed in the absence or presence of consciousness. For this chapter the overall working hypothesis states that all information processing that occurs prior to semantic processing is referred to as unconscious. Again, information that is unconsciously processed can never become conscious. On the other hand, from the very moment, sensory-related information processing leads to semantic processing, we shall label processed information subconscious or conscious depending on the absence or presence of consciousness.

2. Chronology of processes from unconscious to subconscious and conscious

In terms of serial processing in the brain it is interesting to know how long it takes until information related to a physical or chemical stimulus that is translated into neural signals actually reaches cortical areas. Before reaching the cortex, sensory information is already being processed, but as a matter of fact the MEG can hardly measure it. Under the assumption that subcortical structures are not able to process semantic information and according to the above mentioned model we can conclude that any processing before cortical involvement is unconscious. From various MEG studies we know that cortical involvement (at least in the visual domain) starts at about 100 ms post-stimulus (for words: e.g. Hari, 1990; Tarkiainen et al., 1999; Tarkiainen et al., 2002) which according to the above mentioned model means that roughly the first 100 ms after visual stimulation onset are unconscious. The exact time differs between sensory systems and also depends on top-down-processing, but let's use these 100 ms just to have a number to work with. Afterwards, earliest cortical processing is still sensory-related (primary areas and secondary areas). It then roughly takes another 50 to 100 ms until semantic information is being processed resulting in subconscious or even conscious information processing (Walla et al., 2001).

Besides semantic (cognitive) information processing any sensory input is also processed regarding its emotion aspects. Like cognitive information processing also emotion information processing can be but is not necessarily associated with consciousness.

3. Emotion-related information processing

For some reason there is not much literature about MEG and emotion. However, because meanwhile emotion also became an interesting candidate to be divided into non-conscious and conscious, it shall nevertheless be shortly dealt with. According to Peyk et al. (2008), earliest emotion processing in terms of MEG recordings occurs between 120 ms and 310 ms post stimulus in the visual system (pleasant and unpleasant pictures compared to neutral). A two stage model has been proposed with an early and a late activity component within this time window (120 ms to 170 ms and 220 ms to 310 ms). Investigations using faces as emotion stimuli reveal similar time windows within which different brain activity was found to reflect emotion-related information processing (e.g. Streit et al., 1999; Lewis et al., 2003). Only recently, Bröckelmann et al. (2011) described the effect of emotion-associated tones that attract enhanced attention at very early auditory processing (20 ms to 50 ms after stimulus onset). In another study, influences of olfaction on subjective valence intensity ratings of visual presentations were investigated by using the MEG (Walla and Deecke, 2010). Five different emotion categories (pictures: baby, flower, erotic, fear and disgust) were simultaneously associated with different odours. First, a significant interaction was found between odour condition and emotion-picture category in terms of emotion rating performance. Second, around 300 ms after stimulus onset odour-related brain activity effects were found for all emotion picture categories as revealed by MEG. Later, around 700 ms

after stimulus onset, brain activity effects occurred only in the neutral (flower) and both negative (fear and disgust) emotion categories. It was concluded that the earlier time window shows pronounced olfactory and visually induced emotion interaction, whereas the later brain activity effect shows olfaction influences only for specific emotion categories.
Again, it has to be emphasised that the MEG is mainly picking up signals from cortical structures missing out most subcortical information processing.
Although nothing can be said about conscious and non-conscious emotion at this stage in terms of MEG recordings I want to emphasise that this concept makes sense and future MEG studies will provide further insight.
Because there is more to emotion than just subjective feeling, terms such as unconscious emotion have already been introduced to the scientific community (Winkielman and Berridge, 2004). Given the distinction between implicit and explicit memory (see Rugg et al., 1998) it might even be helpful to think of a similar concept for the function of emotion (implicit versus explicit emotion). In this regard, implicit emotion would be understood as the non-conscious processing of emotion-related information influencing behaviour without leading to conscious awareness of it. In contrast, explicit emotion would be understood as conscious emotion, in other words, subjective feeling.
Moving on to cognition as the second major function to control behaviour we can look at non-conscious processes in more detail.

4. Cognition-related information processing

Cognition is a widely used term, but most often it is not clearly defined. In the frame of this chapter, cognition is simply understood as a function that processes semantic information (meaning) in order to guide behaviour based on accumulated knowledge. Strikingly, it is suggested that semantic processing can occur both in the absence or presence of conscious awareness. The phenomenon of intuition might be a good example of subconscious cognition. Also this idea can't be sufficiently supported by existing literature at this stage, but it is suggested as an interesting working hypothesis. Whatever cognition is understood as, in the following you'll find a selection of MEG work about memory-related and olfaction-related phenomena as well as about self awareness that lead to the assumption that much of even highly sophisticated brain functions happen without what we commonly understand as consciousness.

4.1 False recognition depends on prior word encoding

The human brain is a highly sophisticated information processing organ, but as a matter of fact it does make mistakes. Although we usually tend to believe that we know what we know there is convincing evidence to support that this is definitely not the case. It is quite impressive how we trust our conscious evaluations and decisions, but only until some objective evidence proofs us wrong.
One of such mistakes is the well known phenomenon called false recognition (e.g. Walla et al., 2000; for review see Schacter and Slotnick, 2004). It occurs when new items are wrongly classified as already seen. Such wrong classifications are called false alarms. In the laboratory, false recognition happens in test phases of memory experiments where prior presented items from a study list are shown again together with new items. In such test situations some of the new items elicit feelings of familiarity leading to wrong impressions

of being repetitions from the prior study list. Such familiarity arises due to similarity on either sensory or semantic processing (perceptual versus conceptual) levels (see Garoff-Eaton et al., 2007). For example, the new word *fish* in a recognition test list is likely to be judged as repeated if the word *dish* appeared in the prior study list. This would be caused by sensory similarity, because *fish* and *dish* look and sound similar. If instead the word *salmon* appeared in the study list the new word *fish* in the test list would also be judged as repeated above average than without such similarity. This would be caused by semantic similarity. Sensory similarity leads to a higher percentage of false alarms than semantic similarity (figure 1). This is so, because semantic processing is a higher level (more complex) of information processing than sensory processing, thus being less susceptible to mistakes.

On the behavioural level a false alarm can't be distinguished from a hit (correctly recognised repeated item) in terms of response accuracy, but it can be in terms of response time. False alarms are associated with longer response times than hits (Walla et al., 2000). From this it can already be inferred that the brain knows more than it admits, because a longer response time is the result of longer information processing, which obviously isn't known to consciousness. Further, if brain activities are simultaneously recorded to recognition performance one always finds higher frontal brain activity elicited by false alarms (Walla et al., 2000) compared to hits. Thus, longer information processing related to false alarms seems to be due to increased frontal brain activity.

Interestingly, brain activities elicited by false alarms do not only differ from brain activities elicited by hits. They can also differ between false alarms themselves depending only on the level of word processing during the encoding of the prior study list. In particular, false alarms after deep semantic word encoding elicit significantly higher brain activities than false alarms after alphabetical word encoding (figure 2). Respective T-maps are presented in figures 3 and 4. Figure 3 shows t-maps related to raw MEG data. Any differences can be interpreted in terms of amplitude differences. On the other hand, figure 4 shows t-maps related to normalised MEG data. Any differences in these can be interpreted in terms of functional differences. (Anyway, at this point it is important to emphasise a very specific MEG data feature. That is, neural structures eliciting different brain activity are not located underneath the sensors that demonstrate significant differences in these t-maps. This is due to the fact that a neural generator produces a rotating magnetic field which has a maximum ingoing and a maximum outgoing field flux. In a MEG map one neural generator thus results in a red-coloured maximum and a blue-coloured maximum. As a matter of fact, sometimes only one of these two maxima shows significant differences between conditions of interest.) With respect to neural generators being involved in false recognition-related effects figure 5 provides genuine source localisation results. Keeping in mind that false alarms are actually new words without any prior history in the frame of a recognition experiment it seems odd that they elicit different brain activities just depending on how the repeated words they are presented together with were previously processed. The only reason for that must be because something connects false alarms with hits. The idea is that these connections are the above mentioned similarities. If similarities are really causing false alarms it seems plausible that if repeated words that are presented together with new words were semantically encoded during the prior study phase similarities to the new words are rather semantic-related than sensory-related. As a consequence of that the recognition of semantically encoded words influences the processing of any new words intermixed with them. Strikingly, all this happens outside consciousness.

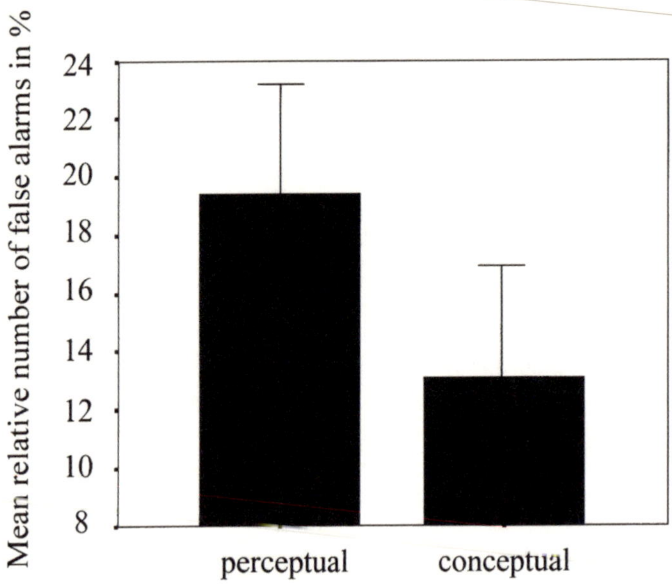

Fig. 1. Different rates of false alarms

Mean number of false alarms for both conditions. Note that the number of false alarms from the perceptual encoding condition is higher. The difference between these two conditions is highly significant (from Walla et al., 2001).

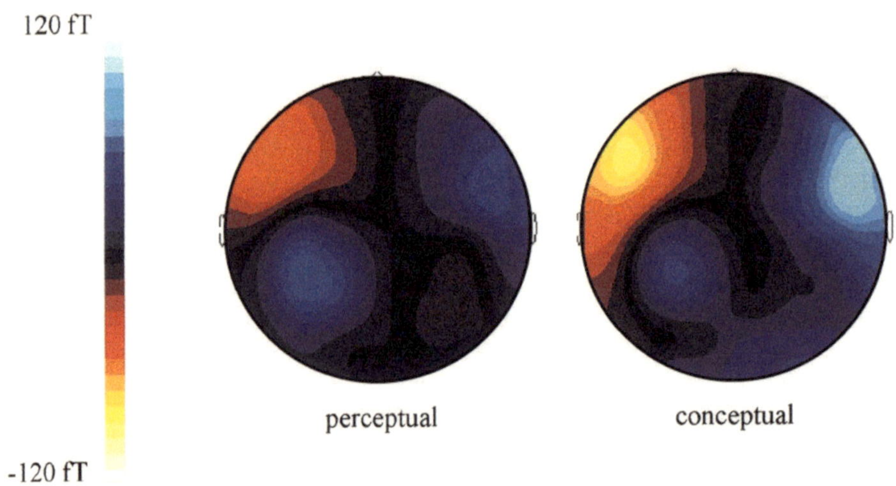

Fig. 2. MEG maps related to false alarms after different levels of encoding

Grand MEG maps of both conditions of false alarms (after perceptual encoding and after conceptual encoding) for the latency region from 300 to 500 ms after stimulus onset averaged over 26 subjects. Note the higher magnetic field flux related to false alarms from the conceptual encoding condition (significant difference) (from Walla et al., 2000).

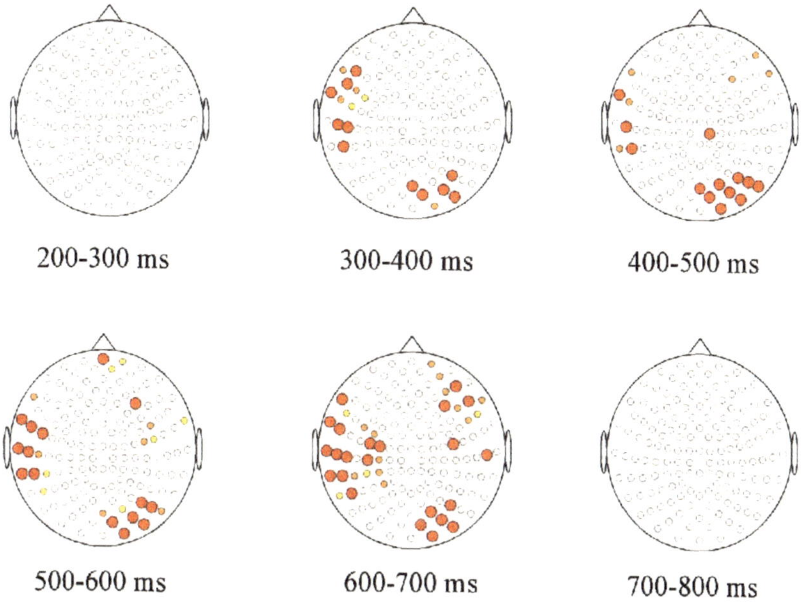

Fig. 3. T-maps (raw data)

Distributions of significant differences (grande average) between the two false alarm conditions (conceptual minus perceptual) as calculated by t-tests for every single sensor location for consecutive time intervals. Red circles represent P values from 0.001 to 0.020, orange circles represent P values from 0.021 to 0.040 and yellow circles represent P values from 0.041 to 0.050 (from Walla et al., 2000).

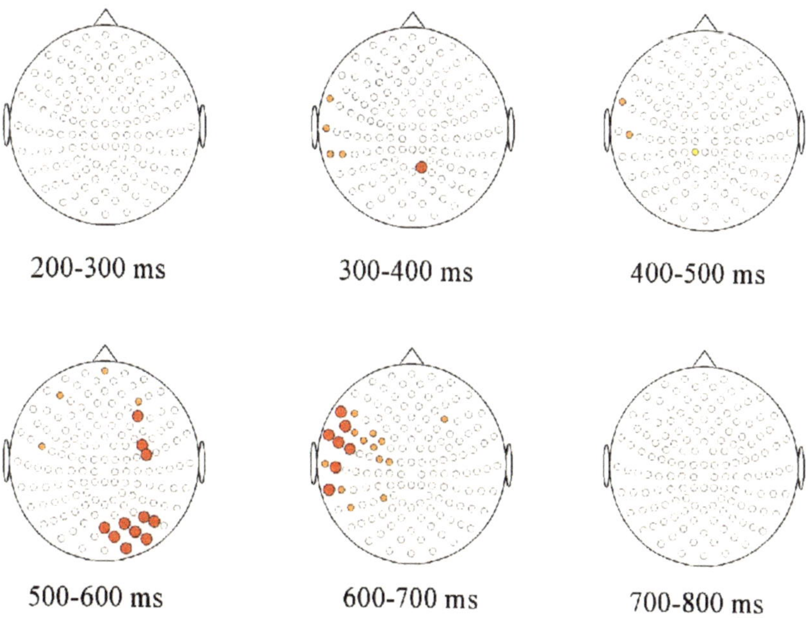

Fig. 4. T-maps (normalised data)

Distributions of significant differences (grande average) between the two false alarm conditions (perceptual and conceptual) as calculated by t-tests for every single sensor location for consecutive time intervals. Red circles represent P values from 0.001 to 0.020, orange circles represent P values from 0.021 to 0.040 and yellow circles represent P values from 0.041 to 0.050 (from Walla et al., 2000).

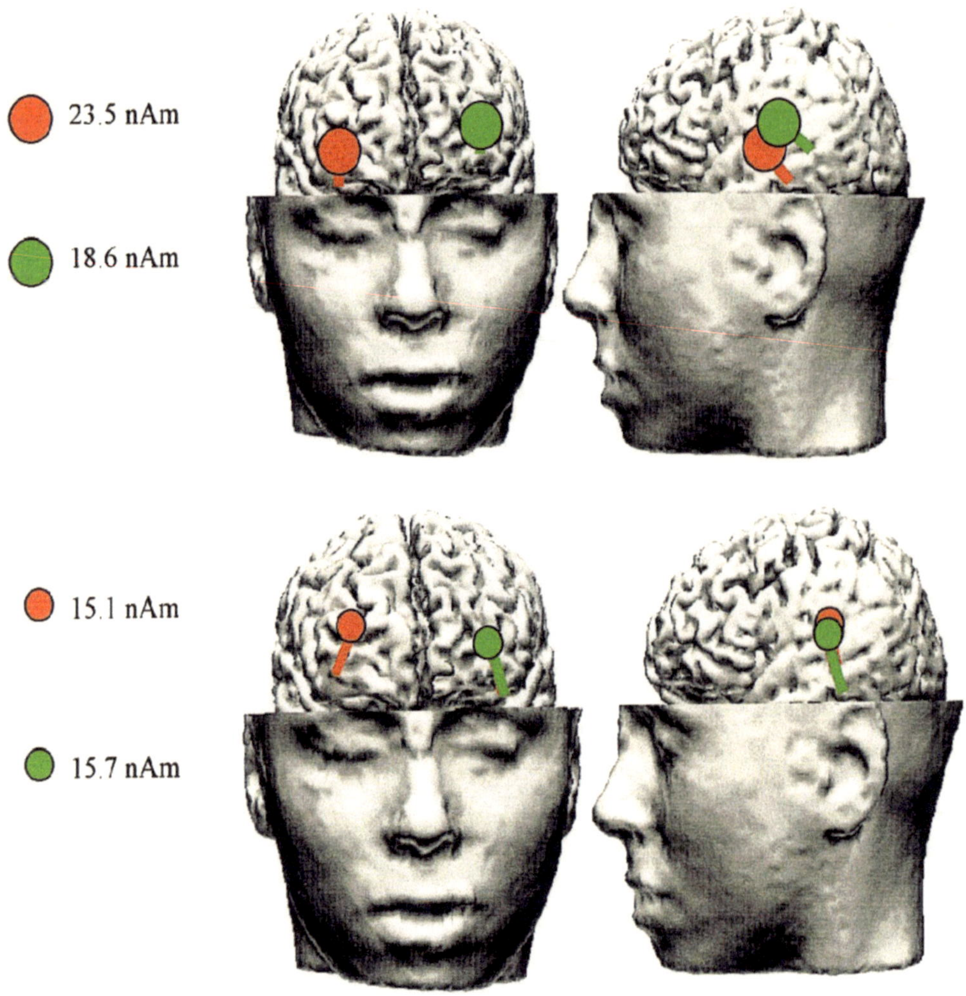

Fig. 5. MRI and function

Source localization results for a single subject including a three-dimensional reconstruction of the brain. The upper line shows the localized dipoles related to false alarms from the conceptual encoding condition and the lower line shows the localized dipoles related to false alarms from the perceptual encoding condition. Note that false alarms from the conceptual encoding condition elicited higher brain activity than false alarms from the perceptual encoding condition in terms of dipole strength (from Walla et al., 2000). The slight difference in right hemisphere dipole localisation between the two conditions has not been further analysed.

4.2 Two stages of olfactory information processing

Early stage olfactory information processing is not associated with consciousness. The human sense of olfaction has long been neglected in terms of scientific investigation. Partly, this may be due to the subjective feeling that the encoding and processing of odours is not important to us. Only people who lost this evolutionary old sense know that not only the appreciation of food is reduced to a minimum but also some abstract feeling of evaluation (see Walla, 2008).

Dynamic influences of olfaction on both word and face processing have been described (Lorig, 1999; Walla et al., 2003a; Walla et al., 2003b; Walla et al., 2005). Most often, it turned out that at least two stages (time windows) of odour-related information processing take place. Within this book chapter we do not go into further detail with respect to the actual influences of olfaction on word and face processing. The recent review by Walla (2008) summarises them anyway. However, what is important to us in relation to this book chapter is the fact that these two stages seem to process different aspects of an odour. In order to better understand these two stages and their functions a further study provides helpful support. Strikingly, that study highlights non-conscious aspects related to olfactory information processing. With MEG and a sophisticated computer-controlled device to accurately deliver olfactory stimuli it was shown that one of these two stages does not lead to conscious awareness, although odour-related brain activity occurred. This finding was revealed by comparing a group of participants who reported conscious odour perception with a group of participants who reported to have had no conscious odour perception during the course of an experiment (Walla et al., 2002). Crucially, both groups confirmed conscious perception of a first test stimulus, but as a matter of fact some participants were not aware of any odour stimulation during the course of the experiment. This might have been caused by the fact that all the attention had to be paid to words being visually presented with the instruction to make a semantic decision for each presentation. As a consequence olfaction was rather incidental anyway.

The main finding was that although no conscious olfaction was reported in the one group MEG data revealed odour-related brain activity (Walla et al., 2002). This brain activity occurred between 200ms and 500ms after stimulus onset and it was also found in the conscious perception group. On the other hand, it was only the conscious perception group that also demonstrated later odour-related brain activity between 600ms and 900ms after stimulus onset. Obviously, regardless of conscious odour perception or not odour-related brain activity occurred. It still remains unclear what aspects of an olfactory stimulus are processed at the early stage and what exactly their effects are, but it seems obvious that consciousness is not essential for them to be processed. Figure 6 demonstrates different magnetic fields (MEG maps) between the group reporting conscious olfaction and the group without conscious olfaction.

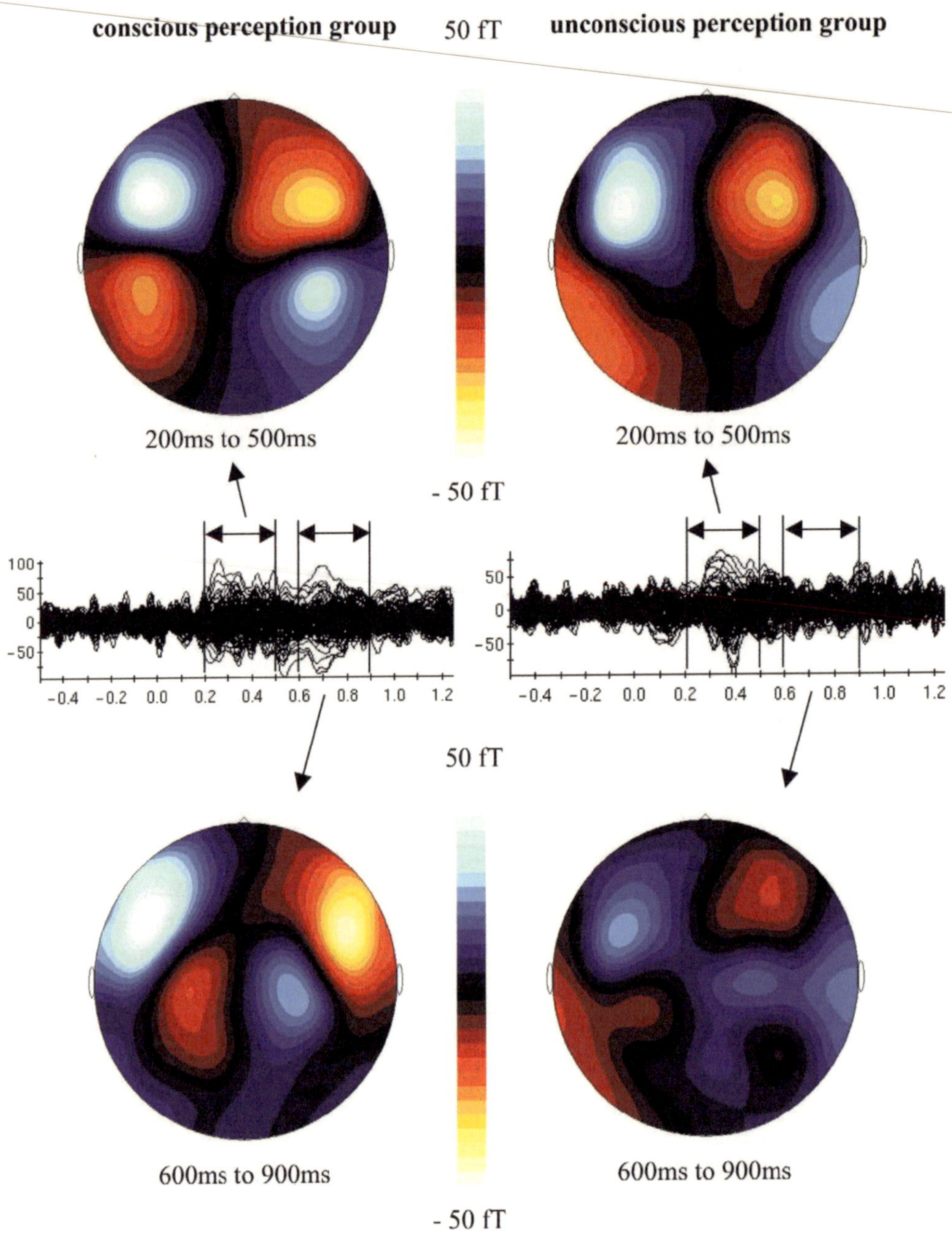

Fig. 6. MEG maps

Brain activity differences between the conditions 'study words with odor' and 'study words without odor' for both the 'unconscious perception' group and the 'conscious perception' group. Note that the activity differences between 200 and 500 ms after stimulus onset are well defined in both groups whereas the activity differences between 600 and 900 ms after stimulus onset are much more conspicuous in the 'conscious perception' group (from Walla et al., 2002).

4.3 The subliminal effect of possessive pronouns

The human self has long been a focus of special interest. It is often treated as one of the most sophisticated and highest forms of neural information processing at all. How can an organ such as the brain become aware of itself?

Braking things down, we begin to realise that our self is in fact a combination of our own body including all its anatomical structures plus our own memories that are stored in our brains. Anatomical structures are processed through the somatosensory system (body representation) and our memories range from simple sensory experiences up to episodes of our own life. The fact that loss of our most personal material possessions (belongings) almost hurt like true physical pain may be linked with the idea that they are processed in our brain like parts of our body. While this seems nothing more than just an interesting idea, recent neuroimaging-research now provides evidence that self awareness at its deepest roots starts with processing the self as a living organism just as any other. On that level the self in our brain is no different from any other human self, perhaps not even different from any other animal. On a higher processing level though, our brain distinguishes between the self and somebody else. Interestingly, all this can happen regardless of consciousness being present or absent.

The respective neuroimaging experiment was conducted with MEG and EEG. Both methods revealed similar findings about brain activities being able to process self- versus other-related information on a non-conscious level. The multiple-aspects-theory of self awareness was developed (Walla et al. 2007, 2008) and is meanwhile confirmed by another research group (Herbert et al. 2010).

The MEG study by Walla et al. (2007) made use of language (German) processing to elicit self- versus other-related processing in the brain. In particular, combinations of possessive pronouns and nouns were used. To give an example, "my garden" and "his garden" versus the neutral condition of "a garden" were thought to ideally elicit self- versus other-related brain activities that can be distinguished from no person engagement such as in the neutral condition. Strikingly, such different word combinations (visually presented) had to be processed under three different conditions in terms of level of consciousness. In one condition, many of these word combinations were encoded following the instruction to only decide whether each noun contained a specific letter or not. This level of encoding is referred to as alphabetical and it does not include conscious semantic information processing and no active pronoun processing at all. In a further condition many new such combinations were encoded following the instruction to decide whether each noun's meaning was living or non-living. This level of processing is referred to as semantic and it does again not include any active pronoun encoding. Finally, in a third condition, another set of pronoun-noun pairs was visually presented, but this time the instruction was to generate a short meaningful sentence (in their minds) containing the noun together with its pronoun. For example, "my garden is nice". In addition, the living/non-living distinction had to be made. Statistical analysis revealed that level of processing had no effect on significant pronoun effects that were found. What did these pronoun effects look like?

Between 200 ms and 300 ms after stimulus onset both "my" and "his" pronoun conditions elicited similar brain activity that was different compared to the neutral condition (figure 7). In contrast, between 500 ms and 800 ms after stimulus onset the "my" pronoun condition differed from both the "his" pronoun condition and the neutral condition (figure 8). It has been suggested that the left insular cortex is involved in processing self-related aspects (Walla et al, 2007).

This is mainly due to source localisation results, which are presented in figure 9 and 10.

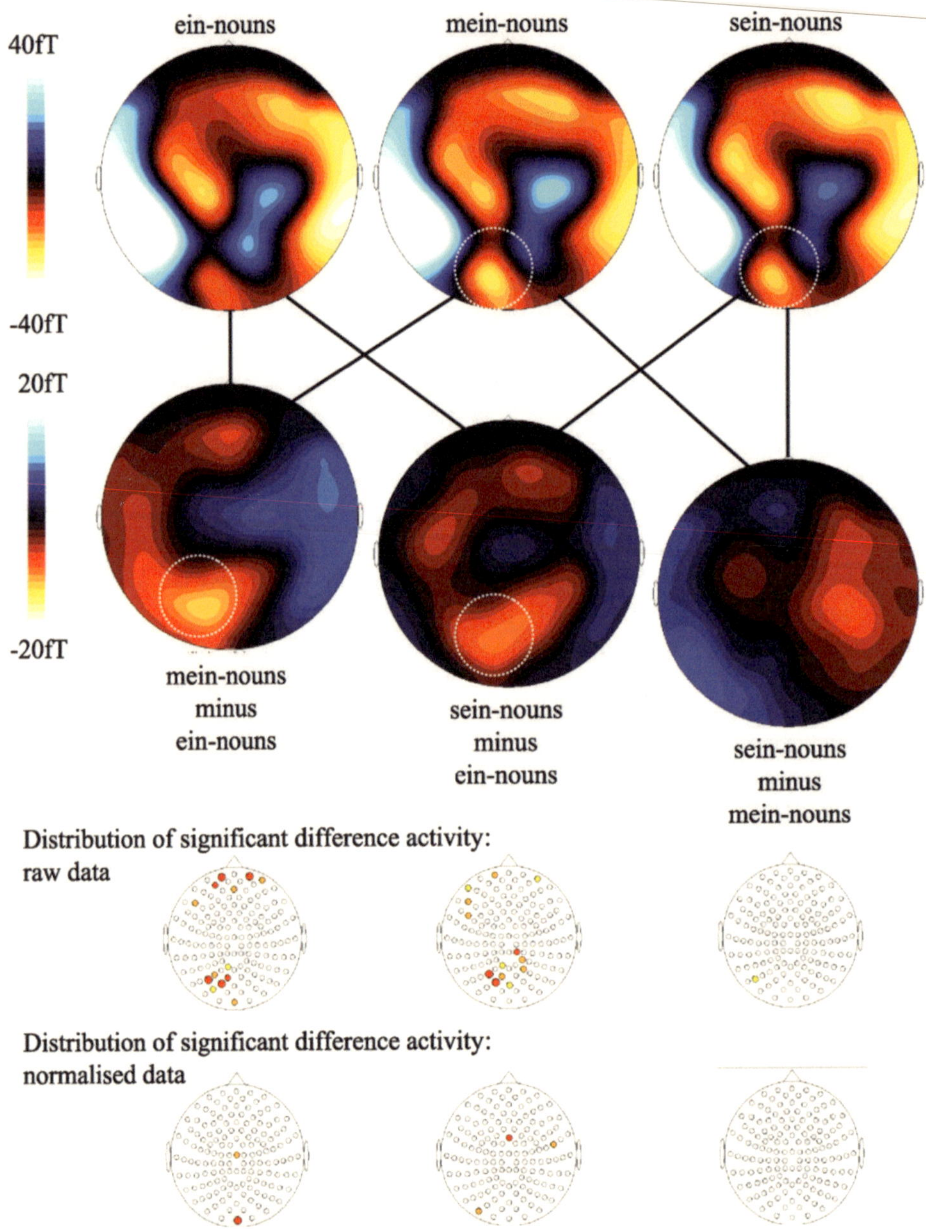

Fig. 7. MEG maps

Early neurophysiological effect: MEG maps (magnetic field distributions) averaged across depth of word processing and across all study participants for the time interval from 200 to 300 ms after stimulus onset. First line: one map for each of the three conditions of pronoun ("ein" ("a"), "mein" ("my"), "sein" ("his")). Second line: difference magnetic field distributions related to comparisons (subtractions) between each possible pair of pronoun condition ("mein" vs. "ein", "sein" vs. "ein", "sein" vs. "mein"). Sensor areas where t-tests resulted in significant differences are marked with a white dotted circle. Third line: t-maps showing the distribution of significant differences for each of the above-mentioned comparisons (raw data). Note that "mein" vs. "ein" and "sein" vs. "ein" both resulted in significant differences, whereas no differences occurred for the comparison "sein" vs. "mein". Fourth line: t-maps showing the distribution of significant differences for each of the above-mentioned comparisons (amplitude-normalized data). Note that hardly any differences occurred (from Walla et al., 2007).

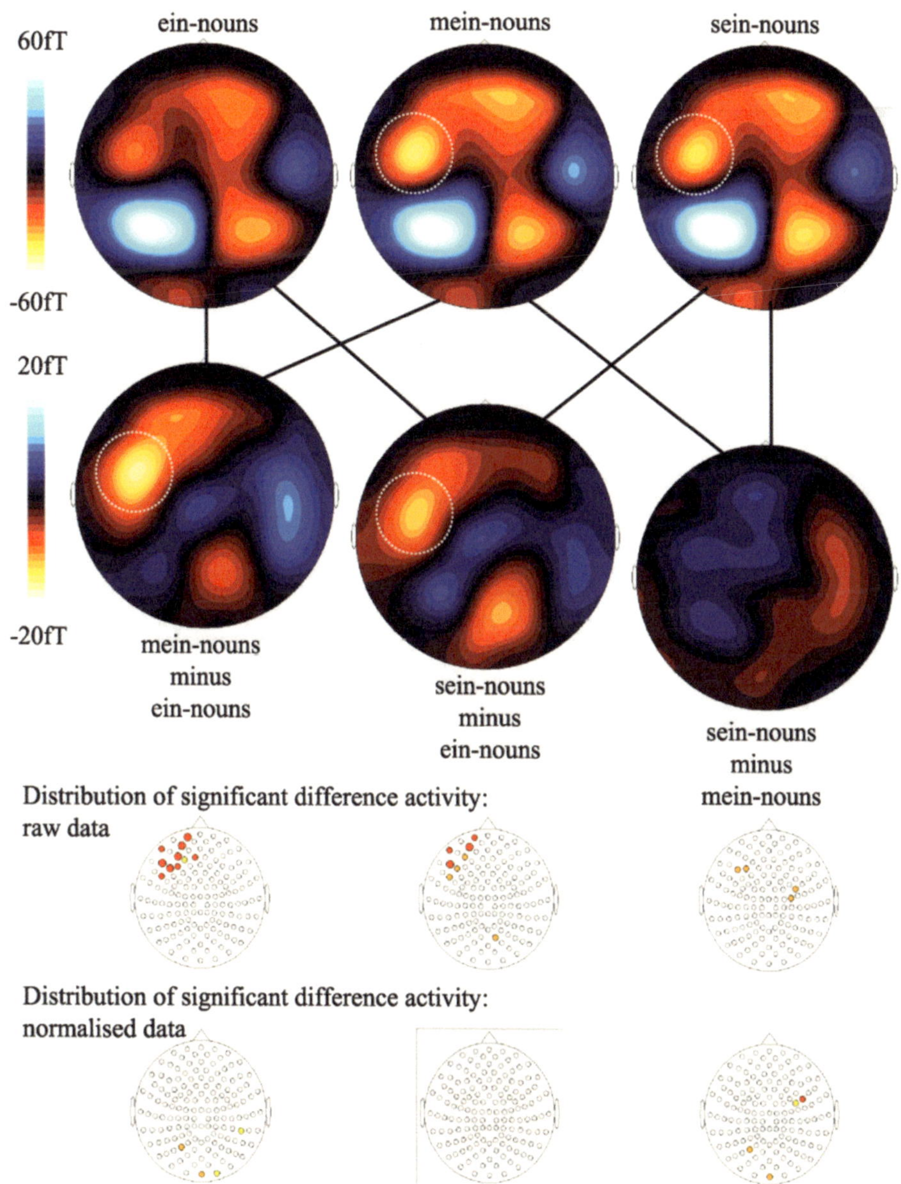

Fig. 8. MEG maps

Later neurophysiological effect: MEG maps (magnetic field distributions) averaged across depth of word processing and across all study participants for the time interval from 500 to 800 ms after stimulus onset. First line: one map for each of the three conditions of pronoun ("ein" ("a"), "mein" ("my"), "sein" ("his")). Second line: difference magnetic field distributions related to comparisons (subtractions) between each possible pair of pronoun condition ("mein" vs. "ein", "sein" vs. "ein", "sein" vs. "mein"). Sensor areas where t-tests resulted in significant differences are marked with a white dotted circle. Third line: t-maps showing the distribution of significant differences for each of the above-mentioned comparisons (raw data). Note that "mein" vs. "ein" and "sein" vs. "ein" both resulted in significant differences. In addition, the comparison between "sein" and "mein" also resulted in significant differences at some of the sensor sites (no such differences were found during the early period of time). Fourth line: t-maps showing the distribution of significant differences for each of the above-mentioned comparisons (normalized data) (from Walla et al., 2007).

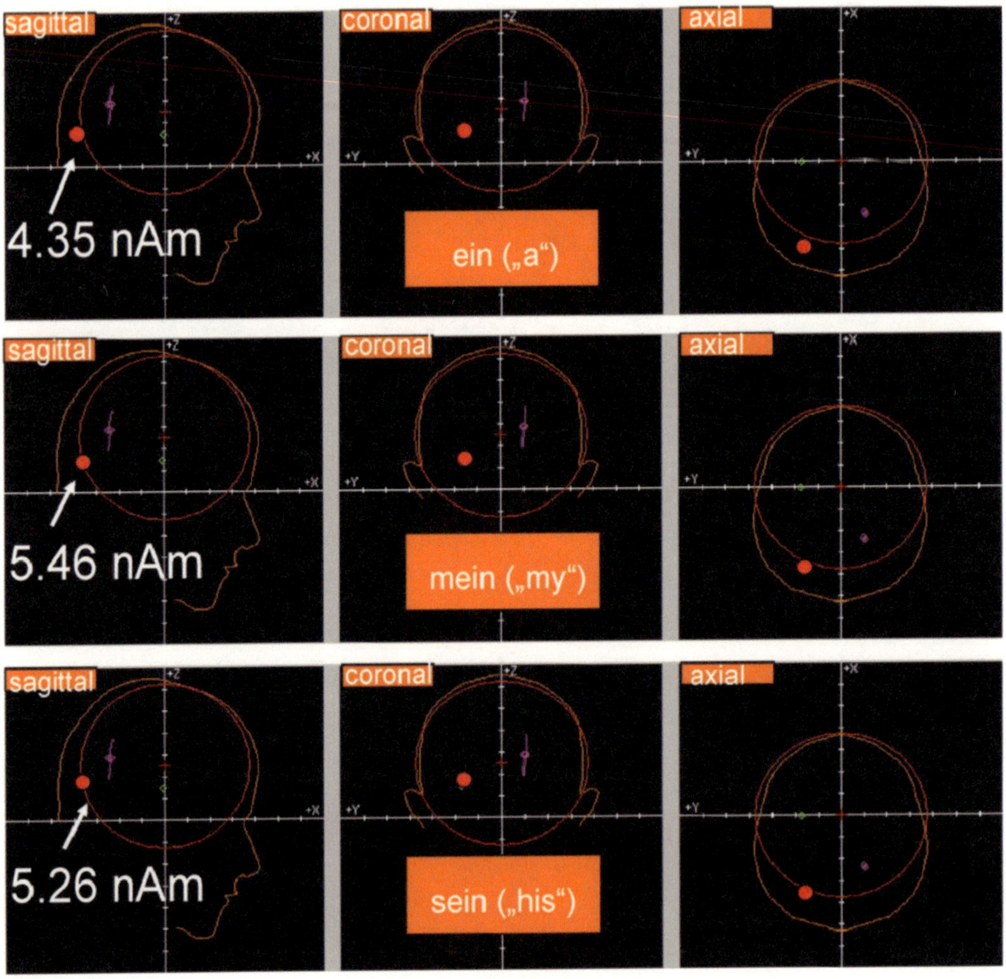

Fig. 9. Source localization for the earlier time range

The localized dipole in this respective region shows stronger brain activity as reflected by dipole strength (nA m) related to both personal pronouns compared to the neutral pronoun. The location of this dipole is interpreted as left occipital (from Walla et al., 2007).

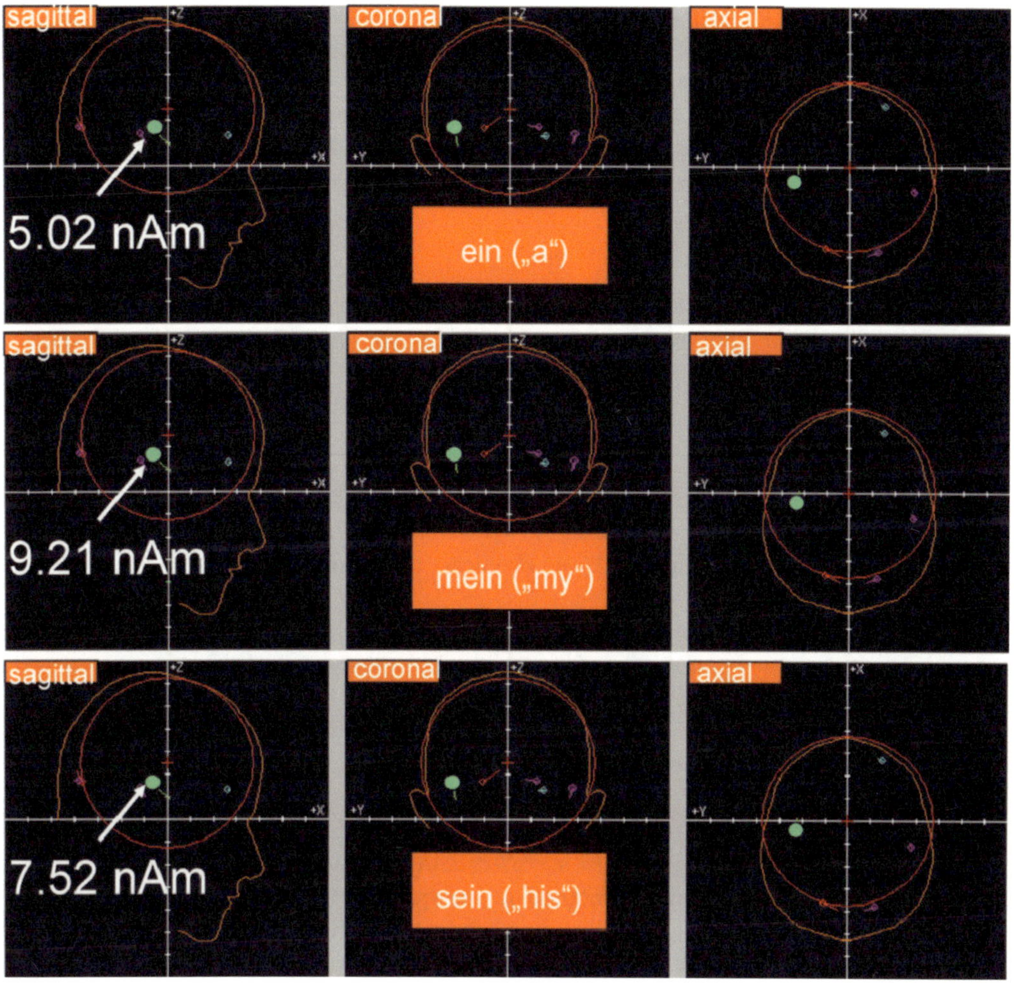

Fig. 10. Source localisation for the later time range

The localized dipole in this respective region shows stronger brain activity as reflected by dipole strength (nA m) related to both personal pronouns compared to the neutral pronoun (strongest activity in the "mein"("my") condition). The location of this dipole is interpreted as left temporal. Most likely it is the left insular cortex that is able to discriminate between self and other. (from Walla et al., 2007).

5. Conclusion

Findings revealed by MEG and other methods clearly demonstrate that only a little fraction of brain processes related to even high cognitive functions such as our self are associated with consciousness. Or in other words, much of our even highest cognitive functions do happen non-consciously. It almost seems as if we mainly run non-conscious with only bits and pieces entering the stream of consciousness. It may be reasonable to believe that around 80 to 90 % of our daily activities are controlled outside our own awareness. However, we should not make the mistake to underestimate consciousness as it arises now in your brain while reading these lines. Consciousness still seems to be inevitable to appreciate a lot of what we are so much used to. The appreciation of music and art, the ability to love and to feel happy are just some of them. In fact, the more we learn about how dominant non-conscious processes guide our behaviour the more we learn to appreciate what our individual consciousness actually means to us.

6. Acknowledgment

The author wants to thank Lüder Deecke for providing the essential equipment and general support, Wilfried Lang for mentorship and general support. Thanks also go to Dennis Balson for helpful financial support.

7. References

Dolan, R.J.; Heinze, H.J.; Hurlemann, R.; Hinrichs, H. (2006). Magnetoencephalography (MEG) determined temporal modulation of visual and auditory sensory processing in the context of classical conditioning to faces. Neuroimage, 15;32(2):778-89.

Van Gaal, S., and Lamme, V.A.F. (2011). Unconscious High-Level Information Processing:Implication for Neurobiological Theories of Consciousness. The Neuroscientist, X: 1-15.

Garoff-Eaton, R.J.; Kensinger, E.A.; & Schacter, D.L. (2007). The neural correlaates of conceptual and perceptual false recognition. Learning and Memory, 14: 684-692.

Hari, R.; Parkkonen, L. & Nangini, C. (2010). The brain in time: insights from neuromagnetic recordings. Annals of the New York Academy of Sciences, 1191: 89-109.

Hari, R. (1990). The neuromagneticmethod in the study of the human auditory cortex. In Auditory Evoked Magnetic Fields and Potentials. Advances in Audiology, Vol. 6. F. Grandori, M. Hoke & G. Romani, Eds.: 222–282. Karger. Basel.

Herbert, C; Herbert, B., Ethofer, T. & Pauli, P. (2010). His or mine? The time course of self-other discrimination in emotion processing. Social Neuroscience, iFirst: 1-12.

Lewis, S.; Thoma, R.J.; Lanoue, M.D.; Miller, G.A.; Heller, W.; Edgar, C.; et al. (2003). Visual processing of facial affect. Neuroreport, 14(14):1841–5.

Lorig, T.S. (1999). On the similarity of odor and language perception. Neurosci. Biobehav. Rev. 23: 391–398.

Peyk, P.; Schupp, H.T.; Elbert, T.; Junghöfer, M. (2008). Emotion processing in the visual brain: a MEG analysis. Brain Topography, 4: 205-215.

Rugg, M.D.; Mark, R.E.; Walla, P.; Schloerscheidt, A.M.; Birch, C.S.; and Allan, K. (1998). Dissociation of the neural correlates of implicit and explicit memory. Nature, 392: 595-598.

Schacter, D.L.; & Slotnick, S.D. (2004). The cognitive neuroscience of memory distortion. Neuron 44: 149–160.

Streit, M.; Ioannides, A.A.; Liu, L.; Wölwer, W.; Dammers, J.; Gross, J.; et al. (1999). Neurophysiological correlates of the recognition of facial expressions of emotion as revealed by magnetoencephalography. Brain research. Cognitive Brain Res, 7(4):481–491.

Tarkiainen, A., Cornelissen, P.L., Salmelin, R., 2002. Dynamics of visual feature analysis and object-level processing in face versus letter-string perception. Brain 125(5), 1125-1136.

Tarkiainen, A., Helenius, P., Hansen, P.C., Cornelissen, P.L., Salmelin, R., 1999. Dynamics of letter string perception in the human occipitotemporal cortex. Brain 122(11), 2119-2132.

Walla, P.; & Deecke, L. (2010). Odours Influence Visually Induced Emotion: Behavior and Neuroimaging. Sensors, 10: 8185-8197.

Walla, P. (2008). Olfaction and its dynamic influence on word and face processing: Cross-modal integration. Progress in Neurobiology, 84: 192-209.

Walla, P.; Duregger, C., Greiner, K., Thurner, S. & Ehrenberger, K. (2008). Multiple aspects related to self awareness and the awareness of others: an Electroencephalography (EEG) study. Journal of Neural Transmission, 115(7):983-92.

Walla, P.; Greiner, K., Duregger, C., Deecke, L. & Thurner, S. (2007). Self awareness and the subconscious effect of personal pronouns on word encoding: a magnetoencephalographic (MEG) study. Neuropsychologia, 45: 796-809.

Walla, P.; Mayer, D., Deecke, L., and Lang, W. (2005). How chemical information processing interferes with face processing: a magnetoencephalographic (MEG) study. Neuroimage, 24(1): 111-117.

Walla, P.; Hufnagl, B., Lehrner, J., Mayer, D., Lindinger, G., Imhof, H., Deecke, L., and Lang, W. (2003a). Olfaction and face encoding in humans: a magnetoencephalographic (MEG) study. Cognitive Brain Research, 15(2): 105-115.

Walla, P.; Hufnagl, B., Lehrner, J., Mayer, D., Lindinger, G., Imhof, H., Deecke, L., and Lang, W. (2003b). Olfaction and depth of word processing: a magnetoencephalographic (MEG) study Neuroimage, 18(1): 104-116.

Walla, P.; Hufnagl, B., Lehrner, J., Mayer, D., Lindinger, G., Deecke, L. & Lang, W. (2002). Evidence of conscious and subconscious olfactory information processing during word encoding: a magnetoencephalographic (MEG) study. Cognitive Brain Research, 14: 309-316.

Walla, P.; Hufnagl, B., Lindinger, G., Deecke, L., Imhof, H. & Lang, W. (2001). False recognition depends on depth of prior word processing: A magnetoencephalographic (MEG) study. Cognitive Brain Research, 11: 249-257.

Walla, P.; Hufnagl, B., Lindinger, G., Imhof, H., Deecke, L. & Lang, W. (2001). Left temporal and temporo-parietal brain activity depends on depth of word encoding: A magnetoencephalographic (MEG) study in healthy young subjects. Neuroimage, 13: 402-409.

Walla, P.; Endl, W.; Lindinger, G.; Deecke, L.; & Lang, W. (2000). False recognition in a verbal memory task: an event-related potential study. Cognitive Brain Research, 9(1): 41-44.

Winkielman, P. & Berridge, K.C. (2004). Unconscious emotion. Current directions in Psychological Science, 13: 120-123.